Chronic Obstructive Pulmonary Disease

Guest Editors

STEPHEN I. RENNARD, MD
BARTOLOME R. CELLI, MD

MEDICAL CLINICS
OF NORTH AMERICA

www.medical.theclinics.com

July 2012 • Volume 96 • Number 4

W.B. SAUNDERS COMPANY
A Division of Elsevier Inc.

1600 John F. Kennedy Boulevard ● Suite 1800 ● Philadelphia, Pennsylvania 19103-2899

http://www.theclinics.com

MEDICAL CLINICS OF NORTH AMERICA Volume 96, Number 4
July 2012 ISSN 0025-7125, ISBN-13: 978-1-4557-3890-8

Editor: Pamela Hetherington
Developmental Editor: Teia Stone

Medical Clinics of North America (ISSN 0025-7125) is published bimonthly by Elsevier Inc., 360 Park Avenue South, New York, NY 10010-1710. Months of issue are January, March, May, July, September, and November. Periodicals postage paid at New York, NY, and additional mailing offices. Subscription prices are USD 232 per year for US individuals, USD 424 per year for US institutions, USD 117 per year for US students, USD 295 per year for Canadian individuals, USD 551 per year for Canadian institutions, USD 184 per year for Canadian students, USD 358 per year for international individuals, USD 551 per year for international institutions and USD 184 per year for international students. To receive student/resident rate, orders must be accompanied by name of affiliated institution, date of term, and the *signature* of program/residency coordinator on institution letterhead. Orders will be billed at individual rate until proof of status is received. Foreign air speed delivery is included in all *Clinics* subscription prices. All prices are subject to change without notice. **POSTMASTER:** Send address changes to *Medical Clinics of North America*, Elsevier Health Sciences Division, Subscription Customer Service, 3251 Riverport Lane, Maryland Heights, MO 63043. **Customer Service: Telephone: 1-800-654-2452** (U.S. and Canada); **1-314-447-8871** (outside U.S. and Canada). **Fax: 1-314-447-8029. E-mail: journalscustomerservice-usa@elsevier.com** (for print support); **journalsonlinesupport-usa@ elsevier.com** (for online support).

Reprints. For copies of 100 or more of articles in this publication, please contact the Commercial Reprints Department, Elsevier Inc., 360 Park Avenue South, New York, NY 10010-1710. Tel.: 212-633-3812; Fax: 212-462-1935; E-mail: reprints@elsevier.com.

Medical Clinics of North America is also published in Spanish by McGraw-Hill Interamericana Editores S. A., P.O. Box 5-237, 06500 Mexico, D.F., Mexico.

Medical Clinics of North America is covered in *MEDLINE/PubMed (Index Medicus), Current Contents, ASCA, Excerpta Medica, Science Citation Index,* and *ISI/BIOMED.*

Printed in the United States of America.

Chronic Obstructive Pulmonary Disease

MEDICAL CLINICS OF NORTH AMERICA

GOAL STATEMENT

The goal of *Medical Clinics of North America* is to keep practicing physicians up to date with current clinical practice by providing timely articles reviewing the state of the art in patient care.

ACCREDITATION

The *Medical Clinics of North America* is planned and implemented in accordance with the Essential Areas and Policies of the Accreditation Council for Continuing Medical Education (ACCME) through the joint sponsorship of the University of Virginia School of Medicine and Elsevier. The University of Virginia School of Medicine is accredited by the ACCME to provide continuing medical education for physicians.

The University of Virginia School of Medicine designates this enduring material activity for a maximum of 15 *AMA PRA Category 1 Credit*(s)™ for each issue, 90 credits per year. Physicians should only claim credit commensurate with the extent of their participation in the activity.

The American Medical Association has determined that physicians not licensed in the US who participate in this CME enduring material activity are eligible for a maximum of 15 *AMA PRA Category 1 Credit*(s)™ for each issue, 90 credits per year.

Credit can be earned by reading the text material, taking the CME examination online at http://www.theclinics.com/home/cme, and completing the evaluation. After taking the test, you will be required to review any and all incorrect answers. Following completion of the test and evaluation, your credit will be awarded and you may print your certificate.

FACULTY DISCLOSURE/CONFLICT OF INTEREST

The University of Virginia School of Medicine, as an ACCME accredited provider, endorses and strives to comply with the Accreditation Council for Continuing Medical Education (ACCME) Standards of Commercial Support, Commonwealth of Virginia statutes, University of Virginia policies and procedures, and associated federal and private regulations and guidelines on the need for disclosure and monitoring of proprietary and financial interests that may affect the scientific integrity and balance of content delivered in continuing medical education activities under our auspices.

The University of Virginia School of Medicine requires that all CME activities accredited through this institution be developed independently and be scientifically rigorous, balanced and objective in the presentation/discussion of its content, theories and practices.

All authors/editors participating in an accredited CME activity are expected to disclose to the readers relevant financial relationships with commercial entities occurring within the past 12 months (such as grants or research support, employee, consultant, stock holder, member of speakers bureau, etc.). The University of Virginia School of Medicine will employ appropriate mechanisms to resolve potential conflicts of interest to maintain the standards of fair and balanced education to the reader. Questions about specific strategies can be directed to the Office of Continuing Medical Education, University of Virginia School of Medicine, Charlottesville, Virginia.

The faculty and staff of the University of Virginia Office of Continuing Medical Education have no financial affiliations to disclose.

The authors/editors listed below have identified no professional or financial affiliations for themselves or their spouse/ partner:

Kristina L. Bailey, MD; Bartolome R. Celli, MD (Guest Editor); Miguel Divo, MD; Marilyn G. Foreman, MD, MS; Pamela Hetherington, (Acquisitions Editor); Bernd Lamprecht, MD; Alex J. Mackay, MBBS, BSc (Hons), MRCP; Carlos H. Martinez, MD, MPH; Victor Pinto-Plata, MD; Cheryl Pirozzi, MD; Sharon R. Rosenberg, MD, MS; Joan B. Soriano, MD; Anthony Tam, BSc; Andrew Wolf, MD (Test Author).

The authors/editors listed below identified the following professional or financial affiliations for themselves or their spouse/ partner:

Michael Campos, MD receives research support from CSL Behring and Grifols.
Juan C. Celedón, MD, DrPH, FCCP served as a consultant for Roche/Genentech, received royalties from UpToDate, and receives research support from NIH.
Francis C. Cordova, MD is on the Advisory Board for Boehringer Ingelheim and is on the Speakers' Bureau for Gilead.
MeiLan K. Han, MD, MS is a consultant for Medimune, UBC, and Novaratis; is on the Speakers' Bureau for Grifols Therapeutics; and is on the Speakers' Bureau and Advisory Committee for Boehringer Ingelheim, Pfizer, Inc., GSK, and Forest Pharmaceuticals.
John R. Hurst, PhD, FRCP is on the Speakers' Bureau and Advisory Board for Astra Zeneca, Boehringer, GSK, Pfizer, and Bayer.
Ravi Kalhan, MD, MS is a consultant for Forest Laboratories and Boehringer-Ingelheim.
Stephen I. Rennard, MD (Guest Editor) is a consultant for ABIM, Align2 Acton, APT, AstraZeneca, Beilenson, Boehringer Ingelheim, Clarus Acuity, Forst, Frankel Group, Gerson Lehman, Globe Life Sciences, GSK, Guidepoint global, Health Advanced, and Leerink Swan; and provides lectures for AARC, Almirall, CME Incite, Forest, HSC Medical Education and Incite.
Mary Beth Scholand, MD receives research support from Internone, Boehringer Ingelheim, and Fibrogen, and is on the Advisory Board for Gilead.
Don D. Sin, MD is on the Advisory Board for Merck Frosst, AstraZeneca, Novartis, and Takeda, and receives research support from AstraZeneca.
Jonathan P. Singer, MD, MS receives research support from Novartis Pharmaceuticals.
George R. Washko, MD, MS's wife is employed by Merck.
Roger D. Yusen, MD, MPH receives research support from Pfizer, Inc. and Bayer Healthcare, is a consultant for Bayer Healthcare and Ortho Pharmaceuticals, and is on the Advisory Board for GSK.

Disclosure of Discussion of Non-FDA Approved Uses for Pharmaceutical Products and/or Medical Devices.

The University of Virginia School of Medicine, as an ACCME provider, requires that all faculty presenters identify and disclose any off-label uses for pharmaceutical and medical device products. The University of Virginia School of Medicine recommends that each physician fully review all the available data on new products or procedures prior to clinical use.

TO ENROLL

To enroll in the Medical Clinics of North America Continuing Medical Education program, call customer service at 1-800-654-2452 or visit us online at http://www.theclinics.com/home/cme. The CME program is available to subscribers for an additional fee of USD 228.

Contributors

GUEST EDITORS

STEPHEN I. RENNARD, MD
Larson Professor, Department of Internal Medicine, University of Nebraska Medical Center, Omaha, Nebraska

BARTOLOME R. CELLI, MD
Lecturer in Medicine, Pulmonary and Critical Care Division, Brigham and Women's Hospital, Harvard Medical School, Boston, Massachusetts

AUTHORS

KRISTINA L. BAILEY, MD
Assistant Professor, Pulmonary, Critical Care, Sleep and Allergy Division, Department of Internal Medicine, University of Nebraska Medical Center, Omaha, Nebraska

MICHAEL CAMPOS, MD
Division of Pulmonary, Critical Care and Sleep Medicine (R-47), Department of Medicine, University of Miami Miller School of Medicine, Miami, Florida

JUAN C. CELEDÓN, MD, DrPH, FACP, FCCP
Division of Pediatric Pulmonary Medicine, Allergy and Immunology, Department of Pediatrics, Children's Hospital of Pittsburgh of UPMC; Division of Pulmonary, Allergy and Critical Care Medicine, Department of Medicine, University of Pittsburgh School of Medicine, Pittsburgh, Pennsylvania

FRANCIS C. CORDOVA, MD
Associate Professor of Medicine, Medical Director, Lung and Heart/Lung Transplant Program, Temple University School of Medicine, Philadelphia, Pennsylvania

MIGUEL DIVO, MD
Pulmonary and Critical Care Medicine Division, Brigham and Women's Hospital, Harvard Medical School, Boston, Massachusetts

MARILYN G. FOREMAN, MD, MS
Division of Pulmonary and Critical Care Medicine, Department of Medicine, Morehouse School of Medicine, Atlanta, Georgia

MEILAN K. HAN, MD, MS
Assistant Professor, Division of Pulmonary and Critical Care Medicine, University of Michigan Health System, Ann Arbor, Michigan

JOHN R. HURST, PhD, FRCP
Clinical Senior Lecturer, Academic Unit of Respiratory Medicine, Royal Free Campus, UCL Medical School, London, United Kingdom

RAVI KALHAN, MD, MS
Assistant Professor in Medicine and Preventive Medicine, Director, Asthma and COPD Program, Northwestern University Feinberg School of Medicine, Chicago, Illinois

BERND LAMPRECHT, MD
Department of Pulmonary Medicine, Paracelsus Private Medical University of Salzburg, Salzburg, Austria

ALEX J. MACKAY, MBBS, BSc (Hons), MRCP
Clinical Research Fellow, Academic Unit of Respiratory Medicine, Royal Free Campus, UCL Medical School, London, United Kingdom

CARLOS H. MARTINEZ, MD, MPH
Division of Pulmonary and Critical Care Medicine, University of Michigan Health System, Ann Arbor, Michigan

VICTOR PINTO-PLATA, MD
Pulmonary and Critical Care Medicine Division, Brigham and Women's Hospital, Harvard Medical School, Boston, Massachusetts

CHERYL PIROZZI, MD
Pulmonary Fellow, Pulmonary Division, Department of Internal Medicine, University of Utah, Salt Lake City, Utah

SHARON R. ROSENBERG, MD, MS
Assistant Professor in Medicine, Co-Director, Asthma and COPD Program, Northwestern University Feinberg School of Medicine, Chicago, Illinois

MARY BETH SCHOLAND, MD
Assistant Professor, Pulmonary Division, Department of Internal Medicine, University of Utah, Salt Lake City, Utah

DON D. SIN, MD
Department of Medicine, The University of British Columbia James Hogg Research Centre, Providence Heart and Lung Centre, University of British Columbia, Vancouver, British Columbia, Canada

JONATHAN P. SINGER, MD, MS
Clinical Instructor, Division of Pulmonary, Critical Care, Allergy and Sleep Medicine and Cardiovascular Research Institute, University of California, San Francisco, San Francisco, California

JOAN B. SORIANO, MD
Program of Epidemiology and Clinical Research, Fundació Caubet-CIMERA Illes Balears, Bunyola, Mallorca, Illes Balears, Spain

ANTHONY TAM, BSc
Department of Medicine, The University of British Columbia James Hogg Research Centre, Providence Heart and Lung Centre, University of British Columbia, Vancouver, British Columbia, Canada

GEORGE R. WASHKO, MD, MS
Assistant Professor of Medicine, Harvard Medical School; Physician, Division of Pulmonary and Critical Care Medicine, Department of Medicine, Brigham and Women's Hospital, Boston, Massachusetts

ROGER D. YUSEN, MD, MPH
Associate Professor, Divisions of Pulmonary and Critical Care Medicine and General Medical Sciences, Washington University, St Louis, Missouri

Contents

> Respiratory diseases receive little attention and funding in comparison with other major causes of global morbidity and mortality. Chronic obstructive pulmonary disease (COPD) has been a major public health problem and will remain a challenge for clinicians within the twenty-first century. Worldwide, COPD is in the spotlight because of its high prevalence, morbidity, and mortality, and creates formidable challenges for health care systems. This review summarizes the magnitude of the COPD problem at the population and individual levels.

> The pathogenesis of chronic obstructive pulmonary disease (COPD) is not fully known. However, it is now well accepted that inflammatory responses to external triggers, such as cigarette smoke and biomass fuel, are important in COPD progression. Protease–antiprotease balance, autoimmunity, mucus hypersecretion, airway wall remodeling, and chronic respiratory infections have all been implicated in disease pathogenesis. This article reviews these and other pathways that have been associated with COPD.

> The marked variability in individual susceptibility to the detrimental effects of smoking on lung function and other findings suggest a significant genetic contribution to chronic obstructive pulmonary disease (COPD). The only known genetic risk factor for COPD, severe a1-antitrypsin (AAT) deficiency, explains only 1% to 2% of cases of this disease. Screening for severe AAT should be done in all cases of COPD. There is considerable interest in identifying susceptibility genes for COPD unrelated to severe AAT deficiency, as this could greatly enhance efforts to prevent, diagnose, and treat COPD by yielding novel insights into its pathogenesis.

> Chronic obstructive pulmonary disease (COPD) is characterized by significant disease heterogeneity. This heterogeneity suggests that various influences, including environmental and biological factors, probably contribute to the disease, but the validation of specific phenotypes has been problematic. This article reviews differences in the presentation and progression of

the evolving field of HRQOL measurement and interpretation. This article defines HRQOL, discusses instruments used to measure HRQOL, and reviews related literature.

The mechanisms of chronic obstructive pulmonary disease exacerbation are complex. Respiratory viruses (in particular rhinovirus) and bacteria play a major role in the cause of these events. A distinct group of patients seems susceptible to frequent exacerbations, irrespective of disease severity, and this phenotype is stable over time. Many current therapeutic strategies help reduce exacerbation frequency. Further work is required to develop novel anti-inflammatory therapies for exacerbation prevention and treatment. This article focuses on the cause of chronic obstructive pulmonary disease exacerbations, and the current preventative and acute interventions available.

Comprehensive medical care of individuals with chronic obstructive pulmonary disease (COPD) requires a detailed evaluation of patients beyond the measurement of lung function. Symptoms should be determined in an objective manner, particular attention should be paid to a history of exacerbations, and the presence of comorbid conditions should be determined. Exercise capacity determined by a 6-minute walk distance can also be informative. Virtually all COPD therapies improve respiratory symptoms, lessen exacerbation frequency, and improve quality of life; selection of COPD pharmacotherapy should be individualized to each patient's symptom and exacerbation burden and their individual response to therapy over time.

Bullectomy, lung volume reduction surgery and lung transplantation have been shown to improve lung function, exercise capacity and quality of life in patients with advanced COPD. Careful patient selection and the use of optimal surgical procedure are important to ensure good clinical outcome. Advances in bronchoscopic techniques have allowed non-surgical lung volume reduction that replicate the clinical benefit of LVRS without its' associated morbidity and mortality. Promising endoscopic lung volume reduction techniques that are in various phases of development include the deployment of unidirectional endobronchial valves, instillation of biodegradable gel, and creation of airways bypass tracts.

Although there are nonmodifiable genetic risk factors for chronic obstructive pulmonary disease (COPD), most known risk factors for development and progression of COPD can be corrected. Continued efforts to encourage smoking cessation and measures to reduce exposure to secondhand smoke, outdoor air pollution, biomass smoke, and occupational and related amateur exposures will have a significant impact on worldwide health.

Preface

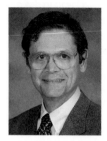 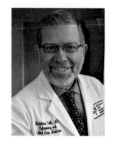

Stephen I. Rennard, MD   Bartolome R. Celli, MD
Guest Editors

Chronic obstructive pulmonary disease (COPD) is a major public health problem. In contrast to most of the other major causes of morbidity and mortality, COPD is increasing in prevalence and impact. In the United States, this is occurring despite the progressive reduction in smoking prevalence. While long recognized as a major health problem, novel diagnostic methods and treatments have only been introduced over the last few decades. However, the thinking about COPD has changed in fundamental ways. Risk factors are better understood and society has implemented preventive approaches that should have an impact on COPD incidence and prevalence. The use of spirometry to detect cases and make the right diagnosis has been gaining acceptance. New complementary diagnostic tools such as imaging techniques and field and laboratory exercise tests have expanded the capacity to better phenotype patients suffering from the disease. Importantly, the impact that treatment can have in ameliorating symptoms and in preventing morbidity and complications has been established. It has been recognized, moreover, that COPD is not just a disease of the lungs but that it has important systemic consequences and that the treatment of the COPD patient requires a holistic and integrated approach.

The current issue of *Medical Clinics of North America* focuses on COPD. This topic was last reviewed in 1996, volume 80, Issue 4. The current issue includes articles that have been selected to bring the clinician up to date with regard to the current impact of COPD in the world, current therapies, and the strategies by which these should be implemented. In addition, diagnostic approaches that are helping to provide novel understanding of the complex spectrum of disease included under the rubric of COPD are discussed. These are changing not only the nature of research studies in COPD but also should be used by the clinician to guide therapy.

Unfortunately, at the present time, COPD is underdiagnosed or misdiagnosed. Even when diagnosed correctly, it is often undertreated or treated with suboptimal strategies. It is our hope that this issue will be useful to the clinician so that the care of COPD patients can be improved to levels easily achievable. Moreover, a concerted effort by all of us involved in the care of patients will help subjects at risk for the disease reduce their risk burden. As shown in the articles in this issue of the *Clinics*, there is

Med Clin N Am 96 (2012) xi–xii
doi:10.1016/j.mcna.2012.05.008
0025-7125/12/$ – see front matter © 2012 Elsevier Inc. All rights reserved.

reason to be optimistic because a lot has been done and will continue to be done for the millions affected by the disease.

Finally, for those of us who have been engaged in the study of COPD and in the care of the COPD patient for over four decades, it is a particular pleasure that the articles in this issue are written by authorities belonging to a younger generation. Some are our students, and of these we are justifiably proud. More importantly, we are delighted that there will be a future generation of COPD experts who can help advance the understanding and guide treatment for this devastating condition.

Stephen I. Rennard, MD
Department of Internal Medicine
University of Nebraska Medical Center
Omaha, NE, USA

Bartolome R. Celli, MD
Pulmonary and Critical Care Division
Brigham and Women's Hospital
Harvard Medical School
Boston, MA, USA

E-mail addresses:
srennard@unmc.edu (S.I. Rennard)
BCelli@copdnet.org (B.R. Celli)

Chronic Obstructive Pulmonary Disease: A Worldwide Problem

Joan B. Soriano, MD[a],*, Bernd Lamprecht, MD[b]

KEYWORDS

- Chronic obstructive pulmonary disease • Epidemiology • Prevalence • Smoking
- Worldwide

KEY POINTS

- Chronic obstructive pulmonary disease (COPD) has been a major public health problem and will remain a challenge for clinicians within the XXIst century.
- COPD causes the death of at least 2.9 million people annually.
- Other than tobacco smoking, risk factors for developing COPD are being increasingly recognized, and include many other environmental exposures like occupational exposures to dust and fumes in the developed and developing countries, and indoor biomass fuel burning in many developing countries.

As of 2012, the world is inhabited by a record 7 billion people. Demographers emphasize that with population increase and hygiene improvements, there will be an epidemic of chronic conditions associated with aging and smoking. Yet, for those who manage patients with COPD, even the simplest of questions, "how many individuals are there in the world with COPD?," was surrounded by a halo of vagueness up to very recently. Estimates have varied by author and publication, and numbers up to 600 million have been widely used and are available elsewhere.[1] It is now agreed that an estimated 210 million people have COPD worldwide.[2] The same expert panel estimated the numbers of other respiratory conditions as 400 million with rhinitis (excluding asthma), 300 million with asthma, 100 million with sleep-disordered breathing

Disclosures: There are no relationships with a commercial company that have a direct financial interest in the subject matter or materials discussed in this article or with a company making a competing product.
Conflict of interest statement: There are no conflicts of interest to report regarding the content of this review.
[a] Program of Epidemiology and Clinical Research, Fundació Caubet-CIMERA Illes Balears, Recinte Hospital Joan March, Carretera Soller Km 12, Bunyola 07110, Mallorca, Illes Balears, Spain; [b] Department of Pulmonary Medicine, Paracelsus Private Medical University of Salzburg, Muellner Hauptstrasse 48, 5020 Salzburg, Austria
* Corresponding author.
E-mail address: jbsoriano@caubet-cimera.es

Med Clin N Am 96 (2012) 671–680
doi:10.1016/j.mcna.2012.02.005
0025-7125/12/$ – see front matter © 2012 Elsevier Inc. All rights reserved.

medical.theclinics.com

disorders, and 50 million with other chronic respiratory diseases, and it is estimated that 1.1 billion people in the world are smokers, more than ever before.

The epidemiology of COPD, or the study of COPD and its determinants at the population level, quantifies the burden of COPD on the society and compares it with other diseases. There is indeed more interest in COPD now than ever before. Describing the epidemiology of any given disease is fundamental to reducing its burden. Despite the well-established public health principle "to measure a health problem is the first step to identify a strategy to tackle it," the spread of the burden of COPD is and will remain a hot topic because the resources for any health intervention are always limited and need to be carefully used. Many initiatives worldwide have aimed at better describing the epidemiology of COPD, including the Global Burden of Disease (GBD) studies,[3] the European Lung White Book,[4] the Global Initiative for Chronic Obstructive Lung Disease (GOLD),[5] the Global Alliance Against Chronic Respiratory Diseases (GARD),[6] and several field studies to be listed subsequently. There are already many recent contributions summarizing the size of the COPD problem and ongoing controversies related with it.[7–9] Furthermore, all major national and international COPD guidelines, both at the primary and specialized care level, also include chapters on related topics, namely the American Thoracic Society/European Respiratory Society (ATS/ERS),[10] the Global Obstructive Lung Disease initiative GOLD,[5] the International Primary Care Research Group (IPCRG),[11] Sociedad Española de Neumología y Cirugía Torácica/Asociación Latinoamericana del Tórax SEPAR/ALAT,[12] and the United Kingdom National Institute for Health and Clinical Excellence (NICE),[13] among others. This article summarizes new developments surrounding the epidemiology of COPD at both the population and clinical levels, and also in comparison with other major burden contributors.

EPIDEMIOLOGY

The highly cited, influential GBD studies estimated that COPD causes the death of at least 2.9 million people annually. Estimates of global mortality in 1990[3] were updated in 2006,[14] and will be next available and expanded in 2012.[15] The GBD highlights that COPD was the sixth leading cause of death in 1990, has been the fourth since 2000, and is projected to be the third by 2020. These estimates are likely to be conservative because they did not account for deaths whereby COPD is a contributory cause, although misclassification can be large.[16] Subsequent to that date, even assuming the most pessimistic scenario regarding the global spread of human immunodeficiency virus (HIV)/AIDS, by 2030 COPD will be the direct underlying cause of 7.8% of all deaths and will represent 27% of deaths related with smoking, only surpassed by 33% for cancer and 29% for cardiovascular disease.[17]

In the absence of population spirometry and with a COPD underdiagnosis of a staggering 80% to 90% in all world regions and scenarios,[18] the number of COPD patients worldwide of 210 million is useful, yet has to be used with caution because its expected geographic distribution (**Fig. 1**) is a result of massive extrapolation from individual limited studies. Overall, the prevalence of COPD in the general population is estimated to be approximately 1% across all ages, increasing steeply to 8% to 10% or higher among those of approximate age 40 years.[19] Both the *Proyecto Latinoamericano de Investigación en Obstrucción Pulmonar* (PLATINO)[20] and the Burden of Obstructive Lung Disease (BOLD)[21] initiatives have expanded our knowledge on the worldwide distribution of COPD. However, the PLATINO initiative involved only 5 Latin American cities whereas the BOLD initiative, as of November 2010, has been completed in 21 centers worldwide plus 15 BOLD

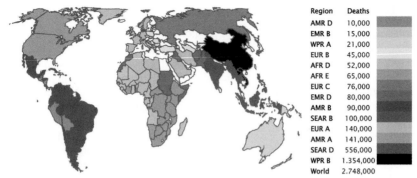

Region	Deaths
AMR D	10,000
EMR B	15,000
WPR A	21,000
EUR B	45,000
AFR D	52,000
AFR E	65,000
EUR C	76,000
EMR D	80,000
AMR B	90,000
SEAR B	100,000
EUR A	140,000
AMR A	141,000
SEAR D	556,000
WPR B	1.354,000
World	2.748,000

Fig. 1. Estimated COPD deaths by World Health Organization (WHO) region in 2002. AFR, Africa; AMR, Americas; SEAR, South-East Asia; EUR, Europe; EMR, Eastern Mediterranean; WPR, Western Pacific. A, very low child and adult mortality; B, low child and adult mortality; C, low child mortality and high adult mortality; D, high child and adult mortality; E, high child mortality and very high adult mortality. The mortality strata (A–E) were used to distinguish groupings of countries likely to be at a similar level of health development among the member states of the WHO regions. (*Adapted from* Lopez AD, Shibuya K, Rao C, et al. The global burden of COPD: future COPD projections. Eur Respir J 2006;27:397–412; with permission.)

subsites in Australia, Canada, and China. There are many areas in the world, especially in Asia and Africa, with an absence of data, not only any type of spirometric data but also data on rates of physician-diagnosed COPD or the old terms chronic bronchitis and emphysema, with all its intrinsic limitations. With diseases changing with time and with an aging population,[22] and countries transitioning within different stages of the tobacco epidemic,[23] current estimates may need to be updated periodically. Contrary to asthma and other conditions, there is a lack of repeated surveys assessing time trends in COPD. Two recent, controversial studies are available, from Spain and Finland,[24,25] and when objective population spirometry is applied it appears that COPD prevalence might have plateaued or even decreased in certain countries. However surprising these conclusions might be, and whether these findings be real or confounded with methodological issues,[26,27] they indicate that perhaps subtle changes in the risk factors or in the way spirometry is performed, apart from the aforementioned demographic changes and with other factors being the same, make spirometry-based measurements difficult to compare over time. The expected geographic homogeneity of COPD estimates (note that all PLATINO and most BOLD estimates are from urban cities from different countries) might also be a complex issue. Also very recently, the IBERPOC (Epidemiologic Study of COPD) in Spain concluded that there were significant variations in the distribution of COPD in the 11 centers participating, up to 3-fold either in prevalence or in underdiagnosis and undertreatment of COPD, and even within 2 neighborhoods of Madrid.[28] A similar magnitude in differences in underdiagnosis and overdiagnosis has been detected within BOLD centers.[29] Current projections up to 2030 indicate that although major vascular diseases will remain leading causes of global disease burden, others such as HIV/AIDS, diarrheal diseases, and lower respiratory infections will be outranked by COPD, in part reflecting the projected increases in death and disability from tobacco use.[30] These factors will be taken into account when producing estimates in GBD III.[15]

DEFINITION OF COPD

Spirometry is the most common of the pulmonary function tests, and enables any health professional to make an objective measurement of airflow limitation and the degree to which it is reversible. As a diagnostic test for COPD, spirometry is a reliable, simple, noninvasive, safe, and nonexpensive procedure to detect airflow limitation. Trained technicians can meet quality goals for spirometry tests about 90% of the time.[31] Early diagnosis of COPD should affect individual and population outcomes, including supporting smoking cessation and reducing the societal burden of COPD. Nevertheless, the thresholds in the diagnosis and staging of COPD have been and are a major setback to many efforts, and many still disagree. The updated NICE guidelines in 2010 have stepped back from using prebronchodilator spirometry alone,[13] and now all major COPD guidelines, at both the primary and secondary levels, recommend the use of postbronchodilator spirometry.[5,10–13] To make things even less simple and more confusing, the historical debate on using a fixed ratio of forced expiration volume in the first second of expiration to forced vital capacity (FEV_1/FVC) of less than 0.70 versus its lower limit of normal or other indices remains a recurrent debate[32–35]; New evidence aimed at making ends meet actually produces more gaps and more questions,[34,36] polarizing all postures even more. Perhaps by learning how other medical specialties have solved similar problems in defining diabetes mellitus, arterial hypertension,[37] or other concomitant disorders might be of help to the COPD definition saga.

RISK FACTORS

There are comprehensive lists of risk factors associated with the development and triggering of COPD exacerbations, available elsewhere.[5,10–13] Some of them are amenable to modification whereas others are not, and some apply at the individual and/or group level, so that in all likelihood any strategy to limit each burden differs.[38] The recent literature is packed with reports aimed at explaining COPD separately from smoking. Risk factors for developing COPD other than smoking tobacco are being increasingly recognized,[3] and include many other environmental exposures such as occupational exposures to dust and fumes in the developed and developing countries[39] and indoor biomass fuel burning in many developing countries.[40] A decade ago, analyses of data from the US population-based Third National Health and Nutrition Examination Survey (NHANES III) suggested that the fraction of COPD attributable to work is 19% overall, and 31% among those who have never smoked.[41] Joint exposure to smoking and occupational factors has been shown to multiply the risk of COPD.[42,43] Reduction of such exposures on a population or an individual might be worthwhile. Factors that seem to be less important in the development of COPD, although they may worsen disease, include outdoor pollutants and passive smoke exposure. Women seem to be more susceptible to the effects of tobacco smoke, and the same might be true for other harmful inhalational substances. A different dose-response relationship for men and women has been shown, especially at lower levels of smoking.[44] Several other factors associated with COPD development may not currently be possible to modify. These include the aging lung, concomitant disorders, and repeated respiratory infections in children or adults. The best-known genetic factor linked to COPD is α_1-antitrypsin deficiency (α_1-ATD), which is present in up to 3% of patients with COPD, and when combined with smoking increases the risk of panlobular emphysema.[45] Several other genes have been implicated in COPD, but the consistency of their effect in the development of COPD is currently unproved. The one concomitant disorder consistently shown to be associated with COPD development is asthma, and it seems that people with asthma who smoke lose lung function more rapidly than individuals without asthma.[46] Recent reports aim also at a direct link with tuberculosis.[47] At present, global climate change, among other health effects, may contribute to increases in respiratory conditions, including COPD, in terms of both increasing incidence and exacerbating prevalent COPD cases.[48]

SPIROMETRY SCREENING

At this early stage, spirometry as a screening tool of disease has been explored in only α_1-ATD probands and their relatives, smokers, and those workers with occupational exposures. Apart from marihuana consumers[49,50] and biomass exposure in selected developing countries,[51] spirometry is unlikely to be successful for other types of exposures.

Although it is important to recognize that COPD does not exclusively affect smokers, it is the authors' opinion that the current emphasis on COPD in nonsmokers[52,53] might distract many (at least in developed countries) from the "elephant in the room." There are now more smokers worldwide than ever before in history; calculating the population-attributable fraction can be tricky, and its interpretation can be misleading. A classic quote from the US Surgeon General Reports was that "90% of COPD can be attributed to smoking."[54] However, by quoting individual studies, these estimates are reduced to a figure of 44% to 45%,[55–57] and it is now suggested that in developed countries cigarette smoking causes COPD in only 50% to 70% of patients.[58] The population-attributable fraction of a given risk factor should only be estimated for causal factors, and the vast amount of available epidemiologic evidence is sufficient to infer a causal relationship between active smoking and COPD. The calculation of the population-attributable fraction of smoking in COPD is proportional to 2 factors: the relative risk of smoking in producing COPD (which should be constant and close to 10) and the prevalence of smoking in the population (which has been decreasing from 60% or more in the 1940s to less than 30% in many Western countries worldwide).[23] The elimination of smoking could largely prevent most COPD. All health care practitioners can be considered Public Health practitioners as well, and tackling tobacco use should be a continued priority. The damage caused by tobacco and other types of smoking on the lungs and other organs of the smoker, as well as on involuntary passive smokers, has been extensively documented.[59] The authors agree that the diagnostic process should start and not stop at the point of a spirometric diagnosis of airflow limitation, as it is simplistic to infer that individuals with airflow limitation who do not smoke constitute cases of nonsmoking COPD.

BURDEN OF COPD IN DEVELOPING COUNTRIES

On a global scale, about 50% of all households and about 90% of those in rural areas of developing countries use solid fuels (coal and biomass) as their main source of energy. Thus, one-half of the world's population (up to 3 billion people) is exposed to the harmful effects of solid-fuel smoke produced by unvented open fires for heating and cooking.[60,61] The use of solid fuels is the most important source of indoor air pollution and is inversely associated with socioeconomic development, because the homes of poor people are places where lung injury caused by smoke from solid fuel is very likely. Whereas the percentage of households using solid fuels for cooking and heating is between 0% and 5% in developed countries, it is as much as 80% in India, China, and sub-Saharan Africa.[62,63] Between 30% and 75% of households in rural areas of Latin America use biomass fuels for cooking.[64] Therefore, the

Table 1
Estimates of worldwide annual deaths (in thousands) due to COPD, comparing the impact of tobacco and biomass by gender

	Men		Women	
Countries	Tobacco	Biomass	Tobacco	Biomass
Poor and middle income	635	309	210	535
Rich	135	0	93	0
All	770	309	302	535

Data from Lopez AD, Mathers CD, Ezzati M, et al, editors. Global burden of disease and risk factors. Washington, DC: World Bank Publications; 2006. p. 1–11. Chapter 1.

World Health Organization estimates that solid-fuel smoke is responsible for about 700,000 deaths due to COPD annually.[65] In conclusion, in developing countries almost 50% of deaths from COPD can be attributed to exposure to biomass, and about 75% of these are in women (**Table 1**).[66,67] However, as previously mentioned, the impact of biomass in COPD in developed countries is negligible.

FUTURE

Several investigators,[68] societies, and nonprofit international initiatives have elegantly outlined some of the burning pending questions on COPD burden now and in the foreseeable future, with an intention either to help funding agencies to prioritize limited resources in competitive decision making or to streamline alternative routes to reduce its overall massive burden. Publications include documents from the ATS/ERS,[10,69] GARD,[6] GOLD,[5] IPCRG,[70] as well as from independent researchers.[68,71,72] Innovative ideas, more brainstorming, and close collaboration of respiratory physicians with primary care and internal medicine colleagues should constitute a formula for success.

ACKNOWLEDGMENTS

The authors thank Professor Michael Studnicka for his helpful comments on the manuscript.

REFERENCES

1. International COPD Coalition. Quick facts about COPD. Available at: http://www.internationalcopd.org/materials/patients/learn/facts.aspx. Accessed September 9, 2011.
2. Bousquet J, Kiley J, Bateman ED, et al. Prioritized research agenda for prevention and control of chronic respiratory diseases. Eur Respir J 2010;36:995–1001.
3. Murray CJ, Lopez AD. Alternative projections of mortality and disability by cause 1990-2020: Global Burden of Disease Study. Lancet 1997;349:1498–504.
4. European Respiratory Society. European lung white book. Huddersfield (UK): European Respiratory Society Journals; 2003.
5. Rabe KF, Hurd S, Anzueto A, et al. Global strategy for the diagnosis, management, and prevention of chronic obstructive pulmonary disease: GOLD executive summary. Am J Respir Crit Care Med 2007;176:532–55.

6. Bousquet J, Khaltaev N. Global surveillance, prevention and control of chronic respiratory diseases. A comprehensive approach. Available at: www.who.int/gard/publications/GARD%20Book%202007.pdf. Date last updated: 2007 [accessed].
7. Stockley RA, Mannino D, Barnes PJ. Burden and pathogenesis of chronic obstructive pulmonary disease. Proc Am Thorac Soc 2009;6:524–6.
8. Mannino DM, Buist AS. Global burden of COPD: risk factors, prevalence, and future trends. Lancet 2007;370:765–73.
9. Chapman KR, Mannino DM, Soriano JB, et al. Epidemiology and costs of chronic obstructive pulmonary disease. Eur Respir J 2006;27:188–207.
10. Celli BR, MacNee W. Standards for the diagnosis and treatment of patients with COPD: a summary of the ATS/ERS position paper. Eur Respir J 2004; 23:932–46.
11. Bellamy D, Bouchard J, Henrichsen S, et al. International Primary Care Respiratory Group (IPCRG) Guidelines: management of chronic obstructive pulmonary disease (COPD). Prim Care Respir J 2006;15(1):48–57.
12. Peces-Barba G, Barberà JA, Agustí A, et al. [Diagnosis and management of chronic obstructive pulmonary disease: joint guidelines of the Spanish Society of Pulmonology and Thoracic Surgery (SEPAR) and the Latin American Thoracic Society (ALAT)]. Arch Bronconeumol 2008;44:271–81 [in Spanish].
13. O'Reilly J, Jones MM, Parnham J, et al. Management of stable chronic obstructive pulmonary disease in primary and secondary care: summary of updated NICE guidance. BMJ 2010;340:c3134.
14. Lopez AD, Shibuya K, Rao C, et al. The Global burden of COPD: future COPD projections. Eur Respir J 2006;27:397–412.
15. Murray CJ, Lopez AD, Black R, et al. Global burden of disease 2005: call for collaborators. Lancet 2007;370:109–10.
16. Jensen HH, Godtfredsen NS, Lange P, et al. Potential misclassification of causes of death from COPD. Eur Respir J 2006;28:781–5.
17. Mathers CD, Roncar D. Projections of global mortality and burden of disease from 2002 to 2030. PLoS Med 2006;3:2011–30.
18. Soriano JB, Zielinski J, Price D. Screening for and early detection of chronic obstructive pulmonary disease. Lancet 2009;29(374):721–32.
19. Halbert RJ, Natoli JL, Gano A, et al. Global burden of COPD: systematic review and meta-analysis. Eur Respir J 2006;28:523–32.
20. Menezes AM, Perez-Padilla R, Jardim JR, et al. Chronic obstructive pulmonary disease in five Latin American cities (the PLATINO study): a prevalence study. Lancet 2005;366:1875–81.
21. Buist AS, McBurnie MA, Vollmer WM, et al, BOLD Collaborative Research Group. International variation in the prevalence of COPD (the BOLD Study): a population-based prevalence study. Lancet 2007;370:741–50.
22. Christensen K, Doblhammer G, Rau R, et al. Ageing populations: the challenges ahead. Lancet 2009;374:1196–208.
23. Shafey O, Erisksen M, Ross H, et al. The tobacco atlas. Geneva: American Cancer Society and the World Lung Foundation; 2009.
24. Soriano JB, Ancochea J, Miravitlles M, et al. Recent trends in COPD prevalence in Spain: a repeated cross-sectional survey 1997-2007. Eur Respir J 2010;36: 758–65.
25. Vasankari TM, Impivaara O, Heliövaara M, et al. No increase in the prevalence of COPD in two decades. Eur Respir J 2010;36:766–73.
26. Celli BR. The light at the end of the tunnel: is COPD prevalence changing? Eur Respir J 2010;36:718–9.

27. Cerveri I, De Marco R. What makes large epidemiological studies comparable? Eur Respir J 2010;36:720–1.
28. Soriano JB, Miravitlles M, Borderías L, et al. [Geographical variations in the prevalence of COPD in Spain: relationship to smoking, death rates and other determining factors]. Arch Bronconeumol 2010;46:522–30 [in Spanish].
29. McBurnie MA, Nizankowska-Mogilnicka E, Nielsen R, et al. Worldwide under- and over-diagnosis of COPD: results from the BOLD study. Abstract Presented at the ERS (European Respiratory Society) Congress 2009. Vienna, 2009. abstract: P1016.
30. Lopez AD, Mathers CD. Measuring the global burden of disease and epidemiological transitions: 2002-2030. Ann Trop Med Parasitol 2006;100:481–99.
31. Enright P, Vollmer WM, Lamprecht B, et al. Quality of Spirometry tests performed by 9893 adults in 14 countries: The BOLD Study. Respir Med 2011;105:1507–15.
32. Celli BR, Halbert RJ. Point: should we abandon FEV_1/FVC <0.70 to detect airway obstruction? No. Chest 2010;138:1037–40.
33. Enright P, Brusasco V. Counterpoint: should we abandon FEV_1/FVC <0.70 to detect airway obstruction? Yes. Chest 2010;138:1040–2.
34. Le groupe Pulmonaria, Quanjer PH, Enright PL, et al. [Open letter to the members of the GOLD committee]. Rev Mal Respir 2010;27:1003–7 [in French].
35. Quanjer P, Enright PL, Ruppel G, et al. GOLD and the fixed ratio. Eur Respir J 2011;38:482–4.
36. García-Rio F, Soriano JB, Miravitlles M, et al. Subjects "over-diagnosed" as COPD by the 0.7 fixed ratio have a poor health-related quality of life. Chest 2011;139: 1072–80.
37. Chobanian AV. Shattuck Lecture. The hypertension paradox—more uncontrolled disease despite improved therapy. N Engl J Med 2009;361:878–87.
38. Rose G. Sick individuals and sick populations. Int J Epidemiol 1985;14:32–8.
39. Blanc PD, Menezes AM, Plana E, et al. Occupational exposures and COPD: an ecological analysis of international data. Eur Respir J 2009;33:298–304.
40. Ezzati M, Hoorn SV, Rodgers A, et al. Estimates of global and regional potential health gains from reducing multiple major risk factors. Lancet 2003;362: 271–80.
41. Hnizdo E, Sullivan PA, Bang KM, et al. Association between chronic obstructive pulmonary disease and employment by industry and occupation in the US population: a study of data from the Third National Health and Nutrition Examination Survey. Am J Epidemiol 2002;156:738–46.
42. Blanc PD, Iribarren C, Trupin L, et al. Occupational exposures and the risk of COPD: dusty trades revisited. Thorax 2009;64:6–12.
43. de Meer G, Kerkhof M, Kromhout H, et al. Interaction of atopy and smoking on respiratory effects of occupational dust exposure: a general population-based study. Environ Health 2004;3(1):6.
44. Sørheim IC, Johannessen A, Gulsvik A, et al. Gender differences in COPD: are women more susceptible to smoking effects than men? Thorax 2010;65(6):480–5.
45. Stoller JK, Aboussouan LS. α1-Antitrypsin deficiency. Lancet 2005;365:2225–36.
46. Lange P, Parner P, Vestbo J, et al. A 15-year follow-up study of ventilatory function in adults with asthma. N Engl J Med 1998;339:1194–200.
47. Menezes AM, Hallal PC, Perez-Padilla R, et al. Tuberculosis and airflow obstruction: evidence from the PLATINO study in Latin America. Eur Respir J 2007;30: 1180–5.
48. Ciscar JC, Iglesias A, Feyen L, et al. Physical and economic consequences of climate change in Europe. Proc Natl Acad Sci U S A 2011;108:2678–83.

49. Tashkin DP. Smoked marijuana as a cause of lung injury. Monaldi Arch Chest Dis 2005;63:93–100.
50. Aldington S, Williams M, Nowitz M, et al. Effects of cannabis on pulmonary structure, function and symptoms. Thorax 2007;62:1058–63.
51. Torres-Duque C, Maldonado D, Pérez-Padilla R, et al. Biomass fuels and respiratory diseases: a review of the evidence. Proc Am Thorac Soc 2008;5:577–90.
52. Anonymous. COPD-more than just tobacco smoke. Lancet 2009;374:663.
53. Eisner MD, Anthonisen N, Coultas D, et al. An official American Thoracic Society public policy statement: novel risk factors and the global burden of chronic obstructive pulmonary disease. Am J Respir Crit Care Med 2010; 182:693–718.
54. U.S. Department of Health and Human Services. The health consequences of smoking: a report of the surgeon general. Atlanta (GA): US Department of Health and Human Services, Centers for Disease Control and Prevention, National Center for Chronic Disease Prevention and Health Promotion, Office on Smoking and Health; 2004.
55. Lundbäck B, Lindberg A, Lindstrom M, et al. Obstructive lung disease in Northern Sweden studies. Not 15 but 50% of smokers develop COPD? Report from the Obstructive Lung Disease in Northern Sweden Studies. Respir Med 2003;97:115–22.
56. Lindberg A, Bjerg-Backlund A, Ronmark E, et al. Prevalence and underdiagnosis of COPD by disease severity and the attributable fraction of smoking. Report from the Obstructive Lung Disease in Northern Sweden Studies. Respir Med 2006; 100:264–72.
57. Mannino DM, Buist AS, Petty TL, et al. Lung function and mortality in the United States: data from the first National Health and Nutrition Examination Survey follow up study. Thorax 2003;58:388–93.
58. Chilvers ER, Lomas DA. Diagnosing COPD in non-smokers: splitting not lumping. Thorax 2010;65:465–6.
59. Brandt AM. FDA regulation of tobacco—pitfalls and possibilities. N Engl J Med 2008;359:445–8.
60. Romieu I, Riojas-Rodríguez H, Marrón-Mares AT, et al. Improved biomass stove intervention in rural Mexico: impact on the respiratory health of women. Am J Respir Crit Care Med 2009;180(7):649–56.
61. Perez-Padilla R, Schilmann A, Riojas-Rodriguez H. Respiratory health effects of indoor air pollution. Int J Tuberc Lung Dis 2010;14:1079–86.
62. Desai M, Mehta S, Smith K. Indoor smoke from solid fuels: assessing the environmental burden of disease at national and local levels. Geneva (Switzerland): World Health Organization; 2004.
63. Smith KR, Metha S, Maeusezahl-Feuz M. Indoor air pollution from household use of solid fuels. In: Ezzati M, Lopez A, Rodgers A, et al, editors. Comparative quantification of health risks. Global and regional burden of disease attributable to selected major risk factors. Geneva (Switzerland): World Health Organization; 2004. p. 1435–9.
64. Bruce N, Perez-Padilla R, Albalak R. Indoor air pollution in developing countries: a major environmental and public health challenge. Bull World Health Organ 2000;78:1078–92.
65. Zhang J, Smith KR. Indoor air pollution: a global health concern. Br Med Bull 2003;68:209–25.
66. World Health Organization. The World Health Report 2002: reducing risks, promoting healthy life. Geneva (Switzerland): World Health Organization; 2002.

67. Lopez AD, Mathers CD, Ezzati M, et al, editors. Global burden of disease and risk factors. Washington, DC: World Bank Publications; 2006. p. 1–11. Chapter 1.
68. Agusti A, Barnes PJ. What the journal would like to publish on chronic obstructive pulmonary disease. Am J Respir Crit Care Med 2010;182(1):1–2.
69. Cazzola M, MacNee W, Martinez FJ, et al. Outcomes for COPD pharmacological trials: from lung function to biomarkers. Eur Respir J 2008;31:416–69.
70. Pinnock H, Thomas M, Tsiligianni I, et al. The International Primary Care Respiratory Group (IPCRG) Research Needs Statement 2010. Prim Care Respir J 2010; 19(Suppl 1):S1–20.
71. Agusti A, Vestbo J. Current controversies and future perspectives in COPD. Am J Respir Crit Care Med 2011;184(5):507–13.
72. Soriano JB, Brusasco V, Dinh-Xuan AT. ERJ makes COPD a priority. Eur Respir J 2011;38(5):999–1001.

Pathobiologic Mechanisms of Chronic Obstructive Pulmonary Disease

Anthony Tam, BSc, Don D. Sin, MD*

KEYWORDS

- Cigarette smoke • COPD • Pathobiologic mechanism • Inflammation • Immunity

KEY POINTS

- External triggers, such as cigarette smoke and biomass fuel, are important in COPD progression.
- Protease–antiprotease balance, autoimmunity, mucus hypersecretion, airway wall remodeling, and chronic respiratory infections have all been implicated in disease pathogenesis.
- The leading candidates for explaining COPD pathogenesis are (1) the protease–antiprotease hypothesis, (2) the Dutch hypothesis, (3) the British hypothesis, and (4) the autoimmunity hypothesis.
- Given the heterogeneity of the disease (and phenotypes), it is unrealistic to believe that one pathway will fully explain COPD pathophysiology.

INTRODUCTION

Chronic obstructive pulmonary disease (COPD) is a common disorder affecting 5% to 15% of the adult population 45 years of age and older across the world. More than 200 million individuals worldwide have COPD and nearly 3 million die from this disorder annually, making COPD the fourth leading cause of mortality in the world. By 2020, COPD will surpass other common causes of mortality and become the third leading cause of mortality, trailing only ischemic heart disease and stroke.[1] Unfortunately, there is a dearth of therapies that can prolong survival in COPD. Cigarette smoke (CS) is the major cause of COPD but there is no consensus on how CS causes COPD.[1,2] Notwithstanding, unless effective regulations are implemented to prevent young people from starting smoking and to help current smokers to quit, global tobacco deaths have

Research Funding: Canadian Institute of Health Research.
Financial interest: AT declared no financial interest. DDS has received honoraria for speaking engagements from GlaxoSmithKine (GSK), AstraZeneca (AZ), and Pfizer. DDS sits on the international advisory board for Merck Frosst and has received research grants in the last 5 years from AZ, GSK, and Merck.
Department of Medicine, The UBC James Hogg Research Centre, Providence Heart and Lung Centre, University of British Columbia, Vancouver, British Columbia, Canada
* Corresponding author. 1081 Burrard Street, Vancouver, BC, Canada.
E-mail address: Don.Sin@hli.ubc.ca

Med Clin N Am 96 (2012) 681–698
doi:10.1016/j.mcna.2012.04.012
0025-7125/12/$ – see front matter © 2012 Elsevier Inc. All rights reserved.
medical.theclinics.com

been projected to approach 1 billion in the twenty-first century.[3] This article reviews some of the postulated pathobiologic mechanisms linking CS to COPD.

PHENOTYPES OF COPD

COPD is characterized by progressive airflow limitation that is not fully reversible.[4] COPD is composed of three major clinical phenotypes: (1) emphysema, (2) chronic bronchitis, and (3) small airways disease. Emphysema is a pathologic diagnosis, defined by abnormal enlargement of airspaces distal to terminal bronchioles that is permanent and accompanied by destruction of alveoli, resulting in a loss of lung elastic recoil pressure without obvious fibrosis and gas exchange abnormalities, such as hypoxemia and hypercapnia.[5,6] In normal lungs, expiration is passive. During expiration, the stored mechanical energy generated in the alveolar walls propels air out of alveoli and into proximal airways. However, in emphysema, there is premature closure of the small airways because of a loss in elastic recoil pressure and increased lung compliance, which leads to overinflation, gas trapping, dynamic hyperinflation, and expiratory flow limitation.[7] During a forced vital capacity (FVC) maneuver, flow is further limited because of early collapse of the small airways from increased pleural pressure.[7]

Chronic bronchitis is characterized clinically by increased mucus production caused by hypertrophy of glandular structures and goblet cell metaplasia in proximal airways, which leads to daily productive cough for at least 3 months for 2 successive years.[4] Approximately 50% of smokers develop chronic bronchitis. Interestingly, some patients with chronic bronchitis do not have airflow limitation, whereas others demonstrate airflow limitation in the absence of chronic bronchitis.[4] Thus, chronic bronchitis represents a distinct phenotype of COPD. Importantly, chronic mucus plugging in the airways is one of the strongest predictor of COPD mortality.[8]

In most cases of COPD, the small airways (<2 mm in diameter) undergo remodeling, which is characterized by increased volume of airway wall tissue including epithelium, lamina propria, smooth muscle, and adventitia located between the epithelial surfaces and muscle layer.[9] These changes are associated with accelerated decline of forced expiratory volume in the first second of expiration (FEV_1).[10] Matsuba and Thurlbeck[11] originally hypothesized that airway remodeling contributes to fixed airflow limitation by preventing adequate dilation in response to bronchodilators, such as β_2 agonists or acetylcholine. With COPD progression, airway remodeling worsens and is accompanied by mucus hypersecretion and poor mucociliary clearance, leading to accumulation of mucus and inflammatory debris in the lumen.[9]

Although most patients with COPD have emphysema and small airway remodeling, some have a clear predominance of emphysema, whereas others have a predominance of airway disease.[12] A recent large-scale genetic study has shown that although emphysema and airway remodeling contribute to airflow limitation in COPD, they demonstrate independent familiar aggregation, suggesting that these phenotypes are influenced by different genetic factors.[13] Consistent with this notion, Gosselink and coworkers[14] showed that there is differential gene expression between airway wall and the surrounding parenchyma by using laser-capture microdissection and Taqman qualitative polymerase chain reaction on lung tissue specimens collected from patients with COPD. In this study, factors that promoted tissue growth and proliferation increased with airway remodeling, whereas factors that enhanced tissue destruction were overrepresented in the surrounding areas of emphysema. The clinical presentations of these two morphologic phenotypes are also different. Patients who are emphysema-predominant tend to be older and thinner, and have a greater smoking history and worse quality of life than those with a predominance of airway disease. Physiologically, the patients who are emphysema-predominant have increased gas exchange abnormalities and lower FEV_1/FVC ratio and poorer FEV_1 reversibility than those with a predominance of airways disease.[15,16] Notwithstanding these different phenotypes, recent data by McDonough and colleagues[17] suggest that the disease begins in the small airways and over time spreads distally into the parenchymal tissue, leading to emphysema. The small airway disease is characterized by airway inflammation and remodeling (defined as thickening of airway wall) and destruction, which in turn results in small airway attrition over time. Even in patients with mild COPD (FEV_1 $\geq$80% of predicted with FEV_1/FVC ratio of <70%), there is significant loss of small airways, suggesting that this process begins early in the pathogenesis of COPD.[17]

PROPERTIES OF CS

CS is the most important risk factor for COPD, responsible for more than 50% of cases worldwide. However, the exact mechanism by which this happens remains largely a mystery. CS consists of sidestream and mainstream smoke. Sidestream smoke is produced by the tips of cigarettes, whereas mainstream smoke is produced by inhaling the mouth end of cigarettes.[18] CS exists in two forms: a gaseous and a particulate phase. The gaseous phase is composed predominantly of carbon monoxide, ammonia, dimethylnitrosamine, formaldehyde, hydrogen cyanide, and acrolein. The main components of the particulate phase are nicotine, tar, benzene, and bezo(a)pyrene. According to the International Agency for Research in Cancer, 10 polycyclic aromatic hydrocarbons (PAH), 8 tobacco-specific nitrosamines, and at least 45 other compounds found in tobacco smoke are possible human carcinogens.[19] Among all chemicals found in CS, nicotine has been the best studied. Nicotine is a powerful alkaloid with highly additive properties and is rapidly absorbed in the body, reaching the brain in 10 to 20 seconds after inhalation.[20] Although nicotine per se is not considered a lung toxin, its metabolites may become carcinogenic through a process called "metabolic bioactivation."[21,22] Nicotine absorption across biologic membranes is maximal at physiologic and at alkaline pH ($\geq$7.4).[23] Lung is an excellent organ for nicotine absorption and delivery because of its large surface area and high perfusion.[23] Once inhaled, approximately 70% to 80% of nicotine is converted to cotinine. Thus, cotinine is a useful biomarker for acute nicotine exposure.[24]

CYTOCHROME P-450 GENE EXPRESSION

After inhalation, the chemicals from CS are rapidly absorbed into the bloodstream and metabolized in two different phases. Phase I is mediated largely by cytochrome P-450 (CYP) enzymes, which are a family of xenobiotic enzymes responsible for detoxifying CS and other environmental irritants into intermediate metabolites. In general, these metabolites are conjugated by phase II enzymes and excreted. The rate-limiting step in most cases is phase II reaction, which involves attachment of glucuronic acid, sulfate, or glycine to intermediate metabolites in forming water-soluble compounds. Thus, if there is underexpression of phase II enzymes or complete saturation of their binding sites, CYP-based metabolites can accumulate in lungs. Because some intermediate metabolites are as toxic as the parent compound or even more toxic than their parent constituents, lungs may suffer oxidant damage from these metabolites unless there is excellent cooperation of phase I and phase II enzymes. For example, benzo(a)pyrene, a relatively harmless PAH, can be oxidized to bezo(a) pyrene-7,8-diol by CYP1A1 and becomes a potent procarcinogen in the lung.[25] In addition, naphthalene, the most abundant PAH in sidestream smoke, can be metabolized by CYP1A2, CYP2E1, and CYP3A4 from naphthalene to naphthalene-1, 2-epoxide and then bioactivated to 1,4-napthoquinole and 1,2-napthoquinone,[26] both of which are known carcinogens to lungs. It has been shown that cells in mice distal airways are three to five times more sensitive to the toxic effects of naphthalene than proximal airways. This may be relevant for COPD because it is generally accepted that airways smaller than 2 mm in diameter are the major site of airflow limitation. There are at least 57 different CYP genes and 24 pseudogenes found in humans[27] and most CYPs are expressed in human liver, but are also expressed on a smaller scale in extrahepatic tissues, such as the skin and lungs.[20]

PATHOBIOLOGIC MECHANISMS
Innate and Adaptive Immunity

The main risk factor for COPD is tobacco smoking; however, other noxious gases, such as biomass smoke, air pollution particles, and marijuana, have also been implicated. When inhaled into lungs, these noxious gases and particles induce an inflammatory reaction in the host that is generally mild and controlled because of several lines of defense including (1) the airway epithelial barrier that allows efficient mucociliary clearance of foreign materials out of the lung,[28] (2) an extensive system of macrophages that take out foreign particles at the bronchial and alveolar surfaces,[29] and (3) a very thin airway surface liquid layer that carries debris from the alveolar surfaces and out of the conducting airways.[30] Epithelial barrier is the first barrier to noxious environmental particles, preventing their penetration into deeper layers. Tight junctions play a critical role in this process. In lumens of the airways, the mucociliary elevator traps incoming particulate matter and carries it back out.[31,32] The next level of defense is the immune system. Resident macrophages and monocytes patrol the lungs for any foreign substances and remove them through phagocytosis. Epithelial cells, macrophages, and dendritic cells also release a cascade of chemokines and cytokines that recruit additional inflammatory cells including neutrophils and monocytes to deal with the foreign substance. Other inflammatory cells involved in the innate immune responses include mast cells, which reside mostly in the connective tissues and mucous membranes; natural killer cells, which destroy tumor cells; basophils; and eosinophils. They, along with epithelial cells, amplify the immune system by activating the complement cascade, pattern recognition receptors, and nucleotide-binding oligomerization domain proteins, such as Nod1 and Nod2, and by releasing defensins. The latter is mostly expressed by neutrophils and macrophages.

Over time, these inflammatory cells orchestrate the shift in the immune response to adaptive immunity by recruiting and activating lymphocytes. B cells are involved in the humoral immune response, whereas T cells are involved in cell-mediated immunity. There are three major types of T cells: (1) cytotoxic, (2) helper, and (3) regulatory. They recognize antigens bound to class I major histocompatibility complex (MHC) molecules of antigen-presenting cells. Once activated, cytotoxic T cells release toxins, such as perforin and granzymes, which induce cellular destruction and lysis. Cytotoxic T cells also express FAS ligand, which on activation can stimulate apoptosis of the targeted cell. Unlike cytotoxic T cells, helper T cells have no intrinsic capacity to destroy cells or antigen. Their primary function is to assist other immune cells to destroy foreign substances and cells. Helper T cells generally respond to MHC class II molecules on antigen-presenting cells. The binding of antigen along with MHC class II molecules to receptors on helper T cells causes activation and proliferation of lymphocytes. Th1 subset of helper T cells secrete predominantly interferon (IFN)-γ and tumor necrosis factor (TNF)-β, whereas the Th2 subset secrete predominantly inter-leukin (IL)-4, 5, 6, 10, and 13. Th1 cells are thought to cause cellular destruction by assisting macrophages and cytotoxic T cells. Th2 cells enhance humoral immune system by promoting B-cell antibody class switching and stimulating antibody production. Th1 and Th2 systems are regulated in a negative feedback loop. Classi-cally, the Th1 system has been associated with bacterial and viral killing, whereas the Th2 system has been associated with allergy and parasite elimination (**Fig. 1**).

Immunity in COPD

The immune responses in COPD are disturbed. Chronic exposure to CS weakens physical barrier and dysregulates mucociliary elevator causing excess penetration of foreign substances into the deeper and more vulnerable layers.[28,33,34] In COPD, for largely unknown reasons, there is excess accumulation of neutrophils and macro-phages in lungs, which unleash a cocktail of proteolytic enzymes, such as serine proteases and matrix metalloproteinases (MMPs), leading to uncontrolled destruction of tissue and perpetuation of the inflammatory cascade.[35] In mice models, the critical molecules involved in the acute inflammatory response related to CS are toll-like receptor (TLR)-4 and its downstream signaling proteins, MyD88 and IL-receptor 1. Stimulation of this signaling pathway induces the production of IL-1β, which in turn recruits inflammatory cells including neutrophils to the lungs.[36] TLR-4 recognizes lipo-polysaccharide (LPS) from gram-negative bacteria, and TLR-2 induces

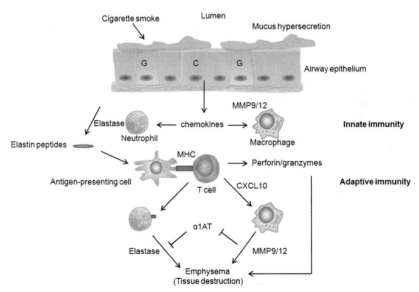

Fig. 1. Dysregulation of immune response by cigarette smoke. Exposure to cigarette smoke leads to the recruitment of inflammatory cells, such as macrophages and neutrophils, by chemokines and cytokines that are released by epithelial and dendritic cells. Proteolytic enzymes including elastase and MMP (9 and 12) lead to the release of elastin peptides, which are phagocytosed by dendritic cells and then the antigen is presented for T-cell acti-vation of the adaptive immune response. Sustained activation of T cells leads to greater production of proteolytic enzymes for tissue destruction, which may ultimately contribute to the development of emphysema. MMP, matrix metalloproteinases.

responsiveness to bacterial lipoproteins and to components of gram-positive bacteria, such as peptidoglycan.[37] TLR-4 and TLR-2 are predominantly expressed by monocyte and macrophage, neutrophils, and bronchial epithelial cells.[38,39] Stimulation of airway epithelial cells with bacterial products triggers these receptors to produce inflammatory mediators, such as chemokine (CXCL8/IL-8) and IFN-γ–inducible protein 10, by activating adaptor protein (MyD88), and subsequent downstream signaling molecules, which include nuclear factor (NF)-κB and extracellular signal-regulated kinase 1/2.[37] In later stages of the disease, there is also increased accumulation of CD8+ T cells, which release granzymes and perforin, causing tissue death and destruction.[40,41] Oxidative stress related to COPD and cigarette smoking may exacerbate the inflammatory state by recruiting additional neutrophils and upregulating the inflammatory transcription factor NF-κB, and neutralizing antiproteases, such as α_1-antitrypsin, secretory leukoprotease inhibitor, and tissue inhibitors of MMPs.[5] Notably, CS alone contains more than 10^{14} free radicals, capable of oxidative damage.

Mucus Hypersecretion

Mucus hypersecretion is one of the most prominent features in COPD and mucus plugging of the airways is the single most powerful histologic predictor of mortality in COPD.[8] Two primary functions of the airway epithelium are mucous production and mucociliary transport where mucous cells and ciliated epithelial cells work in collaboration to trap and remove inhaled foreign materials from the airways.[42] However, in chronic airway diseases, mucus hypersecretion may severely dysregulate the process of normal ciliary clearance. As the predominant form of mucin in the human airway, MUC5AC is produced mainly in goblet cells in the surface epithelium, whereas MUC5B is produced mainly by submucosal glands.[43] MUC5AC may be an acute-response mucin responding directly to environmental insults, whereas MUC5B may play a more prominent role in responding to chronic infection and inflammation.[44] Mucin production has been shown to be regulated by inflammatory mediators, such as LPS,[45] TNF-α,[46] IL-1,[46] IL-17,[47] IL-13,[48] and neutrophil elastase[49]; growth factors, such as epidermal growth factor and transforming growth factor-α[50]; and environmental insults, such as CS[51] and bacteria.[52] In addition, it has been shown that female sex hormones, such as estrogen, can upregulate MUC5B gene expression in normal human nasal epithelial cells.[53]

Inflammatory Mediators

Although gram-negative bacteria endotoxin has long been recognized as the principal ligand for TLR-4,[54] CS-induced airway inflammation has also been shown to be dependent on TLR4/MyD88 with the production of IL-1β, which in turn recruits neutrophils to lungs.[36] This increase in neutrophil influx has been associated with enhanced levels of IL-1, IL-6, keratinocyte-derived chemokine, and MMP-9 activity in the alveolar spaces,[36] suggesting a linkage between CS-induced lung tissue degradation and airway inflammation. Although cigarettes contain small amounts of LPS, it is unlikely that CS-related TLR-4 activation is caused by LPS because only 1% of bioactive LPS remains after combustion.[55]

Exposure of mice to CS has been implicated with increased recruitment of macrophages and neutrophils in lung tissues and bronchoalveolar lavage fluid, MMP, serine protease, and sustained NF-κB translocation.[56] Using quantitative real-time polymerase chain reaction, investigators have shown that CS causes increased expression of chemokines (macrophage inflammatory protein-2, monocyte chemoattractant protein-1); inflammatory mediators (TNF-α, IL-1β); leukocyte growth and survival factors (granulocyte-macrophage colony-stimulating factor, and colony-stimulating factor-1); transforming growth factor-β; and MMP-9 and -12.[56] Moreover, reactive oxygen species from inhaled CS cause cell necrosis or apoptosis of alveolar units.[57] This in turn causes cells to secrete stress markers, such as heat shock protein (HSP70),[36] which may activate TLR2 and TLR4[58] and cause additional apoptosis, which creates a vicious cycle.[59] Collectively, these data suggest that CS can lead to enhanced tissue destruction by activating the inflammatory response by macrophages and neutrophils.

It should be noted that the immune responses to CS are extremely complex. CS extract can upregulate inflammation by increasing the expression of TLR-4 and enhancing LPS binding, NF-κB activation, and the release of CXCL8, which promotes the recruitment of neutrophils into lungs.[60] CS can also paradoxically downregulate innate immune responses, leading to increased risk of respiratory infections.[61] In an in vitro study, Kulkarni and colleagues[61] demonstrated that CS inhibits the production of CXCL8 and IL-6 by reducing NF-κB activation in airway epithelial cell line in response to bacterial stimulation. However, treatment with N-acetylcysteine, which is an antioxidant, reverses the immunomodulatory effects of CS, suggesting that oxidative stress pathways are critical in dampening the innate immune responses by CS.[61] CS can also increase the risk of bacterial infections by inducing physiologic and structural changes to the airways, increasing bacterial virulence, and dysregulating immune responses.[62] For example, CS may play a direct role in bacterial colonization of the respiratory tract by reducing mucociliary clearance of bacteria,[63] while enhancing bacterial binding to airway epithelial cells[64] and decreasing the ability of respiratory phagocytic cells to detect and clear pathogenic microbes.[65] Sayers and Drucker[66] have reported that low levels of nicotine exhibit lethal synergy with toxins produced by several periodontal pathogens, and may also affect the growth of bacteria by causing a population shift in the microbial communities in human tissues. Monocytes exposed to CS are poorly reactive to bacteria and LPS by demonstrating reduced bacterial killing and decreased ability to release reactive-oxygen species.[67] These monocytes also show reduced expression of surface pathogen recognition receptors (TLR-2 and MARCO).[68] Other inflammatory cells are also affected by CS. For example, dendritic cells, whose primary role is to bridge the innate and adaptive immune response by antigen processing and presentation, can be downregulated by CS. Nicotine suppresses the maturation of dendritic cells by reducing the expression of antigen-presenting and costimulatory molecules, such as MHC Class II, CD80, and CD86, and by impairing their capacity for antigen uptake and production of T cell–stimulating cytokines in response to gram-negative bacteria.[69,70] Notwithstanding the complexity of the inflammatory responses in the airways to CS, all smokers (even young adults in their 20s and 30s) demonstrate inflammation in the small airways[71]; however, only 15% to 30% of smokers progress to COPD (usually in their 50s and 60s and beyond),[72] suggesting the contribution of other pathogenic mechanisms in the pathogenesis of COPD.

Structural Damage and Tissue Repair/Remodeling

It is widely accepted that certain inflammatory mediators related to CS exposure can promote emphysema by inducing excess degradation of alveolar units.[73] However, most of the studies providing support for this hypothesis have been performed in rodents, whose lungs differ from humans in several important ways. For example, unlike humans mice do not have respiratory bronchioles. Moreover, in mice the CS-related emphysema is mild and does not resemble the extensive emphysematous destruction found in humans.[74] Nevertheless, animal models of emphysema have provided some important insights to the pathophysiology of CS-induced COPD. For example, CS can induce structural damages in the airway epithelium by unleashing proteases and oxidants and disrupting the barrier function of the airway.[75] Cells in the airway epithelium are held together by tight and gap junctions that play important roles in maintaining structural integrity. When the epithelium is severely damaged, basal cells and Clara cells have stem-cell–like properties that enable them to self-renew and proliferate to repair the damage.[76,77] The upper layer of the basement membrane, the lamina densa, consists of type IV collagen and laminin (predominantly type V), which are laid down by epithelial cells.[78] The lower lamina reticularis layer consists of type III and V collagen and fibronectin, which is synthesized by subepithelial fibroblasts.[79] Increased expression of specific integrins, such as avb1 and avb6, is present on the basal surface of the regenerating epithelium to promote restoration of the physical barrier function after injury.[80] In addition, there is increased expression of fibronectin, collagen IV, and laminin in bovine tracheal epithelial cell culture lesions, which promote the restoration of the basement membrane matrix and allow epithelial cell migration.[81] However, in chronically injured airways, there is marked distortion of the fibroblast architecture and disappearance of the basal laminar layer.[82] Recent studies have demonstrated similar distortion of fibroblasts in the small airways of current smokers, which may promote disruption of the extracellular matrix and tissue remodeling.[83] This process may be mediated by increased synthesis of transforming growth factor-β, which in turn upregulates Smad-2, -3, and -4–mediated signaling, and reduced expression of Smad-7.[84,85]

DUTCH, BRITISH, AND AMERICAN HYPOTHESES

Although the understanding of COPD has improved significantly over the past few decades, knowledge is far from complete. COPD still represents an increasingly important chronic debilitating illness in the United States and worldwide.[86] Because asthma and COPD share many common aspects (ie, epidemiologic characteristics and clinical manifestation), some have posited that COPD is part of the clinical spectrum of asthma. This hypothesis was first proposed in 1961 by Orie and coworkers[87] and became known as the Dutch hypothesis. The Dutch hypothesis encompasses three essential components: (1) different forms of obstructive lung disease (OLD) have overlapping clinical features and phenotypes including cough, breathlessness, allergy, and bronchial hyperresponsiveness (BHR); (2) the development of OLD is influenced by genetic factors, such as atopy, BHR, and environmental triggers, such as exposure to allergens, infections, smoking, and air pollution; and (3) OLD is permissive and malleable such that those with asthma can progress to COPD in the "right" environmental context (eg, smoking).[88] In support of this hypothesis, BHR has been associated with COPD mortality in the general population[89] and in those with established COPD who continue to smoke.[10] A recent study suggests that the population-attributable risk of BHR to the development of COPD is 15% (vs cigarette smoking, which has a population-attributable risk of 39%). Moreover, the Evaluation of COPD Longitudinally to Identify Predictive Surrogate Endpoints study, which recruited and followed more than 2000 patients with COPD for 3 years, demonstrated that bronchodilator reversibility (which is related to BHR) was the second leading risk factor for accelerated progression of COPD (next to cigarette smoking).[90] However, there is little evidence that asthma and COPD share similar genetic factors and to date large genome-wide association studies (GWAS) have failed to identify common genetic loci related to asthma and COPD.[91] Moreover, although there are some overlapping histologic features between asthma and COPD, such as mucus hypersecretion and airway inflammation, there are some fundamentally important pathologic differences between these two disorders.[92] For instance, asthma is associated with an increase in eosinophils, Th2 lymphocytes, and activated mast cells, whereas COPD-associated cell infiltration is characterized by neutrophils, macrophages, and cytotoxic T cells.[1] Asthma is generally responsive to inhaled corticosteroids, whereas COPD is relatively resistant to inhaled corticosteroids.[93]

An alternative hypothesis was proposed by a group of British investigators in the 1960s that recurrent bronchial infections were the reason that some smokers and not others developed progressive airways diseases.[94] Fletcher and Peto[72] tested this hypothesis by examining the frequency of respiratory infections and sputum quantity and quality in relation to the decline in lung function in a group of working male subjects but found no correlation between these parameters. This view was unchallenged for several years; however, recent data suggest that there may be some merit to the British hypothesis. Recurrent respiratory infections have been shown to be associated with an accelerated loss of lung function in patients with COPD[95,96] and that lung function decline is related to bacterial load in sputum.[97] At the very least, some patients with COPD have recurrent exacerbations, characterized by purulence in sputum, cough, and increased breathlessness, and these patients may harbor chronic bacterial infections, which may "flare" periodically, leading to exacerbations.[98] Individuals who have two or more exacerbations per year are now labeled as "frequent exacerbators"[99] and are thought to have a very poor prognosis.

More recently, some have suggested that patients with COPD suffer from abnormal tissue repair in response to CS.[100,101] Emphysema may arise from deficient repair of alveolar structures, whereas small airway remodeling may result from overexuberant repair of peribronchiolar tissues, leading to fibrosis. Consistent with this notion, reduction in circulating blood fibronectin levels (which are critical to injury repair) is associated with rapid progression of COPD and with total mortality in patients with COPD.[102] In recent years, this phenomenon has been referred to as the "American hypothesis."[100]

PROTEASE–ANTIPROTEASE HYPOTHESIS OF EMPHYSEMA

It has long been proposed that proteases break down connective tissue and in particular elastin in lung parenchyma to induce emphysema. Most studies have focused on neutrophil elastase and proteinase 3, which are neutrophil-derived serine proteases that can destroy extracellular matrix through proteolytic attack.[103] Serine proteases are also potent stimulants of mucus production and may induce mucus hypersecretion in patients with chronic bronchitis.[104,105] More recently, there is evidence that MMPs derived from macrophages and neutrophils play a role in extracellular matrix degradation.[106] In patients with emphysema, MMP-1 (collagenase) and MMP-9 (gelatinase B) expression[107] and activities[108] are elevated in bronchoalveolar lavage fluid and in macrophages. Interestingly, mice deficient in MMP-12 (macrophage metalloelastase) are protected against CS-induced emphysema,[109] highlighting the importance of MMPs in the development of emphysema. In normal lungs, all proteolytic activities are counteracted by antiproteases in the lung. The major inhibitors are α-antitrypsin (inhibitors of serine proteases) in lung parenchyma; secretory leukoprotease inhibitor from the airway epithelium; and tissue inhibitors of MMPs (TIMP-1, -2, and -3).[5] In smokers, the neutralizing effects of antiproteases may be inadequate for the chronic production of proteolytic enzymes from various sources including macrophages and neutrophils.[5]

AUTOIMMUNE HYPOTHESIS OF COPD

To add to the complexity of COPD, recent studies have suggested that COPD is an autoimmune disease. Although almost all smokers develop lung inflammation,[71] several studies have shown that inflammation persists even years after smoking cessation.[110–112] Although the underlying mechanisms are not clearly known, this observation raises the possibility of some self-perpetuating process that fuels the inflammatory response.[113] Autoimmune diseases are characterized by the development of immunity to foreign epitopes that cross-react with self-antigens[114] or by the loss of tolerance to self-antigens.[115] COPD shares many pathologic and clinical characteristics of autoimmune diseases, such as rheumatoid arthritis.[115] For example, smoking is a risk factor for COPD[72] and rheumatoid arthritis,[116] and there are similarities in the inflammatory cells (neutrophils, macrophages, T lymphocytes) and cytokines (TNF-α, IL-6) involved in both conditions. Moreover, self-perpetuation of the inflammatory response in rheumatoid arthritis joints[117] is similar to the continuous airway inflammation observed in COPD lungs even after smoking cessation.[110] In support of the "autoimmune" hypothesis, Lee and colleagues[118] demonstrated antielastin antibodies in plasma of patients with COPD but not in control subjects. More importantly, they showed that helper T lymphocytes isolated from peripheral blood of patients with COPD released IFN-γ and IL-10 in the presence of elastin but not in the presence of collagen or albumin, suggesting the involvement of Th1 subset in COPD. The magnitude of INF-γ release by T lymphocytes was significantly related to the extent of emphysema as assessed on thoracic computed tomography. In contrast, similar stimulation in subjects with asthma or control subjects' peripheral T lymphocytes had no effect. The authors thus postulated that in COPD CS causes an initial breakdown in the extracellular matrix of the lung, releasing elastin degradation products. These in turn become antigens, stimulating helper T cells (predominantly Th1 cells) to express autoantibodies against elastin, perpetuating and amplifying the initial inflammatory signal caused by CS. However, more recent studies have failed to replicate these promising data from Lee and coworkers.[119,120] Thus, it remains unsettled whether or not autoimmunity plays any role in the pathogenesis of COPD (**Fig. 2**).

GWAS AND COPD

To date the only established genetic risk factor for COPD is severe deficiency in α_1-antitrypsin, which is present in 1% to 2% of individuals. To identify additional genetic loci associated with COPD a limited number of GWAS in COPD have been completed. GWAS are performed to identify novel genetic variants in the absence of any a priori hypotheses. So far, GWAS have convincingly demonstrated two novel loci: those related to the α-nicotinic receptor (CHRNA 3/5) and the hedgehog interaction protein.[121] Historically, nicotinic receptors are classified as neuronal or muscle-type[122]; however, recent studies have shown the importance of extraneuronal cholinergic signaling in lungs.[123] It remains unclear whether the effects of CHRNA 3/5 are mediated by pulmonary receptors or centrally through the dominergic pathways. The functional effects of hedgehog interaction protein polymorphisms are unknown. There are several limitations of GWAS that deserve emphasis. First, GWAS cannot detect rare variants, which may impart large risks. Second, GWAS may miss multiple common variants that impart small risk but that in concert may produce big effects. Third, GWAS require large sample sizes usually in the tens of thousands of subjects. To date, most COPD GWAS have had relatively small sample sizes. Finally, GWAS in general have not taken into account COPD phenotypes. COPD is a heterogeneous disease with different phenotypes. Each phenotype probably has different pathophysiologies. Thus, without adequate phenotyping, the genetic signal may be difficult to detect. An alternative to GWAS is a candidate approach to gene identification. In smokers with COPD, a rapid decline in FEV$_1$ has been associated with genetic

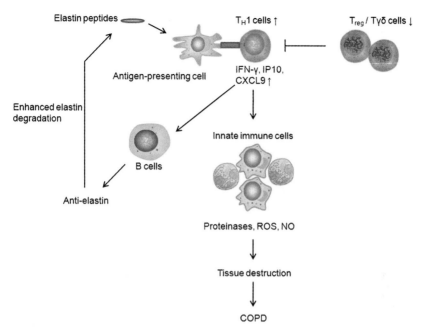

Fig. 2. COPD and autoimmunity. Exposure of cigarette smoke induces secretion of proteolytic enzymes from cells in the innate immune system (ie, neutrophils and macrophages) by liberating elastin fragments. Enhanced accumulation of elastin fragments, which are presented by antigen-presenting cells to T cells, can in turn activate elastin-specific B cells. Reduction in Treg cells leads to clonal expansion of autoreactive elastin-specific T_H1 cells. The autoantibodies generated against elastin are produced by B cells, ultimately leading to massive tissue destruction despite smoking cessation. IP-10, inducible protein 10; NO, nitric oxide; ROS, reactive oxygen species.

polymorphisms in MMP1 (G-1607GG) and MMP12 (Asn357Ser)[124] and several other genetic loci. Unfortunately, many of these "hits" have not been widely replicated. Thus, the clinical relevance of these polymorphisms remains uncertain.

SUMMARY

COPD is a worldwide public health problem that reduces the quality of life. The exact pathways by which CS and other environmental toxins produce COPD are not known. Currently, the leading candidates are (1) the protease-antiprotease hypothesis, (2) the Dutch hypothesis, (3) the British hypothesis, and the (4) autoimmunity hypothesis. Given the heterogeneity of the disease (and phenotypes), it is probably unrealistic that one pathway will fully explain COPD pathophysiology.

REFERENCES

1. Barnes PJ, Shapiro SD, Pauwels RA. Chronic obstructive pulmonary disease: molecular and cellular mechanisms. Eur Respir J 2003;22(4):672–88.
2. Lopez AD, Murray CC. The global burden of disease, 1990-2020. Nat Med 1998;4(11):1241–3.
3. Mackay J, Eriksen M, Shafey O. The tobacco atlas. Atlanta (GA): American Cancer Society; 2006.

4. Standards for the diagnosis and care of patients with chronic obstructive pulmonary disease. American Thoracic Society. Am J Respir Crit Care Med 1995; 152(5 Pt 2):S77–121.

5. Barnes PJ. Chronic obstructive pulmonary disease. N Engl J Med 2000;343(4): 269–80.

6. Snider GL. Chronic obstructive pulmonary disease: a definition and implications of structural determinants of airflow obstruction for epidemiology. Am Rev Respir Dis 1989;140(3 Pt 2):S3–8.

7. Rennard SI. COPD: overview of definitions, epidemiology, and factors influencing its development. Chest 1998;113(Suppl 4):235S–41S.

8. Hogg JC, Chu FS, Tan WC, et al. Survival after lung volume reduction in chronic obstructive pulmonary disease: insights from small airway pathology. Am J Respir Crit Care Med 2007;176(5):454–9.

9. Hogg JC, Chu F, Utokaparch S, et al. The nature of small-airway obstruction in chronic obstructive pulmonary disease. N Engl J Med 2004;350(26):2645–53.

10. Tashkin DP, Altose MD, Connett JE, et al. Methacholine reactivity predicts changes in lung function over time in smokers with early chronic obstructive pulmonary disease. The Lung Health Study Research Group. Am J Respir Crit Care Med 1996;153(6 Pt 1):1802–11.

11. Matsuba K, Thurlbeck WM. The number and dimensions of small airways in emphysematous lungs. Am J Pathol 1972;67(2):265–75.

12. Friedlander AL, Lynch D, Dyar LA, et al. Phenotypes of chronic obstructive pulmonary disease. COPD 2007;4(4):355–84.

13. Patel BD, Coxson HO, Pillai SG, et al. Airway wall thickening and emphysema show independent familial aggregation in chronic obstructive pulmonary disease. Am J Respir Crit Care Med 2008;178(5):500–5.

14. Gosselink JV, Hayashi S, Elliott WM, et al. Differential expression of tissue repair genes in the pathogenesis of chronic obstructive pulmonary disease. Am J Respir Crit Care Med 2010;181(12):1329–35.

15. Kitaguchi Y, Fujimoto K, Kubo K, et al. Characteristics of COPD phenotypes classified according to the findings of HRCT. Respir Med 2006;100(10):1742–52.

16. Papaioannou AI, Mazioti A, Kiropoulos T, et al. Systemic and airway inflammation and the presence of emphysema in patients with COPD. Respir Med 2010;104(2):275–82.

17. McDonough JE, Yuan R, Suzuki M, et al. Small-airway obstruction and emphysema in chronic obstructive pulmonary disease. N Engl J Med 2011;365(17): 1567–75.

18. General US. The health consequences of smoking: chronic obstructive lung disease. Rockville (MD): US Gov Press Office; 1984.

19. Ding YS, Zhang L, Jain RB, et al. Levels of tobacco-specific nitrosamines and polycyclic aromatic hydrocarbons in mainstream smoke from different tobacco varieties. Cancer Epidemiol Biomarkers Prev 2008;17(12):3366–71.

20. Ben-Zaken Cohen S, Pare PD, Man SF, et al. The growing burden of chronic obstructive pulmonary disease and lung cancer in women: examining sex differences in cigarette smoke metabolism. Am J Respir Crit Care Med 2007;176(2): 113–20.

21. Denissenko MF, Pao A, Tang M, et al. Preferential formation of benzo[a]pyrene adducts at lung cancer mutational hotspots in P53. Science 1996;274(5286): 430–2.

22. Hecht SS. Biochemistry, biology, and carcinogenicity of tobacco-specific N-nitrosamines. Chem Res Toxicol 1998;11(6):559–603.

23. Hukkanen J, Jacob P III, Benowitz NL. Metabolism and disposition kinetics of nicotine. Pharmacol Rev 2005;57(1):79–115.
24. Benowitz NL, Jacob P III. Metabolism of nicotine to cotinine studied by a dual stable isotope method. Clin Pharmacol Ther 1994;56(5):483–93.
25. Dix TA, Marnett LJ. Metabolism of polycyclic aromatic hydrocarbon derivatives to ultimate carcinogens during lipid peroxidation. Science 1983;221(4605):77–9.
26. Wilson AS, Davis CD, Williams DP, et al. Characterisation of the toxic metabolite(s) of naphthalene. Toxicology 1996;114(3):233–42.
27. Guengerich FP. Cytochrome P450: what have we learned and what are the future issues? Drug Metab Rev 2004;36(2):159–97.
28. Hulbert WC, Walker DC, Jackson A, et al. Airway permeability to horseradish peroxidase in guinea pigs: the repair phase after injury by cigarette smoke. Am Rev Respir Dis 1981;123(3):320–6.
29. Fels AO, Cohn ZA. The alveolar macrophage. J Appl Physiol 1986;60(2):353–69.
30. Macklin CC. Pulmonary sumps, dust accumulations, alveolar fluid and lymph vessels. Acta Anat (Basel) 1955;23(1):1–33.
31. Knowles MR, Boucher RC. Mucus clearance as a primary innate defense mechanism for mammalian airways. J Clin Invest 2002;109(5):571–7.
32. Green GM, Jakab GJ, Low RB, et al. Defense mechanisms of the respiratory membrane. Am Rev Respir Dis 1977;115(3):479–514.
33. Simani AS, Inoue S, Hogg JC. Penetration of the respiratory epithelium of guinea pigs following exposure to cigarette smoke. Lab Invest 1974;31(1):75–81.
34. Jones JG, Minty BD, Lawler P, et al. Increased alveolar epithelial permeability in cigarette smokers. Lancet 1980;1(8159):66–8.
35. Malhotra S, Man SF, Sin DD. Emerging drugs for the treatment of chronic obstructive pulmonary disease. Expert Opin Emerg Drugs 2006;11(2):275–91.
36. Doz E, Noulin N, Boichot E, et al. Cigarette smoke-induced pulmonary inflammation is TLR4/MyD88 and IL-1R1/MyD88 signaling dependent. J Immunol 2008; 180(2):1169–78.
37. Imler JL, Hoffmann JA. Toll receptors in innate immunity. Trends Cell Biol 2001; 11(7):304–11.
38. Aderem A, Ulevitch RJ. Toll-like receptors in the induction of the innate immune response. Nature 2000;406(6797):782–7.
39. Sha Q, Truong-Tran AQ, Plitt JR, et al. Activation of airway epithelial cells by toll-like receptor agonists. Am J Respir Cell Mol Biol 2004;31(3):358–64.
40. Liu AN, Mohammed AZ, Rice WR, et al. Perforin-independent CD8(+) T-cell-mediated cytotoxicity of alveolar epithelial cells is preferentially mediated by tumor necrosis factor-alpha: relative insensitivity to Fas ligand. Am J Respir Cell Mol Biol 1999;20(5):849–58.
41. Keatings VM, Collins PD, Scott DM, et al. Differences in interleukin-8 and tumor necrosis factor-alpha in induced sputum from patients with chronic obstructive pulmonary disease or asthma. Am J Respir Crit Care Med 1996;153(2):530–4.
42. Kilburn KH. A hypothesis for pulmonary clearance and its implications. Am Rev Respir Dis 1968;98(3):449–63.
43. Hovenberg HW, Davies JR, Carlstedt I. Different mucins are produced by the surface epithelium and the submucosa in human trachea: identification of MUC5AC as a major mucin from the goblet cells. Biochem J 1996;318(Pt 1): 319–24.
44. Thornton DJ, Rousseau K, McGuckin MA. Structure and function of the polymeric mucins in airways mucus. Annu Rev Physiol 2008;70:459–86.

45. Smirnova MG, Guo L, Birchall JP, et al. LPS up-regulates mucin and cytokine mRNA expression and stimulates mucin and cytokine secretion in goblet cells. Cell Immunol 2003;221(1):42–9.

46. Yoon JH, Kim KS, Kim HU, et al. Effects of TNF-alpha and IL-1 beta on mucin, lysozyme, IL-6 and IL-8 in passage-2 normal human nasal epithelial cells. Acta Otolaryngol 1999;119(8):905–10.

47. Chen Y, Thai P, Zhao YH, et al. Stimulation of airway mucin gene expression by interleukin (IL)-17 through IL-6 paracrine/autocrine loop. J Biol Chem 2003; 278(19):17036–43.

48. Danahay H, Atherton H, Jones G, et al. Interleukin-13 induces a hypersecretory ion transport phenotype in human bronchial epithelial cells. Am J Physiol Lung Cell Mol Physiol 2002;282(2):L226–36.

49. Voynow JA, Young LR, Wang Y, et al. Neutrophil elastase increases MUC5AC mRNA and protein expression in respiratory epithelial cells. Am J Physiol 1999;276(5 Pt 1):L835–43.

50. Takeyama K, Dabbagh K, Lee HM, et al. Epidermal growth factor system regulates mucin production in airways. Proc Natl Acad Sci U S A 1999;96(6):3081–6.

51. Shao MX, Nakanaga T, Nadel JA. Cigarette smoke induces MUC5AC mucin overproduction via tumor necrosis factor-alpha-converting enzyme in human airway epithelial (NCI-H292) cells. Am J Physiol Lung Cell Mol Physiol 2004; 287(2):L420–7.

52. Kohri K, Ueki IF, Shim JJ, et al. *Pseudomonas aeruginosa* induces MUC5AC production via epidermal growth factor receptor. Eur Respir J 2002;20(5): 1263–70.

53. Choi HJ, Chung YS, Kim HJ, et al. Signal pathway of 17beta-estradiol-induced MUC5B expression in human airway epithelial cells. Am J Respir Cell Mol Biol 2009;40(2):168–78.

54. Monick MM, Yarovinsky TO, Powers LS, et al. Respiratory syncytial virus up-regulates TLR4 and sensitizes airway epithelial cells to endotoxin. J Biol Chem 2003;278(52):53035–44.

55. Hasday JD, Bascom R, Costa JJ, et al. Bacterial endotoxin is an active component of cigarette smoke. Chest 1999;115(3):829–35.

56. Vlahos R, Bozinovski S, Jones JE, et al. Differential protease, innate immunity, and NF-kappaB induction profiles during lung inflammation induced by sub-chronic cigarette smoke exposure in mice. Am J Physiol Lung Cell Mol Physiol 2006;290(5):L931–45.

57. Dekhuijzen PN. Antioxidant properties of N-acetylcysteine: their relevance in relation to chronic obstructive pulmonary disease. Eur Respir J 2004;23(4): 629–36.

58. Asea A, Rehli M, Kabingu E, et al. Novel signal transduction pathway utilized by extracellular HSP70: role of toll-like receptor (TLR) 2 and TLR4. J Biol Chem 2002;277(17):15028–34.

59. Vayssier M, Banzet N, Francois D, et al. Tobacco smoke induces both apoptosis and necrosis in mammalian cells: differential effects of HSP70. Am J Physiol 1998;275(4 Pt 1):L771–9.

60. Pace E, Ferraro M, Siena L, et al. Cigarette smoke increases Toll-like receptor 4 and modifies lipopolysaccharide-mediated responses in airway epithelial cells. Immunology 2008;124(3):401–11.

61. Kulkarni R, Rampersaud R, Aguilar JL, et al. Cigarette smoke inhibits airway epithelial cell innate immune responses to bacteria. Infect Immun 2010;78(5): 2146–52.

62. Bagaitkar J, Demuth DR, Scott DA. Tobacco use increases susceptibility to bacterial infection. Tob Induc Dis 2008;4:12.
63. Drannik AG, Pouladi MA, Robbins CS, et al. Impact of cigarette smoke on clearance and inflammation after *Pseudomonas aeruginosa* infection. Am J Respir Crit Care Med 2004;170(11):1164–71.
64. El Ahmer OR, Essery SD, Saadi AT, et al. The effect of cigarette smoke on adherence of respiratory pathogens to buccal epithelial cells. FEMS Immunol Med Microbiol 1999;23(1):27–36.
65. Hodge S, Hodge G, Ahern J, et al. Smoking alters alveolar macrophage recognition and phagocytic ability: implications in chronic obstructive pulmonary disease. Am J Respir Cell Mol Biol 2007;37(6):748–55.
66. Sayers NM, Drucker DB. Animal models used to test the interactions between infectious agents and products of cigarette smoked implicated in sudden infant death syndrome. FEMS Immunol Med Microbiol 1999;25(1-2):115–23.
67. Sorensen LT, Nielsen HB, Kharazmi A, et al. Effect of smoking and abstention on oxidative burst and reactivity of neutrophils and monocytes. Surgery 2004; 136(5):1047–53.
68. Baqir M, Chen CZ, Martin RJ, et al. Cigarette smoke decreases MARCO expression in macrophages: implication in *Mycoplasma pneumoniae* infection. Respir Med 2008;102(11):1604–10.
69. Nouri-Shirazi M, Tinajero R, Guinet E. Nicotine alters the biological activities of developing mouse bone marrow-derived dendritic cells (DCs). Immunol Lett 2007;109(2):155–64.
70. Robbins CS, Franco F, Mouded M, et al. Cigarette smoke exposure impairs dendritic cell maturation and T cell proliferation in thoracic lymph nodes of mice. J Immunol 2008;180(10):6623–8.
71. Niewoehner DE, Kleinerman J, Rice DB. Pathologic changes in the peripheral airways of young cigarette smokers. N Engl J Med 1974;291(15):755–8.
72. Fletcher C, Peto R. The natural history of chronic airflow obstruction. Br Med J 1977;1(6077):1645–8.
73. Churg A, Zay K, Shay S, et al. Acute cigarette smoke-induced connective tissue breakdown requires both neutrophils and macrophage metalloelastase in mice. Am J Respir Cell Mol Biol 2002;27(3):368–74.
74. Hogg JC, Timens W. The pathology of chronic obstructive pulmonary disease. Annu Rev Pathol 2009;4:435–59.
75. Rennard SI. Cigarette smoke in research. Am J Respir Cell Mol Biol 2004;31(5): 479–80.
76. Hackett TL, Shaheen F, Johnson A, et al. Characterization of side population cells from human airway epithelium. Stem Cells 2008;26(10):2576–85.
77. Chen H, Matsumoto K, Stripp BR. Bronchiolar progenitor cells. Proc Am Thorac Soc 2009;6(7):602–6.
78. Knight DA, Holgate ST. The airway epithelium: structural and functional properties in health and disease. Respirology 2003;8(4):432–46.
79. Paulsson M. Basement membrane proteins: structure, assembly, and cellular interactions. Crit Rev Biochem Mol Biol 1992;27(1-2):93–127.
80. Horiba K, Fukuda Y. Synchronous appearance of fibronectin, integrin alpha 5 beta 1, vinculin and actin in epithelial cells and fibroblasts during rat tracheal wound healing. Virchows Arch 1994;425(4):425–34.
81. Rickard KA, Taylor J, Rennard SI, et al. Migration of bovine bronchial epithelial cells to extracellular matrix components. Am J Respir Cell Mol Biol 1993;8(1): 63–8.

82. Sirianni FE, Milaninezhad A, Chu FS, et al. Alteration of fibroblast architecture and loss of basal lamina apertures in human emphysematous lung. Am J Respir Crit Care Med 2006;173(6):632–8.

83. Van Der Geld YM, Van Straaten JF, Postma DS, et al. Role of proteoglycans in development and pathogenesis of emphysema. In: Garg HG, Roughly PJ, Hales CA, editors. Proteoglycans in lung disease. New York: Marcel Dekker; 2002. p. 241–67.

84. Zandvoort A, Postma DS, Jonker MR, et al. Altered expression of the Smad signalling pathway: implications for COPD pathogenesis. Eur Respir J 2006;28(3): 533–41.

85. Springer J, Scholz FR, Peiser C, et al. SMAD-signaling in chronic obstructive pulmonary disease: transcriptional down-regulation of inhibitory SMAD 6 and 7 by cigarette smoke. Biol Chem 2004;385(7):649–53.

86. National Heart, Lung, and Blood Institute. Morbidity and mortality: 2000 chartbook on cardiovascular, lung, and blood diseases. Bethesda (MD): US Department of Health and Human Services, Public Health Service, National Institutes of Health; 2000.

87. Orie NGM, Sluiter HJ, de Vries K, et al. The host factor in bronchitis. In: Orie NGM, Sluiter HJ, editors. Bronchitis. Assen (The Netherlands): Royal van Gorcum; 1961. p. 43–59.

88. Silverman EK, Palmer LJ, Mosley JD, et al. Genomewide linkage analysis of quantitative spirometric phenotypes in severe early-onset chronic obstructive pulmonary disease. Am J Hum Genet 2002;70(5):1229–39.

89. Hospers JJ, Postma DS, Rijcken B, et al. Histamine airway hyperresponsiveness and mortality from chronic obstructive pulmonary disease: a cohort study. Lancet 2000;356(9238):1313–7.

90. Vestbo J, Edwards LD, Scanlon PD, et al. Changes in forced expiratory volume in 1 second over time in COPD. N Engl J Med 2011;365(13):1184–92.

91. Postma DS, Kerkhof M, Boezen HM, et al. Asthma and chronic obstructive pulmonary disease: common genes, common environments? Am J Respir Crit Care Med 2011;183(12):1588–94.

92. Barnes PJ. Against the Dutch hypothesis: asthma and chronic obstructive pulmonary disease are distinct diseases. Am J Respir Crit Care Med 2006; 174(3):240–3 [discussion: 243–4].

93. Barnes PJ, Ito K, Adcock IM. Corticosteroid resistance in chronic obstructive pulmonary disease: inactivation of histone deacetylase. Lancet 2004; 363(9410):731–3.

94. Fletcher CM. Chronic bronchitis. Its prevalence, nature, and pathogenesis. Am Rev Respir Dis 1959;80:483–94.

95. Kanner RE, Anthonisen NR, Connett JE. Lower respiratory illnesses promote FEV(1) decline in current smokers but not ex-smokers with mild chronic obstructive pulmonary disease: results from the lung health study. Am J Respir Crit Care Med 2001;164(3):358–64.

96. Donaldson GC, Seemungal TA, Bhowmik A, et al. Relationship between exacerbation frequency and lung function decline in chronic obstructive pulmonary disease. Thorax 2002;57(10):847–52.

97. Wilkinson TM, Patel IS, Wilks M, et al. Airway bacterial load and FEV1 decline in patients with chronic obstructive pulmonary disease. Am J Respir Crit Care Med 2003;167(8):1090–5.

98. Sethi S, Evans N, Grant BJ, et al. New strains of bacteria and exacerbations of chronic obstructive pulmonary disease. N Engl J Med 2002;347(7):465–71.

99. Hurst JR, Vestbo J, Anzueto A, et al. Susceptibility to exacerbation in chronic obstructive pulmonary disease. N Engl J Med 2010;363(12):1128–38.

100. Rennard SI. Chronic obstructive pulmonary disease: linking outcomes and pathobiology of disease modification. Proc Am Thorac Soc 2006;3(3): 276–80.

101. Soriano JB, Agusti A. The yin and yang of COPD: or balancing repair (yang) and inflammation (yin). Eur Respir J 2008;32(6):1426–7.

102. Man SF, Xing L, Connett JE, et al. Circulating fibronectin to C-reactive protein ratio and mortality: a biomarker in COPD? Eur Respir J 2008;32(6):1451–7.

103. Stockley RA. Neutrophils and protease/antiprotease imbalance. Am J Respir Crit Care Med 1999;160(5 Pt 2):S49–52.

104. Sommerhoff CP, Nadel JA, Basbaum CB, et al. Neutrophil elastase and cathepsin G stimulate secretion from cultured bovine airway gland serous cells. J Clin Invest 1990;85(3):682–9.

105. Witko-Sarsat V, Halbwachs-Mecarelli L, Schuster A, et al. Proteinase 3, a potent secretagogue in airways, is present in cystic fibrosis sputum. Am J Respir Cell Mol Biol 1999;20(4):729–36.

106. Shapiro SD, Senior RM. Matrix metalloproteinases. Matrix degradation and more. Am J Respir Cell Mol Biol 1999;20(6):1100–2.

107. Finlay GA, O'Driscoll LR, Russell KJ, et al. Matrix metalloproteinase expression and production by alveolar macrophages in emphysema. Am J Respir Crit Care Med 1997;156(1):240–7.

108. Ohnishi K, Takagi M, Kurokawa Y, et al. Matrix metalloproteinase-mediated extracellular matrix protein degradation in human pulmonary emphysema. Lab Invest 1998;78(9):1077–87.

109. Hautamaki RD, Kobayashi DK, Senior RM, et al. Requirement for macrophage elastase for cigarette smoke-induced emphysema in mice. Science 1997; 277(5334):2002–4.

110. Turato G, Di Stefano A, Maestrelli P, et al. Effect of smoking cessation on airway inflammation in chronic bronchitis. Am J Respir Crit Care Med 1995;152(4 Pt 1): 1262–7.

111. Rutgers SR, Postma DS, ten Hacken NH, et al. Ongoing airway inflammation in patients with COPD who do not currently smoke. Thorax 2000;55(1):12–8.

112. Retamales I, Elliott WM, Meshi B, et al. Amplification of inflammation in emphysema and its association with latent adenoviral infection. Am J Respir Crit Care Med 2001;164(3):469–73.

113. Van Parijs L, Abbas AK. Homeostasis and self-tolerance in the immune system: turning lymphocytes off. Science 1998;280(5361):243–8.

114. Albert LJ, Inman RD. Molecular mimicry and autoimmunity. N Engl J Med 1999; 341(27):2068–74.

115. Davidson A, Diamond B. Autoimmune diseases. N Engl J Med 2001;345(5): 340–50.

116. Hutchinson D, Moots R. Coffee consumption, RF, and the risk of RA. Ann Rheum Dis 2001;60(5):540–1.

117. Toivanen P. From reactive arthritis to rheumatoid arthritis. J Autoimmun 2001; 16(3):369–71.

118. Lee SH, Goswami S, Grudo A, et al. Antielastin autoimmunity in tobacco smoking-induced emphysema. Nat Med 2007;13(5):567–9.

119. Greene CM, Low TB, O'Neill SJ, et al. Anti-proline-glycine-proline or antielastin autoantibodies are not evident in chronic inflammatory lung disease. Am J Respir Crit Care Med 2010;181(1):31–5.

120. Wood AM, de Pablo P, Buckley CD, et al. Smoke exposure as a determinant of autoantibody titre in alpha-antitrypsin deficiency and COPD. Eur Respir J 2011; 37(1):32–8.
121. Pillai SG, Ge D, Zhu G, et al. A genome-wide association study in chronic obstructive pulmonary disease (COPD): identification of two major susceptibility loci. PLoS Genet 2009;5(3):e1000421.
122. Caulfield MP, Birdsall NJ. International Union of Pharmacology. XVII. Classification of muscarinic acetylcholine receptors. Pharmacol Rev 1998;50:279–90.
123. Wessler I, Kirkpatrick CJ, Racke K. Non-neuronal acetylcholine, a locally acting molecule, widely distributed in biological systems: expression and function in humans. Pharmacol Ther 1998;77(1):59–79.
124. Joos L, He JQ, Shepherdson MB, et al. The role of matrix metalloproteinase polymorphisms in the rate of decline in lung function. Hum Mol Genet 2002; 11(5):569–76.

Genes and Chronic Obstructive Pulmonary Disease

Marilyn G. Foreman, MD, MS[a,1], Michael Campos, MD[b,1],
Juan C. Celedón, MD, DrPH, FCCP[c,d,*]

KEYWORDS

• COPD • Genetics • α_1-antitrypsin deficiency

KEY POINTS

- Severe a1-antitrypsin (AAT) deficiency is the only well-established genetic risk factor for chronic obstructive pulmonary disease (COPD).
- Severe AAT deficiency explains only a small proportion of cases of COPD (1%–2%), and genes other than PI type (genetic modifiers) likely influence lung function in PI Z subjects.
- Current guidelines thus recommend screening for severe AAT deficiency in all patients with COPD.

Severe α_1-antitrypsin (AAT) deficiency is the only well-established genetic risk factor for chronic obstructive pulmonary disease (COPD). Patients with severe AAT deficiency (most commonly, protease inhibitor [PI] Z) are at increased risk for developing COPD, particularly if they smoke.[1,2] However, severe AAT deficiency explains only a small proportion of cases of COPD (1%–2%), and genes other than PI type (genetic modifiers) likely influence lung function in PI Z subjects.[3,4]

Burrows and colleagues[5] noted that the development of chronic airflow obstruction in response to cigarette smoking is highly variable in the general population, suggesting that individuals vary in their genetic susceptibility to the detrimental effects of smoking on lung function. Several studies have since confirmed a genetic contribution

Sources of support: Grants from the US National Institutes of Health (HL073373 and HL029601) and The Alpha 1 Foundation.
[a] Division of Pulmonary and Critical Care Medicine, Department of Medicine, Morehouse School of Medicine, 720 Westview Drive SW, Atlanta, GA 30310-1495, USA; [b] Division of Pulmonary, Critical Care and Sleep Medicine (R-47), Department of Medicine, University of Miami Miller School of Medicine, 1600 NW 10th Avenue, RMSB 7052, Miami, FL 33136, USA; [c] Division of Pediatric Pulmonary Medicine, Allergy and Immunology, Department of Pediatrics, Children's Hospital of Pittsburgh of UPMC, 4401 Penn Avenue, Pittsburgh, PA 15224, USA; [d] Division of Pulmonary, Allergy and Critical Care Medicine, Department of Medicine, University of Pittsburgh School of Medicine, 3459 Fifth Avenue, 628 NW, Pittsburgh, PA 15213, USA
[1] These authors contributed equally to this manuscript.
* Division of Pediatric Pulmonary Medicine, Allergy and Immunology, Children's Hospital of Pittsburgh of UPMC, 4401 Penn Avenue, Pittsburgh, PA 15224.
E-mail address: juan.celedon@chp.edu

to the pathogenesis of COPD in cigarette smokers without severe AAT deficiency.[6–8] A search for COPD susceptibility genes other than PI type has included genome-wide linkage analyses; candidate-gene studies; and, more recently, genome-wide association studies (GWASs).

In this article, the authors review the genetics, diagnosis, and treatment of severe AAT deficiency. They then assess findings from recent genetic studies of COPD and its intermediate phenotypes (eg, lung function). The authors then briefly discuss future directions in this field.

COPD DUE TO SEVERE AAT DEFICIENCY

Severe deficiency of AAT was first recognized as a risk factor for COPD in 1963.[9] Since then, many studies have characterized the genetics and role of this protein in the pathogenesis of COPD.

Genetics

The AAT protein is encoded by a 12.2-kilobase gene located on chromosome 14q32.1 called *SERPINA1* or *PI*.[10] The gene has 7 exons and 6 introns, is inherited in an autosomal codominant manner, and has more than 120 single-nucleotide polymorphisms (SNPs).[11] Numerous AAT protein variants can be differentiated by their speed of migration on gel electrophoresis using isoelectric focusing. The most common alleles are M, S, and Z. The M variants (M1, M2, M3) result in proteins with a medium rate of migration and a normal level of AAT, the S variant is associated with mild reductions in serum AAT level, and the Z variant has the slowest rate of migration and leads to severe reduction of AAT level. Null alleles also occur, with undetectable protein levels. Combinations of the M, S, and Z variants are seen in more than 95% of the population. Serum AAT levels in subjects with the MZ and ZZ phenotypes are 60% and 10%, respectively, of those in (normal) subjects with the MM phenotype.

The most common forms of severe AAT deficiency with a high risk of COPD involve combinations of 2 Z alleles (Glu342Lys) and a Z allele with a null allele (both referred as phenotype PI*Z) or a combination of 2 null alleles. Combinations of a Z allele and an S allele (Glu264Val) also confer a moderate risk of COPD.[12] The phenotype MZ has also been associated with a lower but still increased risk of COPD, whereas the MS phenotype has been associated with only mild reductions in AAT level and no risk of COPD.[13] AAT deficiency has been described in all races, although the highest frequencies of the Z allele have been described in whites. In the United States, the frequency of the ZZ phenotype is 1 in 4775 individuals, SZ phenotype 1 in 1124, and MZ phenotype 1 in 36.[14] Worldwide, severe AAT deficiency affects approximately 3.4 million individuals.[15]

Pathophysiology

SERPINA1 codes a 52-kDa glycoprotein with 394 amino acids that contains a reactive loop with an active site at methionine 358. Although AAT is an acute phase reactant synthesized mostly by liver cells, it is also produced by local synthesis by cells such as neutrophils, monocytes, macrophages, and epithelial cells.[16,17] The major function of AAT is the neutralization of serine proteases, particularly neutrophil elastase (NE); other targets include cathepsin G, trypsin, and proteinase 3.[18,19] Severe deficiency of AAT results in excess protease activity in the lungs, particularly during periods of inflammation, and leads to progressive degradation of the lung parenchyma (emphysema) and accelerated decline in lung function over time.[20] Although protease-antiprotease imbalance is the most important cause of COPD in severe AAT deficiency, the loss of other functions of AAT likely contributes to COPD pathogenesis. These include endothelial cell protection against apoptosis by binding to caspases,[21] regulation of airway epithelial lining fluid balance by binding to matryptase,[22] and inflammatory response modulation. For example, AAT modulates endotoxin-induced inflammation,[23] reduces tumor necrosis factor (TNF) α–induced lung injury in rabbits,[24] inhibits super-oxide production by neutrophils,[25] and regulates the response of macrophages to proinflammatory stimuli.[26]

Z-AAT has reduced capacity to inhibit NE,[27] as well as a conformational protein change that enables a loop-sheet polymerization process and its accumulation in the endoplasmic reticulum (ER) with loss of secretion into the circulation.[28] The Z-polymers are degraded by ER-associated degradation pathways via proteasomes and by autophagy as part of the ER overload response.[29] If these cellular mechanisms fail, gain-of-toxic function and ER stress occur, which can lead to inflammation via nuclear factor κβ activation,[30] hepatocyte death by apoptosis,[31] and ultimately liver disease, both during childhood and later in life; a similar process may occur in the lung but has not been as well characterized.

AAT polymers can also further worsen protease-antiprotease imbalance. When instilled in the trachea of mice, Z-polymers produce a significant concentration-dependent influx of neutrophils that is not mediated by chemokines.[32] The polymers can be detected in the circulation[33] and bronchoalveolar lavage fluid of patients with severe AAT deficiency, in whom these polymers may also induce inflammation by a direct effect on epithelial cells.[34]

Diagnosis

Compared with young subjects who have a PI*ZZ phenotype but do not smoke, those who have a PI*ZZ phenotype and do smoke have a significantly lower forced expiratory volume in the first second of expiration to forced vital capacity ratio (FEV_1/FVC) and diffusing capacity of carbon monoxide.[35] At age 30 years, Pi*Z subjects who smoke have significantly more shortness of breath, sputum production, and wheezing than Pi*MM smokers; among nonsmokers, Pi*ZZ subjects report only more wheezing than nonaffected controls.[35]

Not uncommonly, clinicians stereotype the presentation of severe AAT deficiency as that of a young (<40 years old) white nonsmoker who presents with COPD and pan-acinar emphysema predominantly in the lower lobes. Although some affected individuals present this way, most symptomatic individuals have features that resemble those of COPD not due to severe AAT deficiency. About one-third of affected subjects have a more indolent presentation and are diagnosed after age 50 years,[36] about one-third have emphysema predominantly located in the upper lobes,[37] and more than 80% have a significant smoking history[38]; bronchiectasis of variable severity are also common.[39] Current guidelines thus recommend screening for severe AAT deficiency in all patients with COPD.[40] Screening of relatives of affected subjects may find nonsmokers with the PI*ZZ phenotype but no respiratory symptoms.[41]

Genetic Modifiers

The significant variability observed in the development, progression, and manifestations of COPD due to severe AAT deficiency strongly suggests that genetic and/or environmental factors modify disease expression. Studies of familial aggregation and heritability suggest that genetic factors other than PI type influence lung function and airflow obstruction in PI*Z individuals.[3,42] Although no genetic modifiers of severe AAT deficiency have been confidently identified, candidate genes have been examined. In a case-control study, 2 coding polymorphisms in NOS3 were associated with severe airflow obstruction in PI*Z individuals.[43] In a family-based association study of 10 genes previously associated with asthma and/or COPD, variants in the genes for TNF and interleukin 10 were associated with lung function measures.[44]

In subjects with severe AAT deficiency, the development of airflow obstruction is associated with age; male sex; bronchodilator responsiveness and chronic bronchitis; and, most strongly, cigarette smoke.[45–47]

Treatment

A detailed description of how to treat lung disease in severe AAT deficiency is beyond the scope of this article. The pharmacologic and nonpharmacologic treatment of COPD due to AAT deficiency follows the same guidelines as those for COPD in general.[48] Interventions showing benefit in subjects with severe AAT deficiency include disease management programs (which improve quality of life and decrease health care use[49]), lung volume reduction surgery (which improves 6-minute walking test and dyspnea scores[50]), and inhaled steroids (which reduce airflow obstruction and hyperinflation).[51]

Intravenous augmentation therapy with donor-derived purified AAT is the only Food and Drug Administration–approved specific treatment of lung disease due to severe AAT deficiency (defined as a baseline serum AAT level below 11 μM).[40] The recommended dose (60 mg/kg once a week) is intended to keep trough serum AAT level above 11 μM. Studies supporting this therapy are mostly observational.[52] Whereas results from a recent meta-analysis of observational studies suggest that augmentation therapy with AAT slows lung function decline in subjects with moderately reduced lung function,[53] a meta-analysis of the only 2 published randomized placebo-controlled trials concluded that there was not sufficient evidence to recommend this therapy.[54] In spite of this controversy, augmentation therapy should be used while the effectiveness, optimal dosage, therapeutic goals, and target populations for this treatment are further studied. Additional potential treatments for severe AAT deficiency are being examined, including gene therapy[55] and correction of the underlying genetic defect using inducible stem cells.[56]

GENETICS OF COPD UNRELATED TO SEVERE AAT DEFICIENCY

Findings from studies of candidate genes for COPD susceptibility, reviewed in detail elsewhere,[57] have yielded additional insight into the understanding of COPD pathobiology, particularly for certain pathways (eg, transforming growth factor β, matrix metalloproteinases).[57,58] In contrast to studies of 1 or few genes selected on the basis of known biology, GWASs are hypothesis-free studies that leverage information from markers genotyped along the entire genome and can thus yield unanticipated discoveries and insights into disease pathogenesis. Findings from recent GWASs and other new approaches to study COPD genetics are the focus of this review.

GWAS of COPD

Published GWASs of COPD are summarized in **Table 1**. In 2009, Pillai and colleagues[59] performed the first GWAS of COPD using a multistage replication design. The discovery (primary or initial) cohort comprised 823 subjects with COPD (cases) and 810 unaffected smokers (controls) from Bergen, Norway. The 100 SNPs with the lowest P values in the GWAS of this cohort were then tested for association with COPD in 1891 members of 606 white families from the family-based International COPD Genetics Network (ICGN). Seven of the 100 SNPs tested in ICGN showed significant evidence of association and were then tested for association with COPD in 389 cases from the National Emphysema Treatment Trial (NETT) and 472 smoking controls from the

Table 1
GWAS of COPD and COPD-related phenotypes

References	Study Design	Results	Limitations
Pillai et al,[59] 2009	GWAS of COPD in 1633 participants in a case-control study in Norway, with subsequent replication of top results in additional cohorts (ICGN, NETT-NAS, and BEOCOPD)	1. Two SNPs in the *CHRNA3/CHRNA5/IREB2* locus on chromosome 15 (rs803491 and rs1051730) were significantly associated with COPD in 2 replication cohorts (ICGN and NETT-NAS) and in a combined analysis including the discovery (Norway) cohort 2. These SNPs were also associated with lung function in ICGN and BEOCOPD	1. No genome-wide significant association with any SNP in the discovery cohort 2. No functional data
Cho et al,[63] 2010	GWAS of COPD in 4320 subjects in 3 case-control studies: Norway, NETT-NAS, and ECLIPSE. Replication was attempted in the COPDGene, BEOCOPD, and ICGN studies	An SNP in *FAM13A*, rs7671167, was significantly associated with COPD in the discovery cohort and in 2 of 3 replication cohorts (combined $P = 1.2 \times 10^{-11}$, combined odds ratio for case-control studies, 0.76; 95% confidence interval, 0.69–0.83)	No functional data
Kong et al,[65] 2011	GWAS of percent emphysema detected by computed tomography in the Norway, ECLIPSE, and NETT studies	1. An SNP (rs10844154) in *BICD1* on chromosome 12 was significantly associated with emphysema in the meta-analysis of the 3 cohorts (OR for at least mild emphysema = 1.46, $P = 5.2 \times 10^{-7}$, and OR for at least moderate emphysema = 1.56, $P = 4.8 \times 10^{-8}$) 2. Strongest signals came from radiologist scoring rather than density mask analysis	1. No genome-wide significant association with emphysema in any of the 3 individual cohorts 2. No functional data
Wan et al,[72] 2011	GWAS of BMI in approximately 3000 subjects with COPD in 3 cohorts: ECLIPSE, Norway, and NETT, with replication attempted in 502 subjects in COPDGene. A GWAS of fat-free mass index in COPD subjects was conducted in ECLIPSE and Norway	SNP rs8050136, located in the intron of the fat mass and obesity-associated gene (*FTO*), was significantly associated with BMI ($P = 4.97 \times 10^{-7}$) and FFMI ($P = 1.19 \times 10^{-7}$) in the discovery cohort. Findings for BMI were replicated in COPDGene ($P = 6 \times 10^{-3}$)	No functional data

Abbreviations: BEOCOPD, Boston Early-Onset COPD; BMI, body mass index; COPDGene Study, Genetic Epidemiology of COPD Study; ECLIPSE, Evaluation of COPD Longitudinally to Identify Predictive Surrogate Endpoints; FFMI, fat-free mass index; HRCT, high-resolution computed tomography of the thorax; ICGN, International COPD Genetics Network; NAS, Normative Aging Study; NETT, National Emphysema Treatment Trial; SNP, single-nucleotide polymorphism.

Normative Aging Study (NAS). Of these 7 SNPs, 6 were also tested for association with lung function measures in 949 members of 127 families in the Boston Early-Onset COPD Study (BEOCOPD).[60] Two SNPs (rs8034191 and rs1051730) in the α-nicotinic acetylcholine receptor (*CHRNA3/CHRNA5/IREB2*) locus on chromosome 15 showed significant evidence of association with COPD susceptibility in ICGN and NETT-NAS and reached genome-wide (GW) statistical significance in the analysis of 3 combined cohorts (Norway, ICGN and NETT-NAS) but were not GW significant in the discovery cohort. Nominal evidence of significant associations with FEV_1 was also noted in BEO-COPD ($P = .03$ for each polymorphism) and ICGN ($P = 1.04 \times 10^{-4}$ for rs8034191 and $P = 1.75 \times 10^{-5}$ for rs1051730). Polymorphisms in the gene for hedgehog interacting protein (*HHIP*) on chromosome 4 were consistently replicated but did not reach GW statistical significance in the discovery cohort or the combined analysis. The hedgehog signaling pathway has received continued attention (see later) because of its involvement in branching morphogenesis of the lung.[61]

Family with sequence similarity 13, member A, (*FAM13A*) was identified as a susceptibility gene for COPD in a GWAS of a cohort comprising 4320 subjects enrolled in 3 case-control studies: Norway, NETT-NAS, and the multicenter Evaluation of COPD Longitudinally to Identify Predictive Surrogate Endpoints (ECLIPSE[62]).[63] Replication was then attempted in 502 cases and 504 controls from COPDGene (a multicenter study of the genetics and epidemiology of COPD),[64] BEOCOPD, and ICGN. A polymorphism in *FAM13A* (rs7671167) on chromosome 4q22.1 was associated with COPD in the discovery cohort and in 2 of the 3 replication cohorts (combined P value = 1.2×10^{-11}, combined odds ratio [OR] in the case-control studies = 0.76, 95% confidence interval [CI] = 0.69–0.83). This SNP was also associated with prebronchodilator FEV_1 in BEOCOPD ($P = .02$) and with prebronchodilator ($P = 5.3 \times 10^{-5}$) and post-bronchodilator FEV_1 in ICGN.

Intermediate phenotypes offer several advantages for genetic studies of complex diseases such as COPD because they are objectively defined and may be influenced by fewer genes than the disease per se. Kong and colleagues[65] conducted a meta-analysis of GWAS results from the Norway, ECLIPSE, and NETT cohorts on percent emphysema from computed tomography (CT) (defined by densitometry as the percentage of lung voxels at −950 Hounsfield units and also qualitatively by visual scoring). Although no SNPs in any of the 3 cohorts were significantly associated with emphysema, an SNP (rs10844154) in the gene for bicaudal homolog 1 (*BICD1*) on chromosome 12 reached genome-wide significance for association in the meta-analysis of emphysema (OR for at least mild emphysema = 1.46, $P = 5.2 \times 10^{-7}$, and OR for at least moderate emphysema = 1.56, $P = 4.8 \times 10^{-8}$) in CT. The strongest signal in this study came from radiologist scoring rather than density mask analysis, although the investigators stressed that this did not imply superiority of one method over the other. The investigators noted that variants in *BICD1* are associated with length of telomeres, suggesting that a mechanism linked to accelerated aging may be involved in the pathogenesis of emphysema.

Five SNPs in loci previously associated with COPD (*HHIP*, *CHRNA3/CHRNA5/IREB2*, and *FAM13A*) were tested for association with COPD-related phenotypes (smoking behavior, lung function, body mass index [BMI], fat-free body mass, BODE index [BMI index, degree of airflow obstruction, dyspnea, and exercise capacity],[66] emphysema and airway wall thickness determined by CT) in ECLIPSE and then validated in ICGN.[67] An SNP in the *CHRNA3/CHRNA5* locus (rs8034191) was associated with increased smoking intensity (expressed as pack-years), radiologist's assessment of emphysema on high-resolution CT of the chest, and airflow obstruction in the ECLIPSE and ICGN cohorts. In ECLIPSE, subjects with COPD who were current or former smokers and homozygous for the rs8034191 risk allele had 7.5 more cumulative pack-years of smoking ($P = .002$) than those who were heterozygous or homozygous for the nonrisk allele; this association was confirmed in the ICGN. SNPs in *HHIP* or *FAM13A* loci were not associated with smoking intensity. An SNP in *HHIP* was associated with FEV_1/FVC in the ECLIPSE and ICGN cohorts; this SNP was also significantly associated with fat-free body mass and COPD exacerbations in ECLIPSE. *FAM13A* SNPs were associated with lung function, but this association was not consistently significant across cohorts. These findings, taken together with others, suggest that (1) the *CHRNA3/CHRNA5* locus, which has also been associated lung cancer,[68] influences COPD-related phenotypes, at least partly, through its effects on smoking behavior[69]; (2) the *HHIP* locus, which has also been associated with lung cancer[70] and lung function in subjects with asthma,[71] has effects on lung function and the systemic components of COPD; and (3) *FAM13A* influences lung function and airflow obstruction.

Cachexia, common in subjects with advanced COPD, is associated with increased severity of airflow obstruction and increased mortality. Wan and colleagues[72] conducted a GWAS of BMI in 2950 subjects with COPD in 3 cohorts (ECLIPSE, Norway, and NETT), with replication attempted in 502 subjects from COPDGene. A GWAS of fat-free mass index (FFMI) was also conducted in the ECLIPSE and Norway cohorts. SNP rs8050136, located in the intron of the fat mass and obesity-associated gene (*FTO*), was significantly associated with BMI ($P = 4.97 \times 10^{-7}$) and FFMI ($P = 1.19 \times 10^{-7}$) in the discovery cohort. Findings for BMI were replicated in COPDGene ($P = 6 \times 10^{-3}$). These findings suggest that *FTO* influences anthropometric measures in subjects with COPD.

GWAS of Lung Function: Relevance to COPD

Spirometric measures of lung function such as FEV_1 and FEV_1/FVC are key intermediate phenotypes of COPD. Thus, some genes that influence lung function in the general population may also be relevant to the pathogenesis of COPD. Wilk and colleagues[73] conducted a GWAS of lung function measures in 7691 participants in the Framingham Heart Study (FHS) with validation in an independent cohort of 835 subjects in the Family Heart Study that was enriched for airflow obstruction. Four SNPs in tight linkage disequilibrium (eg, highly correlated) on chromosome 4q31were significantly associated with FEV_1/FVC percent predicted in the discovery (FHS) cohort. The association between 1 of the 4 SNPs (rs13147758) and FEV_1/FVC was replicated in the Family Heart Study, in which significant associations were also shown with FEV_1 and binary airflow obstruction phenotypes (particularly in smokers). The associated SNPs were not in a gene transcript but were near *HHIP*, a candidate gene for COPD susceptibility (mentioned earlier).

In a meta-analysis of GWAS results for lung function in 20,890 participants from 4 CHARGE consortium studies (Atherosclerosis Risk in Communities, Cardiovascular Heath Study, FHS, and the Rotterdam Study), *HHIP* and *FAM13A* (mentioned earlier) were among the 8 loci associated with FEV_1/FVC (the other 6 were *GPR126*, *ADAM19*, *AGER-PPT2*, *PTCH1*, *PID1*, and *HTR4*) at or near the threshold for genome-wide statistical significance.[74] In a separate study, a GWAS of lung function measures was conducted in 20,288 subjects of European ancestry in the SpiroMeta Consortium (discovery cohort); this GWAS was then followed by a meta-analysis of data for the top signals from the discovery cohort and 32,184 subjects in the CHARGE consortium, as well as in silico summary association data from 21,209 individuals from the CHARGE consortium and 883 individuals in the Health 2000 Survey.[75] This study confirmed the previously reported locus on chromosome 4q31 near *HHIP* (mentioned earlier) and identified 5 novel loci for FEV_1 or FEV_1/FVC: 2q35 in *TNS1*, 4q24 in *GSTCD*, 5q33 in *HTR4*, 6p21 in *AGER*, and 15q23 in *THSD4*.

Two recent studies have assessed whether loci identified by GWAS on lung function also influence COPD. Soler Artigas and colleagues[76] studied a large sample of subjects of European ancestry (including individuals with and without COPD) and constructed a risk score including 6 SNPs in *HTR4, GSTCD, TNS1, AGER, THSD4*, and near *HHIP*. Compared with subjects in a common baseline group, those in the highest risk category (estimated as approximately 5% or Europeans) had a 1.6-fold increased risk of developing COPD.[76] In another study, Castaldi and colleagues[77] tested whether 32 SNPs in or near 11 loci associated with lung function in prior GWAS were associated with COPD in 5362 subjects in 4 cohorts (NETT-NAS, ECLIPSE, Norway, and the first 1000 subjects in COPDGene). Of the previously identified susceptibility loci for lung function, 3 genomic regions harbored polymorphisms associated with susceptibility to COPD at a 5% false discovery rate: the *FLJ20184/INTS12/ GSTCD/NPNT* locus on chromosome 4q24, the chromosome 6p21 locus including AGER and PPT2, and the chromosome 5q33 locus that includes ADAM19.

Beyond GWAS

As with other complex diseases, GWASs have identified susceptibility loci that explain a modest fraction of the heritability (the proportion of variation in a phenotype due to genetic factors) of COPD, with nominal explanation of disease risk.[78] Additional work is needed for functional characterization and full assessment of variation in these susceptibility loci, as well as for understanding their individual and combined (eg, gene-by-gene and gene-by-environment [ie, smoking]) effects on COPD-related phenotypes.

Beyond GWAS, additional approaches to the study of COPD genetics include sequencing exomes and/or the whole genome to identify rare susceptibility variants and conducting studies of integrative genomics (where genetic variants are evaluated for their contribution to gene expression) and epigenetics (heritable changes in gene expression that occur without changes in DNA sequence).

Genetic variants that are uncommon (minor allele frequency [MAF] = 1%–4%) or rare (MAF <1%) may confer greater susceptibility to COPD in certain individuals and/or ethnic groups. Because the genotyping platforms used for GWAS of COPD predominantly include variants with MAF greater than or equal to 5%, they would not be able to detect these uncommon/rare variants with moderate to strong genetic effects. Next-generation sequencing technologies provide this capability.[79] Exome sequencing allows investigators to detect rare variants in protein-coding regions of the genome. Compared with whole-genome sequencing, exome sequencing is less expensive and thus allows studying a larger number of subjects.[80] Exome sequencing has been successful in identifying the genetic etiology of a rare mendelian disorder[81] and is currently being applied to the investigation of COPD. As prices of whole-genome sequencing decrease, this will become a feasible and attractive method to detect rare variants with strong effects on COPD, particularly regulatory (noncoding) variants. Integration of data from GWAS and sequencing studies with those from studies of gene expression and proteomics should allow researchers to focus on the most promising candidate genes for COPD susceptibility.

Studying epigenetic mechanisms (including DNA methylation, histone modification, and micro-RNA) provides a unique opportunity to examine the potential impact of demographic, environmental, and lifestyle factors (eg, diet, aging, and cigarette smoking)[82] on gene expression in the lung and COPD. Whole-genome studies of DNA methylation, the best characterized epigenetic mechanism, and COPD are now in progress.

SUMMARY

Although much remains to be done, recent advances and the advent of new methodologies are promising and should yield increased understanding of the genetic and epigenetic mechanisms influencing the pathogenesis of COPD, both related and unrelated to severe AAT deficiency. Such understanding should ultimately be translated into novel approaches to prevent, diagnose, and treat COPD.

REFERENCES

1. Janus ED, Phillips NT, Carrell RW. Smoking, lung function, and alpha 1-antitrypsin deficiency. Lancet 1985;1:152–4.
2. Tobin MJ, Cook PJL, Hutchison DC. Alpha 1-antitrypsin deficiency: the clinical and physiological features of pulmonary emphysema in subjects homozygous for Pi type Z. Br J Dis Chest 1983;77:14–27.
3. Silverman EK, Pierce JA, Province MA, et al. Variability of pulmonary function in alpha 1-antitrypsin deficiency: clinical correlates. Ann Intern Med 1989;111: 982–91.
4. Silverman EK, Province MA, Campbell EJ, et al. Variability of pulmonary function in alpha-1-antitrypsin deficiency: residual family resemblance beyond the effect of the Pi locus. Hum Hered 1990;40:340–55.
5. Burrows B, Knudson RJ, Cline MG, et al. Quantitative relationships between cigarette smoking and ventilatory function. Am Rev Respir Dis 1977;115:195–205.
6. Celedon JC, Speizer FE, Drazen JM, et al. Bronchodilator responsiveness and serum total IgE levels in families of probands with severe early-onset COPD. Eur Respir J 1999;14:1009–14.
7. McCloskey SC, Patel BD, Hinchliffe SJ, et al. Siblings of patients with severe chronic obstructive pulmonary disease have a significant risk of airflow obstruction. Am J Respir Crit Care Med 2001;164:1419–24.
8. Silverman EK, Chapman HA, Drazen JM, et al. Genetic epidemiology of severe, early-onset chronic obstructive pulmonary disease: risk to relatives for airflow obstruction and chronic bronchitis. Am J Respir Crit Care Med 1998;157:1770–8.
9. Laurell CB, Eriksson S. The electrophoretic a_1-globulin pattern of serum in a_1-antitrypsin deficiency. Scand J Clin Lab Invest 1963;15:132–40.
10. Schroeder WT, Miller MF, Woo SL, et al. Chromosomal localization of the human alpha 1-antitrypsin gene (PI) to 14q31-32. Am J Hum Genet 1985;37:868–72.
11. DeMeo DL, Silverman EK. Alpha1-antitrypsin deficiency. 2: genetic aspects of alpha(1)-antitrypsin deficiency: phenotypes and genetic modifiers of emphysema risk. Thorax 2004;59:259–64.
12. Turino GM, Barker AF, Brantly ML, et al. Clinical features of individuals with PI*SZ phenotype of alpha 1-antitrypsin deficiency. Am J Respir Crit Care Med 1996; 154:1718–25.
13. Dahl M, Tybjaerg-Hansen A, Lange P, et al. Change in lung function and morbidity from chronic obstructive pulmonary disease in a_1-antitrypsin MZ heterozygotes; a longitudinal study of the general population. Ann Intern Med 2002;136:270–9.
14. de Serres FJ, Blanco I, Fernandez-Bustillo E. Genetic epidemiology of alpha-1 antitrypsin deficiency in North America and Australia/New Zealand: Australia, Canada, New Zealand and the United States of America. Clin Genet 2003;64:382–97.
15. de Serres FJ. Worldwide racial and ethnic distribution of alpha1-antitrypsin deficiency: summary of an analysis of published genetic epidemiologic surveys. Chest 2002;122:1818–29.

16. Cichy J, Potempa J, Travis J. Biosynthesis of alpha1-proteinase inhibitor by human lung-derived epithelial cells. J Biol Chem 1997;272:8250–5.
17. Perlmutter DH, Cole FS, Kilbridge P, et al. Expression of the alpha 1-proteinase inhibitor gene in human monocytes and macrophages. Proc Natl Acad Sci U S A 1985;82:795–9.
18. Rao NV, Wehner NG, Marshall BC, et al. Characterization of proteinase-3 (PR-3), a neutrophil serine proteinase. Structural and functional properties. J Biol Chem 1991;266:9540–8.
19. Vercaigne-Marko D, Davril M, Laine A, et al. Interaction of human alpha 1-proteinase inhibitor with human leukocyte cathepsin G. Biol Chem Hoppe Seyler 1985;366:655–61.
20. Taggart C, Cervantes-Laurean D, Kim G, et al. Oxidation of either methionine 351 or methionine 358 in alpha 1-antitrypsin causes loss of anti-neutrophil elastase activity. J Biol Chem 2000;275:27258–65.
21. Petrache I, Fijalkowska I, Medler TR, et al. Alpha-1 antitrypsin inhibits caspase-3 activity, preventing lung endothelial cell apoptosis. Am J Pathol 2006;169: 1155–66.
22. Malhotra D, Thimmulappa R, Vij N, et al. Heightened endoplasmic reticulum stress in the lungs of patients with chronic obstructive pulmonary disease: the role of Nrf2-regulated proteasomal activity. Am J Respir Crit Care Med 2009; 180:1196–207.
23. Nita I, Hollander C, Westin U, et al. Prolastin, a pharmaceutical preparation of purified human alpha1-antitrypsin, blocks endotoxin-mediated cytokine release. Respir Res 2005;6:12.
24. Jie Z, Cai Y, Yang W, et al. Protective effects of alpha 1-antitrypsin on acute lung injury in rabbits induced by endotoxin. Chin Med J (Engl) 2003;116:1678–82.
25. Bucurenci N, Blake DR, Chidwick K, et al. Inhibition of neutrophil superoxide production by human plasma alpha 1-antitrypsin. FEBS Lett 1992;300:21–4.
26. Janciauskiene S, Larsson S, Larsson P, et al. Inhibition of lipopolysaccharide-mediated human monocyte activation, in vitro, by alpha1-antitrypsin. Biochem Biophys Res Commun 2004;321:592–600.
27. Dafforn TR, Mahadeva R, Elliott PR, et al. A kinetic mechanism for the polymerization of alpha1-antitrypsin. J Biol Chem 1999;274:9548–55.
28. Lomas DA, Evans DL, Finch JT, et al. The mechanism of Z alpha 1-antitrypsin accumulation in the liver [see comments]. Nature 1992;357:605–7.
29. Teckman JH, Perlmutter DH. Retention of mutant alpha(1)-antitrypsin Z in endoplasmic reticulum is associated with an autophagic response. Am J Physiol Gastrointest Liver Physiol 2000;279:G961–74.
30. Hidvegi T, Schmidt BZ, Hale P, et al. Accumulation of mutant alpha1-antitrypsin Z in the endoplasmic reticulum activates caspases-4 and -12, NFkappaB, and BAP31 but not the unfolded protein response. J Biol Chem 2005;280: 39002–15.
31. Hultcrantz R, Mengarelli S. Ultrastructural liver pathology in patients with minimal liver disease and alpha 1-antitrypsin deficiency: a comparison between heterozygous and homozygous patients. Hepatology 1984;4:937–45.
32. Mahadeva R, Atkinson C, Li Z, et al. Polymers of Z alpha1-antitrypsin co-localize with neutrophils in emphysematous alveoli and are chemotactic in vivo. Am J Pathol 2005;166:377–86.
33. Lomas DA, Elliott PR, Sidhar SK, et al. alpha 1-Antitrypsin Mmalton (Phe52-deleted) forms loop-sheet polymers in vivo. Evidence for the C sheet mechanism of polymerization. J Biol Chem 1995;270:16864–70.

34. Mulgrew AT, Taggart CC, Lawless MW, et al. Z alpha1-antitrypsin polymerizes in the lung and acts as a neutrophil chemoattractant. Chest 2004;125:1952–7.

35. Bernspang E, Sveger T, Piitulainen E. Respiratory symptoms and lung function in 30-year-old individuals with alpha-1-antitrypsin deficiency. Respir Med 2007;101: 1971–6.

36. Campos MA, Wanner A, Zhang G, et al. Trends in the diagnosis of symptomatic patients with alpha1-antitrypsin deficiency between 1968 and 2003. Chest 2005; 128:1179–86.

37. Parr DG, Stoel BC, Stolk J, et al. Pattern of emphysema distribution in alpha1-antitrypsin deficiency influences lung function impairment. Am J Respir Crit Care Med 2004;170:1172–8.

38. Campos MA, Alazemi S, Zhang G, et al. Effects of a disease management program in individuals with alpha-1 antitrypsin deficiency. COPD 2009;6:31–40.

39. Parr DG, Guest PG, Reynolds JH, et al. Prevalence and impact of bronchiectasis in alpha1-antitrypsin deficiency. Am J Respir Crit Care Med 2007;176:1215–21.

40. American Thoracic Society/European Respiratory Society statement: standards for the diagnosis and management of individuals with alpha-1 antitrypsin deficiency. Am J Respir Crit Care Med 2003;168:818–900.

41. Silverman EK, Miletich JP, Pierce JA, et al. Alpha-1-antitrypsin deficiency: high prevalence in the St. Louis area determined by direct population screening. Am Rev Respir Dis 1989;140:961–6.

42. DeMeo DL, Campbell EJ, Brantly ML, et al. Heritability of lung function in severe alpha-1 antitrypsin deficiency. Hum Hered 2009;67:38–45.

43. Novoradovsky A, Brantly ML, Waclawiw MA, et al. Endothelial nitric oxide synthase as a potential susceptibility gene in the pathogenesis of emphysema in alpha1-antitrypsin deficiency. Am J Respir Cell Mol Biol 1999;20:441–7.

44. Demeo DL, Campbell EJ, Barker AF, et al. IL10 polymorphisms are associated with airflow obstruction in severe alpha1-antitrypsin deficiency. Am J Respir Cell Mol Biol 2008;38:114–20.

45. Castaldi PJ, DeMeo DL, Kent DM, et al. Development of predictive models for airflow obstruction in alpha-1-antitrypsin deficiency. Am J Epidemiol 2009;170: 1005–13.

46. Carp H, Miller F, Hoidal JR, et al. Potential mechanism of emphysema: alpha1-proteinase inhibitor recovered from lungs of cigarette smokers contains oxidized methionine and has decreased elastase inhibitory capacity. Proc Natl Acad Sci U S A 1982;79:2041–5.

47. Alam S, Li Z, Janciauskiene S, et al. Oxidation of Z {alpha}1-antitrypsin by cigarette smoke induces polymerization: a novel mechanism of early-onset emphysema. Am J Respir Cell Mol Biol 2011;45:261–9.

48. Rabe KF, Hurd S, Anzueto A, et al. Global strategy for the diagnosis, management, and prevention of chronic obstructive pulmonary disease: GOLD executive summary. Am J Respir Crit Care Med 2007;176:532–55.

49. Bourbeau J, Nault D, Dang-Tan T. Self-management and behaviour modification in COPD. Patient Educ Couns 2004;52:271–7.

50. Donahue JM, Cassivi SD. Lung volume reduction surgery for patients with alpha-1 antitrypsin deficiency emphysema. Thorac Surg Clin 2009;19:201–8.

51. Corda L, Bertella E, La Piana GE, et al. Inhaled corticosteroids as additional treatment in alpha-1-antitrypsin-deficiency-related COPD. Respiration 2008;76:61–8.

52. Petrache I, Hajjar J, Campos M. Safety and efficacy of alpha-1-antitrypsin augmentation therapy in the treatment of patients with alpha-1-antitrypsin deficiency. Biologics 2009;3:193–204.

53. Chapman KR, Stockley RA, Dawkins C, et al. Augmentation therapy for alpha1 antitrypsin deficiency: a meta-analysis. COPD 2009;6:177–84.
54. Gotzsche PC, Johansen HK. Intravenous alpha-1 antitrypsin augmentation therapy for treating patients with alpha-1 antitrypsin deficiency and lung disease. Cochrane Database Syst Rev 2010;7:CD007851.
55. Brantly ML, Spencer LT, Humphries M, et al. Phase I trial of intramuscular injection of a recombinant adeno-associated virus serotype 2 alpha1-antitrypsin (AAT) vector in AAT-deficient adults. Hum Gene Ther 2006;17:1177–86.
56. Somers A, Jean JC, Sommer CA, et al. Generation of transgene-free lung disease-specific human induced pluripotent stem cells using a single excisable lentiviral stem cell cassette. Stem Cells 2010;28:1728–40.
57. Smolonska J, Wijmenga C, Postma DS, et al. Meta-analyses on suspected COPD genes—a summary of 20 years' research. Am J Respir Crit Care Med 2009; 180(7):618–31.
58. Hunninghake GM, Cho MH, Tesfaigzi Y, et al. MMP12, lung function, and COPD in high-risk populations. N Engl J Med 2009;361:2599–608.
59. Pillai SG, Ge D, Zhu G, et al. A genome-wide association study in chronic obstructive pulmonary disease (COPD): identification of two major susceptibility loci. PLoS Genet 2009;5(3):e1000421.
60. Silverman EK, Palmer LJ, Mosley JD, et al. Genomewide linkage analysis of quantitative spirometric phenotypes in severe early-onset chronic obstructive pulmonary disease. Am J Hum Genet 2002;70:1229–39.
61. Warburton D, Bellusci S, De Langhe S, et al. Molecular mechanisms of early lung specification and branching morphogenesis. Pediatr Res 2005;57:26R–37R.
62. Vestbo J, Anderson W, Coxson HO, et al. Evaluation of COPD Longitudinally to Identify Predictive Surrogate End-points (ECLIPSE). Eur Respir J 2008;31: 869–73.
63. Cho MH, Boutaoui N, Klanderman BJ, et al. Variants in FAM13A are associated with chronic obstructive pulmonary disease. Nat Genet 2010;42:200–2.
64. Regan EA, Hokanson JE, Murphy JR, et al. Genetic epidemiology of COPD (COPDGene) study design. COPD 2010;7:32–43.
65. Kong X, Cho MH, Anderson W, et al. Genome-wide association study identifies BICD1 as a susceptibility gene for emphysema. Am J Respir Crit Care Med 2011;183:43–9.
66. Celli BR, Cote CG, Marin JM, et al. The body-mass index, airflow obstruction, dyspnea, and exercise capacity index in chronic obstructive pulmonary disease. N Engl J Med 2004;350:1005–12.
67. Pillai SG, Kong X, Edwards LD, et al. Loci identified by genome-wide association studies influence different disease-related phenotypes in chronic obstructive pulmonary disease. Am J Respir Crit Care Med 2010;182:1498–505.
68. Amos CI, Wu X, Broderick P, et al. Genome-wide association scan of tag SNPs identifies a susceptibility locus for lung cancer at 15q25.1. Nat Genet 2008;40: 616–22.
69. Saccone NL, Culverhouse RC, Schwantes-An TH, et al. Multiple independent loci at chromosome 15q25.1 affect smoking quantity: a meta-analysis and comparison with lung cancer and COPD. PLoS Genet 2010;6(8):e1001053.
70. Young RP, Whittington CF, Hopkins RJ, et al. Chromosome 4q31 locus in COPD is also associated with lung cancer. Eur Respir J 2010;36:1375–82.
71. Li X, Howard TD, Moore WC, et al. Importance of hedgehog interacting protein and other lung function genes in asthma. J Allergy Clin Immunol 2011;127: 1457–65.

72. Wan ES, Cho MH, Boutaoui N, et al. Genome-wide association analysis of body mass in chronic obstructive pulmonary disease. Am J Respir Cell Mol Biol 2011; 45:304–10.
73. Wilk JB, Chen TH, Gottlieb DJ, et al. A genome-wide association study of pulmonary function measures in the Framingham Heart Study. PLoS Genet 2009;5(3): e1000429.
74. Hancock DB, Eijgelsheim M, Wilk JB, et al. Meta-analyses of genome-wide association studies identify multiple loci associated with pulmonary function. Nat Genet 2010;42:45–52.
75. Repapi E, Sayers I, Wain LV, et al. Genome-wide association study identifies five loci associated with lung function. Nat Genet 2010;42:36–44.
76. Soler Artigas M, Wain LV, Repapi E, et al. Effect of 5 genetic variants associated with lung function on the risk of COPD, and their joint effects on lung function. Am J Respir Crit Care Med 2011;184(7):786–95.
77. Castaldi PJ, Cho MH, Litonjua AA, et al. The association of genome-wide significant spirometric loci with COPD susceptibility. Am J Respir Cell Mol Biol 2011; 45(6):1147–53.
78. Cookson WO, Moffatt MF. Genetics of complex airway disease. Proc Am Thorac Soc 2011;8:149–53.
79. Cirulli ET, Goldstein DB. Uncovering the roles of rare variants in common disease through whole-genome sequencing. Nat Rev Genet 2010;11:415–25.
80. Ng SB, Turner EH, Robertson PD, et al. Targeted capture and massively parallel sequencing of 12 human exomes. Nature 2009;461:272–6.
81. Ng SB, Bigham AW, Buckingham KJ, et al. Exome sequencing identifies MLL2 mutations as a cause of Kabuki syndrome. Nat Genet 2010;42:790–3.
82. Yang IV, Schwartz DA. Epigenetic control of gene expression in the lung. Am J Respir Crit Care Med 2011;183:1295–301.

Contribution of the Environment and Comorbidities to Chronic Obstructive Pulmonary Disease Phenotypes

Carlos H. Martinez, MD, MPH, MeiLan K. Han, MD, MS*

KEYWORDS

- Emphysema • Chronic bronchitis • Inflammation • Systemic disease

KEY POINTS

- The heterogeneity implicit to COPD suggests that a wide variety of influences including environmental and biologic factors likely contribute to an individual's disease presentation and progression.
- Certain comorbid conditions such as cardiovascular disease and osteoporosis also contribute to the heterogeneity of the patient population.
- Systemic inflammation may be pathogenically related to many of the comorbidities seen in COPD including cardiovascular disease, osteoporosis, metabolic syndrome and depression.
- New research in COPD using large patient populations with extensive clinical and biologic characterization along with advanced analytic methods will hopefully further expand our potential to identify disease phenotypes such that targeted therapies can be developed.

Chronic obstructive pulmonary disease (COPD) is a syndrome characterized by significant disease heterogeneity.[1] Whereas the presence of airflow obstruction that is not completely reversible is a hallmark of the disease, in the individual patient this obstruction may be caused by airway inflammation and remodeling, emphysema, or both. Clinicians have identified 2 basic subtypes of COPD: "pink puffers" characterized by emphysema, significant dyspnea, hyperinflation, and weight loss but with adequate oxygenation; and "blue bloaters" characterized by chronic bronchitis, hypoventilation, and obesity. It is likely that many other phenotypes exist in COPD but their relevance has not been adequately validated.[2] To provide some clarity, a recent consensus

Disclosures: C.H.M None. M.K.H Dr Han has received lecture fees from Boehringer-Ingelheim, Pfizer and GlaxoSmithKline. She has received consulting fees from Novartis, Genentech, GlaxoSmithKline, Pfizer, Boehringer-Ingelheim and Medimmune.
Division of Pulmonary and Critical Care Medicine, University of Michigan Health System, 1500 East Medical Center Drive, 3916 Taubman Center, Ann Arbor, MI 48109-5360, USA
* Corresponding author.
E-mail address: mrking@umich.edu

group defined COPD phenotypes as, "a single or combination of disease attributes that describe differences between individuals with COPD as they relate to clinically meaningful outcomes (symptoms, exacerbations, response to therapy, rate of disease progression, or death)."[2] The validation of phenotypes will ultimately require an iterative process (**Fig. 1**) so that groups of patients may initially be identified either by similar clinical outcome, radiologic or physiologic characteristics, biological or molecular signature, or response to therapy. Ultimately, the hope is that these patient subgroups share similar pathophysiologic processes, so that specific therapies can be developed. The goal of this article is to highlight the accumulated data regarding environmental and host factors, in particular comorbid diseases, that may help to identify and refine patient phenotypes in COPD.

ENVIRONMENT

Tobacco is the principal risk factor and environmental toxin responsible for the development of the disease in most patients with COPD. Most of what we know about the natural history of COPD is in tobacco smokers. The prevalence of COPD in smokers is approximately 20% as compared with 4% in nonsmokers.[3] This association is supported by the acceptance of the preventive effects of smoking cessation. The Lung Health Study, an interventional smoking cessation study in smokers with COPD with mild airflow obstruction, demonstrated that the decline in the rate of forced expiratory volume in 1 second (FEV_1) was greatest in patients who smoked the most and least in those who achieved sustained smoking cessation.[4] However, the fact that only one in five smokers develops COPD, points towards additional factors that contribute to its development. The importance of second-hand smoke exposure, also known as environmental tobacco smoke (ETS), should not be overlooked. Higher cumulative lifetime ETS at home and work has been associated with increased risk of COPD, even after adjustment for personal smoking history and occupational exposure.[5]

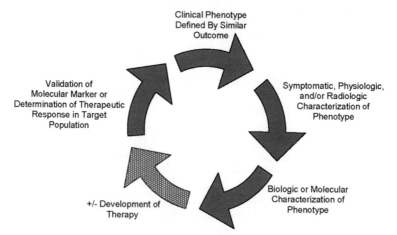

Fig. 1. Ideal phenotyping construct wherein candidate phenotypes are validated once their relevance to clinical outcomes is established. There are multiple potential points of entry into this iterative process of phenotype identification. For instance, similar clinical outcomes may define a subpopulation that leads to the identification of a biologic target and focused therapy. Alternatively, the process might begin with the differentiation of subgroups based on a biologic marker that is then validated by similar clinical response within subgroups. (*From* Han MK, Agusti A, Calverley PM, et al. Chronic obstructive pulmonary disease phenotypes: the future of COPD. Am J Respir Crit Care Med 2010;182(5):598–4; with permission.)

The prevalence of COPD in nonsmokers in the United States, according to data from the Third National Health and Nutrition Epidemiologic Survey is approximately 6.6%.[6] Worldwide figures for nontobacco related COPD vary around 20% to 25% of all COPD cases, with estimates as high as 40% to 50% in countries such as Colombia and South Africa.[7] The risk factors associated with COPD in nonsmokers are numerous and incompletely understood, but a history of asthma or tuberculosis, exposure to traffic and outdoor pollution, and exposure to biomass smoke show the strongest associations.[8,9] How disease presentation and course differs by risk factor is not well described. One study has suggested that life expectancy for nonsmokers with COPD is only modestly reduced (0.7 years for the Global Initiative for Chronic Obstructive Lung Disease (GOLD) stage 2 patients, and 1.3 years for GOLD stages 3–4) compared with substantially reduced life expectancy in current smokers with COPD (2.2 years for GOLD stage 2, and 5.8 years for GOLD stages 3–4) and former smokers with COPD (1.4 years for GOLD stage 2 and 5.6 years for GOLD stages 3–4).[10]

Whereas it has been estimated that COPD attributable to cigarette smoking is between 80% and 90%, COPD attributed to occupational exposures (vapors, gas, dust, or fumes) is close to 15%.[11] Whereas specific industries, such as coal mining, have been related to the development of airflow obstruction, increasing data from across various industries and occupations are being collected.[11] Outdoor air pollution also probably contributes to the development of COPD. A 1958 study of postmen in the United Kingdom documented the prevalence of COPD to be higher in those working in more polluted areas, independent of personal smoking history.[12] Data from other population studies of individuals living close to roads with heavy motor vehicle traffic also support these findings.[13]

In the developing world, exposure to smoke from biomass fuels is an important cause of COPD, particularly in women who use biomass fuels for cooking.[14] It is unclear whether the phenotype of COPD in this group of nonsmokers differs from that of tobacco-exposed individuals, although studies of women exposed to biomass fuel smoke suggest that disease presentation and mortality are similar to those with COPD attributable to tobacco smoking.[15]

Nutrition may also be an important factor that influences the development of COPD. Vitamin D levels, in particular, demonstrate an inverse relationship with pulmonary function in COPD.[16] Genetic polymorphisms in vitamin D metabolic pathways have also been associated with COPD.[17] An association has also been described between higher levels of vitamin C in plasma and protection against incident COPD.[18] Similar information has been reported between vitamin A intake and prevalence of COPD.[19] Lately, a protective function has been attributed to a diet high in cereal fiber.[20] Further studies of the relationship between nutritional factors and COPD may offer mechanistic insights into the pathogenesis and treatment of this disease.

HOST FACTORS

Gender is an important factor that also may affect disease phenotype.[14] Conflicting data exist on whether women are more susceptible to developing COPD for a similar amount of tobacco smoke exposure.[14] However, women with COPD report more dyspnea, similar degrees of cough, but less sputum compared with men with similar degrees of airflow obstruction.[21] It has been suggested that women are more likely to display a chronic bronchitic phenotype of COPD whereas men display a more emphysematous phenotype.[14] Radiologic data from the National Emphysema Treatment Trial among patients with severe emphysema supports this hypothesis whereby women demonstrated less overall emphysema, particularly in the peripheral portions of the lung.[22] Histologic data from the same study revealed that the bronchioles of women have significantly thicker airway walls and smaller lumen than the bronchioles of men.[22] Recent data also suggest that COPD exacerbations are more frequent in women but it is unknown whether this represents a difference in disease biology or reporting patterns.[23,24]

Whereas genetic and epigenetic contributions to COPD are discussed in more detail elsewhere, genetics must also play a role in disease phenotype. The best known genetic risk factor for development of COPD is alpha-1 anti-trypsin (AAT) deficiency, whereby patients are more likely to develop lower lobe predominant emphysema patterns compared with patients without AAT deficiency, who are more likely to present with upper lobe emphysema. More data in this regard are likely to come from the ongoing COPDGene Study, a genome-wide association study of more than 10000 subjects, with the goal of identifying the genetic determinants of specific disease phenotypes (http://www.copdgene.org). Information derived from such studies may help determine the reason for these phenotypic expressions of the disease and their clinical relevance.

Another host factor that probably contributes to the COPD phenotype but is often over-looked is the lung microbiome. Alteration in the lung and the gut microbiomes has been associated with the development of asthma.[25–27] This leads to the consideration of the role of the microbiome in COPD, wherein bacterial colonization has been associated with FEV_1 decline and increased rates of acute exacerbations of COPD (AECOPD).[28] Recent data also support a similar process with the genesis of emphysema and airway structural abnormality.[28,29] Although investigations of COPD using advanced, culture-independent techniques are limited, a predominance of Pseudomonas species in patients with more impaired lung function in COPD has been reported.[30]

COMORBIDITIES

Accumulating data suggest that comorbidities must be included in the assessment of patients with COPD. Some comorbid conditions, such as cardiovascular disease and osteoporosis, are more common in patients with COPD compared with the general population. Although comorbidities such as obstructive sleep apnea may not be more prevalent in COPD, they are important because they may modify the course of the disease.[31] Because comorbid conditions can alter the course of the disease or the need for specific therapies in COPD, they remain important considerations in the development and refinement of COPD phenotypes. Systemic inflammation may be pathogenically related to many comorbidities seen in COPD including cardiovascular disease, osteoporosis, metabolic syndrome, and depression.[32,33] There is not enough confirmatory data to support the specific treatment of systemic inflammation in patients with COPD but current studies aimed at capturing the nature and extent of the importance of this pathobiological mechanism, may lead to the development of specific therapy for patients presenting with this phenotype.

Cardiovascular Disease

Ischemic cardiovascular disease continues to be a leading cause of death in COPD.[34] Whereas shared risk factors, such as tobacco use, contribute to this association, epidemiologic evidence suggests that impaired lung function itself is an independent risk factor for increased cardiovascular mortality. Data from the National Health and Nutrition Examination Survey demonstrated that patients in the lowest FEV_1 quintile had the highest risk of cardiovascular mortality (risk ratio [RR] of 3.36), even after adjustment for pertinent risk factors including smoking status, blood pressure, body mass index (BMI), and diabetes.[35] In a meta-analysis of studies relating cardiovascular mortality to reduced FEV_1 adjusted for smoking status, the RR of death for patients with COPD was 1.77 (95% confidence interval [CI], 1.46–1.97).[35] In the Lung Health Study, cardiovascular events accounted for 42% of first hospitalizations and 48% of second hospitalizations in patients with mild to moderate COPD.[36] An inverse relationship between FEV_1 and the presence of atherosclerosis has also been documented.[37] In addition to the degree of airflow obstruction in COPD, the actual rate of FEV_1 decline is also an independent predictor of cardiovascular mortality.[38,39]

Because atherosclerosis, like COPD, is a disease of systemic inflammation,[40] an increase in systemic inflammation may explain the association between the two diseases. Elevated C-reactive protein (CRP) levels correlate not only with the presence of COPD but also with the presence of exacerbations, severity of lung function, and risk for hospitalization and death.[41] The interaction between COPD and cardiovascular disease may also have important therapeutic implications. In one study, the withdrawal of inhaled steroids in patients with COPD with moderate-to-severe disease was associated with a 71% increase in serum CRP levels.[42] Subsequent treatment with inhaled corticosteroids resulted in a 50% reduction in CRP levels (95% CI, 9%–73%); prednisone-treated patients had a reduction of CRP levels of 63% (95% CI, 29%–81%) whereas the patients receiving placebo experienced no significant change in CRP levels. Medications used to treat cardiovascular disease may affect COPD outcomes. In an analysis of a large Canadian database of patients with COPD, the combination of statin and either angiotensin-converting inhibitor or angiotensin receptor blocker therapy was associated with a reduction in hospitalization (RR 0.66; 95% CI, 0.51–0.85) and total mortality (RR 0.42; 95% CI, 0.33–0.52).[43] A separate cohort study also found that statin therapy in COPD was associated with reduced risk of death, (hazard ratio 0.57; 95% CI, 0.38–0.87).[44] Although beta-blockers have been used with caution in obstructive lung disease, a retrospective analysis of a COPD cohort recently reported that there was a 22% overall reduction in all-cause mortality in patients with COPD using beta-blockers.[45]

Musculoskeletal Disease

Although prevalence estimates vary, low BMI is clearly associated with COPD, and in particular with disease severity.[46] Low BMI is also an important independent prognostic factor for increased mortality in patients with COPD.[47] A relationship between low fat-free mass index (FFMI) and increased mortality in COPD has been demonstrated, even in subjects with a normal BMI, after controlling for age and spirometric severity.[48] The prognostic effect of the BMI is further supported by its importance in the calculation of the BMI, obstruction, dyspnea, exercise capacity (BODE) index, one of the best mortality prediction indices in COPD.[49]

Low BMI has been recognized as a distinguishing feature of pink puffers for many years and several studies correlating low BMI with greater extent of emphysema on high resolution computed tomography (HRCT) help to confirm this association.[50] The fat-free mass index (FFMI) has also been demonstrated to have an inverse association with extent of emphysema on HRCT, the six minute walk test distance, and CRP levels.[51] In contrast to the observed association between low BMI and emphysema, the presence of chronic bronchitis has been statistically associated not only with higher BMI but also with HRCT indicators of airway disease.[52] Different mechanisms have been postulated for the loss of body mass in COPD including systemic inflammation and oxidative stress, tissue hypoxia, disuse atrophy, energy imbalance, hormone insufficiency, and genetic factors but no definitive explanation has been identified.[53] There have been several attempts to reverse the cachexia observed in a significant proportion of patients with COPD. The results have been disappointing with nutrition-based interventions, the use of nocturnal ventilation to decrease energy expenditure, and the use of growth-hormone releasing factors.[53] However, there are data supporting the capacity of COPD patients with low FFI (<17 kg/m^2) to remodel muscle and improve cachexia in response to exercise training.[54]

Whereas estimates vary, the prevalence of osteoporosis is increased in patients with COPD. Estimates ranging between two- and fivefold increase have been made for patients with COPD compared with age-matched controls without airflow obstruction.[55,56] The frequency of osteoporosis also seems to be correlated to the severity of airflow obstruction. Vertebral fractures are more prevalent as the severity of spirometrically-defined COPD increases.[55,57] Whereas there are multiple shared-risk factors such as the use of oral steroids, smoking, and low BMI that may contribute to osteoporosis in COPD, these risk factors do not appear to completely explain the association, as several studies have documented lower bone mineral density (BMD) even in the absence of systemic steroids.[57,58]

As with low BMI, osteoporosis and low BMD also seem to be more strongly related to the presence and severity of emphysema but not related to the severity of chronic bronchitis or airway wall thickness as assessed by HRCT.[59] Whereas an adequate understanding of this association at the cellular and molecular level is incomplete, better insights could lead to novel diagnostic and therapeutic interventions. Although matrix metallopeptidase-9 (MMP-9), interleukin-6 (IL-6) and adipokines have all been implicated, no clear causal link has emerged.[60–62] Participation in pulmonary rehabilitation is an option to improve the functional status of patients with advanced COPD. Whereas exercise programs have not been demonstrated to increase BMD in COPD, they may diminish the risk of fracture by decreasing the risk of falls.[63]

Diabetes

Diabetes is another frequent comorbidity in COPD. Many studies have reported a relationship between increased risk of the development of diabetes and the presence of COPD. Lung function impairment, measured either by a low FEV_1 or a low forced vital capacity (FVC), has been associated with the coexistence of the metabolic syndrome, the development of insulin resistance, and development of diabetes.[64–66] The association between lung-function impairment and metabolic syndrome remains, even after adjustment for BMI and smoking history. The independent risk for metabolic syndrome conferred by a low FEV_1 was estimated to be 1.28 (95% CI, 1.20–1.37) in a study of more than 121,000 cases.[64] In the Nurse's Health Study, the RR of incident diabetes among participants with COPD was 1.8 (95% CI, 1.1–2.8),[67] a value very similar to that reported in the Women's Health Study cohort, wherein the relative risk of incident diabetes after a diagnosis of COPD was 1.38 (95% CI, 1.14–1.67).[65]

The link between COPD and diabetes is not clear. Certainly the role of therapies, such as inhaled corticosteroids (ICS) frequently used by patients with COPD, must be considered. At least two independent studies point toward the existence of a dose-dependent association between the use of ICS and diabetes control or new-onset diabetes,[68] but this is unlikely to be the sole explanation responsible for the association. Certain inflammatory mediators, Interleukin 6 (IL-6) and tumor necrosis factor-alpha (TNF-α) in particular, have been implicated in both bronchial inflammation and insulin resistance. In a study of the HRCT characteristics of patients with COPD who experienced exacerbations, a higher prevalence of diabetes was associated with an airway-disease-predominant COPD phenotype compared with an emphysema-predominant disease phenotype.[69] Not surprisingly, patients with predominant airway disease also demonstrated higher BMI and less frequent osteoporosis. These data support a possible relationship between certain metabolic pathways and COPD phenotypes, although the exact pathways and potential therapeutic implications are yet to be defined.

Anemia

Because COPD is a disease of chronic inflammation, it is not surprising to find that anemia is another common comorbidity. The prevalence of anemia in COPD has been reported to be between 7% and 17% in outpatients,[70,71] 12% in patients receiving long-term oxygen therapy,[72] and 23% in hospitalized patients.[73] Anemia in COPD patients has significant implications, and is particularly associated with increased health-care related costs.[71,74] Anemia also has an independent impact on 3-year survival[72] and all-cause mortality.[74] The pathophysiology of anemia in COPD patients is probably similar to that of other chronic inflammatory diseases.[75] The mediators responsible for the airway and pulmonary parenchymal inflammation, especially IL-6, can interfere with the intestinal absorption of iron.[75] Interleukin 1 (IL-1) and TNF-α have been implicated in abnormalities in the production and peripheral effect (or resistance) of erythropoietin.[75] There are no specific recommendations for the treatment of the anemia seen in patients with COPD.

Gastroesophageal Reflux Disease

The association between gastroesophageal reflux disease (GERD) and COPD has been long recognized. In cross-sectional studies using validated questionnaires, the prevalence of heartburn, regurgitation, and dysphagia have been found with higher frequency in patients with COPD compared with controls.[76,77] In one series using 24-h continuous esophageal pH monitoring, acid reflux was recorded in 62% of patients with COPD compared with 19% of controls.[78] This study highlighted the fact that the actual proportion of reflux in the COPD patient population was probably higher than estimates based on symptoms alone. However, even GERD detected by symptoms in the COPD patient population has been associated with poorer outcomes. Both cross-sectional and longitudinal studies have reported associations between the presence of reflux and poor quality of life in COPD.[79] GERD has also been identified as a risk factor for COPD exacerbations[23,80] and seems to be specifically associated with the chronic bronchitic phenotype in COPD.[52]

One hypothesis attempting to explain the association between GERD and COPD is that aspiration may lead to persistent airway inflammation resulting in bronchial remodeling. In support of this hypothesis is human data demonstrating a relationship between elevated C-reactive protein levels and swallowing dysfunction in patients with COPD.[81] An association between lower exhaled breath condensate pH, and GERD symptoms in COPD has also been documented.[77] Whether COPD precedes GERD or vice versa is still open to debate, although epidemiologic evidence supports the idea that a diagnosis of COPD is a risk factor for the development of GERD.[82] Whereas robust evidence that GERD treatment alters COPD outcomes is lacking, in a small, randomized, single-blind, study the proton pump inhibitor lansoprazole reduced the risk of COPD exacerbations and adjusted the odds ratio of 0.23, $P = .004$.[83] Thus, common sense suggests that GERD should be suspected in patients with COPD and once diagnosed it should be treated because there are effective treatments for this condition.

Neuropsychiatric Disorders

Like patients afflicted with other chronic diseases, patients with COPD tend to have a significant burden of coexistent depression and anxiety. Assessments of the prevalence of neuropsychiatric disorders demonstrate wide variation, given the difficulty of exploring this sensitive issue in large population samples, the diversity of the instruments available for assessment, and variations in the severity of the disease detected in different surveys.[84] Conservative estimates suggest that the prevalence of anxiety and depression is at least 10% in the nonhospitalized, general, COPD patient population. Higher estimates have been reported of the prevalence of symptoms of depression (37%–71%) and anxiety (51%–75%) in patients with severe COPD.[85]

Factors associated with increased risk for depression in COPD include disease severity, limited mobility, low body mass, coexistent comorbid conditions, and the need for supplementary oxygen therapy.[86,87] Women are particularly susceptible, with the frequency of depression and anxiety being nearly two times greater in women compared with men.[88] More importantly, depression and anxiety have also been associated with poorer disease outcomes in patients with COPD. Anxiety has been associated with lower functional capacity measured by the six minute walk test[89] Anxiety and depression are also associated with greater dyspnea at rest, worse scores in quality of life questionnaires, and reduced exercise performance at both the beginning and end of pulmonary rehabilitation.[90] Anxiety has been associated with increased risk for COPD exacerbations and greater mortality.[91] Depressive symptoms have been associated with two to three times greater risk of death in COPD.[92,93] Unfortunately, only a small proportion of COPD patients with anxiety and depression receive effective treatment.[86] Specific note should be made that pulmonary rehabilitation can also improve symptoms of anxiety and depression, although its effects beyond the treatment period are not well defined.[86]

A frequently overlooked comorbidity in COPD is cognitive dysfunction. Data on the prevalence of cognitive dysfunction in COPD is limited by methodological issues, including the need for normative data, the use of different cognitive evaluation instruments, and the interaction of shared risk factors. Even with these limitations, the finding of abnormal cognitive function in COPD has been consistent and includes decreased cognitive performance (story recall, addition tests) compared with healthy controls, lower scores on the Mini-Mental State Examination, slower reaction time, and impaired verbal and logical thinking.[94–96] Common factors associated with cognitive dysfunction in cross-sectional studies of patients with COPD include low FEV1, coexistent cardiovascular disease, diabetes, depression, and also obstructive sleep apnea (OSA), hypoxemia, and hypercapnia, all with the potential to affect the cerebral metabolism.[97] COPD exacerbations may also affect cognitive dysfunction, in particular those requiring mechanical ventilation.[97] The mechanisms behind cognitive dysfunction probably vary with each of these associations; some studies have demonstrated that participation in rehabilitation programs and the use of supplementary oxygen in patients with hypoxemia may decrease the risk of cognitive abnormalities.[94,98]

Obstructive Sleep Apnea

The coexistence of COPD and OSA, commonly described as overlap syndrome, has gained significant attention in recent years. Poor sleep quality, decreased sleep efficiency, and difficulties in initiating and maintaining sleep have been reported in more than 40% of patients with COPD.[99] The frequency of sleep-disordered breathing in the general population has been estimated to be 9% for women and 24% for men.[100] In patients with COPD, the prevalence of OSA been estimated to be about 16%.[101] In general, COPD patients with OSA are more severely hypercapnic, demonstrate more profound and frequent nocturnal oxygen desaturation, and have higher risk of pulmonary hypertension.[102] Untreated OSA is also a risk factor for poor quality of life, development of AECOPD, and increased all-cause mortality.[31,103] COPD and OSA share some pathophysiological characteristics and risk factors, including hyperinflation with parenchymal destruction and increased traction on the upper airway, the presence of systemic inflammation, particularly TNF-α, IL-6 and Interleukin-8 and increased oxidative stress.[102] The importance of OSA assessment in COPD is underscored by the recent finding that continuous positive airway pressure (CPAP) therapy during sleep in patients with overlap syndrome, was associated with both decreased risk of death (RR 1.79; 95% CI, 1.16–2.77) and decreased risk of severe AECOPD leading to a hospitalization (RR 1.70; 95% CI, 1.21–2.38).[31]

PROGRESS IN DISEASE PHENOTYPES

Only a few of the proposed phenotypes in COPD meet the premise that these phenotypes relate to clinically relevant outcomes or response to therapy. One such example is the subgroup of patients with upper-lobe-predominant emphysema and low exercise tolerance. This unique group benefits from lung-volume-reduction surgery with significant improvements in functional status, quality of life, and survival, although the mechanism of benefit in this specific group is not well understood.[104] Another phenotype is composed of patients with frequent exacerbations who produce significant sputum at baseline. These patients specifically demonstrate reduction of exacerbation in response to the phosphodiesterase-4 inhibitor, roflumilast.[105] The premise that combinations of comorbid conditions help define disease phenotypes is supported by the data presented here. Two general patterns of clinical features and comorbidities that share some association include (1) emphysema, low BMI and osteoporosis and (2) chronic bronchitis, airway disease, high BMI, OSA, and diabetes. It remains unknown whether these associations are related to specific mechanistic pathways that will lead to the development of targeted therapies.

SUMMARY

- COPD is a heterogeneous disease, modified by environmental and intrinsic host factors. The interaction between COPD and its comorbidities is complex and bidirectional.
- It has been estimated that the proportion of patients with COPD caused by cigarette smoking is between 80% and 90%. Risk factors associated with COPD in nonsmokers are numerous and incompletely understood, but a history of asthma or tuberculosis, exposure to traffic and outdoor pollution, and exposure to biomass smoke show the strongest associations. Other factors that may contribute to COPD phenotypes include gender, genetics, and the lung microbiome.
- Certain comorbid conditions, such as cardiovascular disease and osteoporosis, are more common in the COPD patient population. Other comorbidities, such as overlap syndrome, the coexistence of COPD, and obstructive sleep apnea may not be as prevalent in COPD but are important because they may modify disease course.
- Systemic inflammation may be pathogenically related to many comorbidities seen in COPD including cardiovascular disease, osteoporosis, metabolic syndrome, and depression.
- Based on the data presented here, two general patterns of clinical features and comorbidities that share some associations are (1) emphysema, low BMI and osteoporosis and (2) chronic bronchitis, airway disease, high BMI, OSA, and diabetes.
- The classification of patients with COPD into subgroups with shared characteristics and outcomes offers the potential for specific interventions. New research tools from the fields of epidemiology, immunology, imaging, and data analysis will be helpful in accomplishing this goal.

REFERENCES

1. Agusti A, Calverley PM, Celli B, et al. Characterisation of COPD heterogeneity in the ECLIPSE cohort. Respir Res 2010;11:122.
2. Han MK, Agusti A, Calverley PM, et al. Chronic obstructive pulmonary disease phenotypes: the future of COPD. Am J Respir Crit Care Med 2010;182: 598–604.
3. Lokke A, Lange P, Scharling H, et al. Developing COPD: a 25 year follow up study of the general population. Thorax 2006;61:935–9.
4. Anthonisen NR, Connett JE, Kiley JP, et al. Effects of smoking intervention and the use of an inhaled anticholinergic bronchodilator on the rate of decline of FEV1. The Lung Health Study. JAMA 1994;272:1497–505.
5. Eisner MD, Balmes J, Katz PP, et al. Lifetime environmental tobacco smoke exposure and the risk of chronic obstructive pulmonary disease. Environ Health 2005;4:7.
6. Behrendt CE. Mild and moderate-to-severe COPD in nonsmokers: distinct demographic profiles. Chest 2005;128:1239–44.
7. Salvi SS, Barnes PJ. Chronic obstructive pulmonary disease in non-smokers. Lancet 2009;374:733–43.
8. Lamprecht B, McBurnie MA, Vollmer WM, et al. COPD in never smokers: results from the population-based burden of obstructive lung disease study. Chest 2011;139:752–63.
9. Silva GE, Sherrill DL, Guerra S, et al. Asthma as a risk factor for COPD in a longitudinal study. Chest 2004;126:59–65.
10. Shavelle RM, Paculdo DR, Kush SJ, et al. Life expectancy and years of life lost in chronic obstructive pulmonary disease: findings from the NHANES III Follow-up Study. Int J Chron Obstruct Pulmon Dis 2009;4:137–48.
11. Blanc PD, Eisner MD, Earnest G, et al. Further exploration of the links between occupational exposure and chronic obstructive pulmonary disease. J Occup Environ Med 2009;51:804–10.
12. Fairbairn AS, Reid DD. Air pollution and other local factors in respiratory disease. Br J Prev Soc Med 1958;12:94–103.
13. Andersen ZJ, Hvidberg M, Jensen SS, et al. Chronic obstructive pulmonary disease and long-term exposure to traffic-related air pollution: a cohort study. Am J Respir Crit Care Med 2011;183:455–61.
14. Han MK, Postma D, Mannino DM, et al. Gender and chronic obstructive pulmonary disease: why it matters. Am J Respir Crit Care Med 2007;176:1179–84.
15. Ramirez-Venegas A, Sansores RH, Perez-Padilla R, et al. Survival of patients with chronic obstructive pulmonary disease due to biomass smoke and tobacco. Am J Respir Crit Care Med 2006;173:393–7.
16. Janssens W, Lehouck A, Carremans C, et al. Vitamin D beyond bones in chronic obstructive pulmonary disease: time to act. Am J Respir Crit Care Med 2009; 179:630–6.
17. Wood AM, Bassford C, Webster D, et al. Vitamin D-binding protein contributes to COPD by activation of alveolar macrophages. Thorax 2011;66:205–10.
18. Sargeant LA, Jaeckel A, Wareham NJ. Interaction of vitamin C with the relation between smoking and obstructive airways disease in EPIC Norfolk. European prospective investigation into cancer and nutrition. Eur Respir J 2000;16:397–403.
19. Hirayama F, Lee AH, Binns CW, et al. Do vegetables and fruits reduce the risk of chronic obstructive pulmonary disease? A case-control study in Japan. Prev Med 2009;49:184–9.

20. Varraso R, Willett WC, Camargo CA. Prospective study of dietary fiber and risk of chronic obstructive pulmonary disease among US women and men. Am J Epidemiol 2010;171:776–84.
21. Watson L, Vestbo J, Postma DS, et al. Gender differences in the management and experience of chronic obstructive pulmonary disease. Respir Med 2004; 98:1207–13.
22. Martinez FJ, Curtis JL, Sciurba F, et al. Sex differences in severe pulmonary emphysema. Am J Respir Crit Care Med 2007;176:243–52.
23. Hurst JR, Vestbo J, Anzueto A, et al. Susceptibility to exacerbation in chronic obstructive pulmonary disease. N Engl J Med 2010;363:1128–38.
24. Tashkin D, Celli B, Kesten S, et al. Effect of tiotropium in men and women with COPD: results of the 4-year UPLIFT trial. Respir Med 2010;104:1495–504.
25. Bjorksten B, Sepp E, Julge K, et al. Allergy development and the intestinal microflora during the first year of life. J Allergy Clin Immunol 2001;108:516–20.
26. Kalliomaki M, Kirjavainen P, Eerola E, et al. Distinct patterns of neonatal gut microflora in infants in whom atopy was and was not developing. J Allergy Clin Immunol 2001;107:129–34.
27. Penders J, Thijs C, van den Brandt PA, et al. Gut microbiota composition and development of atopic manifestations in infancy: the KOALA Birth Cohort Study. Gut 2007;56:661–7.
28. Martinez F, Han M, Flaherty K, et al. Role of infection and antimicrobial therapy in acute exacerbations of chronic obstructive pulmonary disease. Expert Rev Anti Infect Ther 2006;4:101–24.
29. Sethi S, Murphy T. Infection in the pathogenesis and course of chronic obstructive pulmonary disease. N Engl J Med 2008;359:2355–65.
30. Erb-Downward JR, Thompson DL, Han MK, et al. Analysis of the lung microbiome in the "healthy" smoker and in COPD. PLoS One 2011;6:e16384.
31. Marin JM, Soriano JB, Carrizo SJ, et al. Outcomes in patients with chronic obstructive pulmonary disease and obstructive sleep apnea: the overlap syndrome. Am J Respir Crit Care Med 2010;182:325–31.
32. Agusti AG, Noguera A, Sauleda J, et al. Systemic effects of chronic obstructive pulmonary disease. Eur Respir J 2003;21:347–60.
33. Fabbri LM, Rabe KF. From COPD to chronic systemic inflammatory syndrome? Lancet 2007;370:797–9.
34. Hansell AL, Walk JA, Soriano JB. What do chronic obstructive pulmonary disease patients die from? A multiple cause coding analysis. Eur Respir J 2003;22:809–14.
35. Sin DD, Wu L, Man SF. The relationship between reduced lung function and cardiovascular mortality: a population-based study and a systematic review of the literature. Chest 2005;127:1952–9.
36. Anthonisen NR, Connett JE, Enright PL, et al. Hospitalizations and mortality in the Lung Health Study. Am J Respir Crit Care Med 2002;166:333–9.
37. Beaty TH, Newill CA, Cohen BH, et al. Effects of pulmonary function on mortality. J Chronic Dis 1985;38:703–10.
38. Speizer FE, Fay ME, Dockery DW, et al. Chronic obstructive pulmonary disease mortality in six U.S. cities. Am Rev Respir Dis 1989;140:S49–55.
39. Hospers JJ, Postma DS, Rijcken B, et al. Histamine airway hyper-responsiveness and mortality from chronic obstructive pulmonary disease: a cohort study. Lancet 2000;356:1313–7.
40. Ross R. Atherosclerosis–an inflammatory disease. N Engl J Med 1999;340: 115–26.

41. Han MK, McLaughlin VV, Criner GJ, et al. Pulmonary diseases and the heart. Circulation 2007;116:2992–3005.
42. Sin DD, Lacy P, York E, et al. Effects of fluticasone on systemic markers of inflammation in chronic obstructive pulmonary disease. Am J Respir Crit Care Med 2004;170:760–5.
43. Mancini GB, Etminan M, Zhang B, et al. Reduction of morbidity and mortality by statins, angiotensin-converting enzyme inhibitors, and angiotensin receptor blockers in patients with chronic obstructive pulmonary disease. J Am Coll Cardiol 2006;47:2554–60.
44. Soyseth V, Brekke PH, Smith P, et al. Statin use is associated with reduced mortality in COPD. Eur Respir J 2007;29:279–83.
45. Short PM, Lipworth SI, Elder DH, et al. Effect of beta blockers in treatment of chronic obstructive pulmonary disease: a retrospective cohort study. BMJ 2011; 342:d2549.
46. Chailleux E, Laaban JP, Veale D. Prognostic value of nutritional depletion in patients with COPD treated by long-term oxygen therapy: data from the ANTADIR observatory. Chest 2003;123:1460–6.
47. Landbo C, Prescott E, Lange P, et al. Prognostic value of nutritional status in chronic obstructive pulmonary disease. Am J Respir Crit Care Med 1999;160: 1856–61.
48. Vestbo J, Prescott E, Almdal T, et al. Body mass, fat-free body mass, and prognosis in patients with chronic obstructive pulmonary disease from a random population sample: findings from the Copenhagen City Heart Study. Am J Respir Crit Care Med 2006;173:79–83.
49. Celli BR, Cote CG, Marin JM, et al. The body-mass index, airflow obstruction, dyspnea, and exercise capacity index in chronic obstructive pulmonary disease. N Engl J Med 2004;350:1005–12.
50. Marquez-Martin E, Ramos PC, Lopez-Campos JL, et al. Components of physical capacity in patients with chronic obstructive pulmonary disease: relationship with phenotypic expression. Int J Chron Obstruct Pulmon Dis 2011;6:105–12.
51. Kurosaki H, Ishii T, Motohashi N, et al. Extent of emphysema on HRCT affects loss of fat-free mass and fat mass in COPD. Intern Med 2009;48:41–8.
52. Kim V, Han MK, Vance GB, et al. The chronic bronchitic phenotype of chronic obstructive pulmonary disease: an analysis of the COPDGene Study. Chest 2011;140(3):626–33.
53. Wagner PD. Possible mechanisms underlying the development of cachexia in COPD. Eur Respir J 2008;31:492–501.
54. Vogiatzis I, Simoes DC, Stratakos G, et al. Effect of pulmonary rehabilitation on muscle remodelling in cachectic patients with COPD. Eur Respir J 2010;36: 301–10.
55. Nuti R, Siviero P, Maggi S, et al. Vertebral fractures in patients with chronic obstructive pulmonary disease: the EOLO Study. Osteoporos Int 2009;20: 989–98.
56. Bolton CE, Ionescu AA, Shiels KM, et al. Associated loss of fat-free mass and bone mineral density in chronic obstructive pulmonary disease. Am J Respir Crit Care Med 2004;170:1286–93.
57. Sin DD, Man JP, Man SF. The risk of osteoporosis in Caucasian men and women with obstructive airways disease. Am J Med 2003;114:10–4.
58. Dam TT, Harrison S, Fink HA, et al. Bone mineral density and fractures in older men with chronic obstructive pulmonary disease or asthma. Osteoporos Int 2010;21: 1341–9.

59. Bon J, Fuhrman CR, Weissfeld JL, et al. Radiographic emphysema predicts low bone mineral density in a tobacco-exposed cohort. Am J Respir Crit Care Med 2011;183:885–90.
60. Bolton CE, Stone MD, Edwards PH, et al. Circulating matrix metalloproteinase-9 and osteoporosis in patients with chronic obstructive pulmonary disease. Chron Respir Dis 2009;6:81–7.
61. Bon JM, Leader JK, Weissfeld JL, et al. The influence of radiographic phenotype and smoking status on peripheral blood biomarker patterns in chronic obstructive pulmonary disease. PLoS One 2009;4:e6865.
62. Vondracek SF, Voelkel NF, McDermott MT, et al. The relationship between adipokines, body composition, and bone density in men with chronic obstructive pulmonary disease. Int J Chron Obstruct Pulmon Dis 2009;4:267–77.
63. Beauchamp MK, O'Hoski S, Goldstein RS, et al. Effect of pulmonary rehabilitation on balance in persons with chronic obstructive pulmonary disease. Arch Phys Med Rehabil 2010;91:1460–5.
64. Leone N, Courbon D, Thomas F, et al. Lung function impairment and metabolic syndrome: the critical role of abdominal obesity. Am J Respir Crit Care Med 2009;179:509–16.
65. Song Y, Klevak A, Manson JE, et al. Asthma, chronic obstructive pulmonary disease, and type 2 diabetes in the Women's Health Study. Diabetes Res Clin Pract 2010;90:365–71.
66. Lazarus R, Sparrow D, Weiss ST. Baseline ventilatory function predicts the development of higher levels of fasting insulin and fasting insulin resistance index: the Normative Aging Study. Eur Respir J 1998;12:641–5.
67. Rana JS, Mittleman MA, Sheikh J, et al. Chronic obstructive pulmonary disease, asthma, and risk of type 2 diabetes in women. Diabetes Care 2004;27:2478–84.
68. Suissa S, Kezouh A, Ernst P. Inhaled corticosteroids and the risks of diabetes onset and progression. Am J Med 2010;123:1001–6.
69. Han MK, Kazerooni EA, Lynch DA, et al. Chronic obstructive pulmonary disease exacerbations in the COPDGene Study: associated radiologic phenotypes. Radiology 2011;261(1):274–82.
70. Cote C, Zilberberg MD, Mody SH, et al. Haemoglobin level and its clinical impact in a cohort of patients with COPD. Eur Respir J 2007;29:923–9.
71. Ershler WB, Chen K, Reyes EB, et al. Economic burden of patients with anemia in selected diseases. Value Health 2005;8:629–38.
72. Chambellan A, Chailleux E, Similowski T. Prognostic value of the hematocrit in patients with severe COPD receiving long-term oxygen therapy. Chest 2005;128:1201–8.
73. John M, Lange A, Hoernig S, et al. Prevalence of anemia in chronic obstructive pulmonary disease: comparison to other chronic diseases. Int J Cardiol 2006;111:365–70.
74. Halpern MT, Zilberberg MD, Schmier JK, et al. Anemia, costs and mortality in chronic obstructive pulmonary disease. Cost Eff Resour Alloc 2006;4:17.
75. Weiss G, Goodnough LT. Anemia of chronic disease. N Engl J Med 2005;352:1011–23.
76. Mokhlesi B, Morris AL, Huang CF, et al. Increased prevalence of gastroesophageal reflux symptoms in patients with COPD. Chest 2001;119:1043–8.
77. Terada K, Muro S, Sato S, et al. Impact of gastrooesophageal reflux disease symptoms on COPD exacerbation. Thorax 2008;63:951–5.
78. Casanova C, Baudet JS, del Valle Velasco M, et al. Increased gastrooesophageal reflux disease in patients with severe COPD. Eur Respir J 2004;23:841–5.

79. Rascon-Aguilar IE, Pamer M, Wludyka P, et al. Poorly treated or unrecognized GERD reduces quality of life in patients with COPD. Dig Dis Sci 2011;56: 1976–80.
80. Rascon-Aguilar IE, Pamer M, Wludyka P, et al. Role of gastroesophageal reflux symptoms in exacerbations of COPD. Chest 2006;130:1096–101.
81. Terada K, Muro S, Ohara T, et al. Abnormal swallowing reflex and COPD exacerbations. Chest 2010;137:326–32.
82. Garcia Rodriguez LA, Ruigomez A, Martin-Merino E, et al. Relationship between gastroesophageal reflux disease and COPD in UK primary care. Chest 2008; 134:1223–30.
83. Sasaki T, Nakayama K, Yasuda H, et al. A randomized, single-blind study of lansoprazole for the prevention of exacerbations of chronic obstructive pulmonary disease in older patients. J Am Geriatr Soc 2009;57:1453–7.
84. Yohannes AM, Willgoss TG, Baldwin RC, et al. Depression and anxiety in chronic heart failure and chronic obstructive pulmonary disease: prevalence, relevance, clinical implications and management principles. Int J Geriatr Psychiatry 2010;25:1209–21.
85. Solano JP, Gomes B, Higginson IJ. A comparison of symptom prevalence in far advanced cancer, AIDS, heart disease, chronic obstructive pulmonary disease and renal disease. J Pain Symptom Manage 2006;31:58–69.
86. Maurer J, Rebbapragada V, Borson S, et al. Anxiety and depression in COPD: current understanding, unanswered questions, and research needs. Chest 2008;134:43S–56S.
87. Hanania NA, Mullerova H, Locantore NW, et al. Determinants of depression in the ECLIPSE chronic obstructive pulmonary disease cohort. Am J Respir Crit Care Med 2011;183:604–11.
88. Laurin C, Lavoie KL, Bacon SL, et al. Sex differences in the prevalence of psychiatric disorders and psychological distress in patients with COPD. Chest 2007;132:148–55.
89. Giardino ND, Curtis JL, Andrei AC, et al. Anxiety is associated with diminished exercise performance and quality of life in severe emphysema: a cross-sectional study. Respir Res 2010;11:29.
90. von Leupoldt A, Taube K, Lehmann K, et al. The impact of anxiety and depression on outcomes of pulmonary rehabilitation in patients with COPD. Chest 2011;140(3):730–6.
91. Eisner MD, Blanc PD, Yelin EH, et al. Influence of anxiety on health outcomes in COPD. Thorax 2010;65:229–34.
92. de Voogd JN, Wempe JB, Koeter GH, et al. Depressive symptoms as predictors of mortality in patients with COPD. Chest 2009;135:619–25.
93. Fan VS, Ramsey SD, Giardino ND, et al. Sex, depression, and risk of hospitalization and mortality in chronic obstructive pulmonary disease. Arch Intern Med 2007;167:2345–53.
94. Thakur N, Blanc PD, Julian LJ, et al. COPD and cognitive impairment: the role of hypoxemia and oxygen therapy. Int J Chron Obstruct Pulmon Dis 2010;5: 263–9.
95. Liesker JJ, Postma DS, Beukema RJ, et al. Cognitive performance in patients with COPD. Respir Med 2004;98:351–6.
96. Klein M, Gauggel S, Sachs G, et al. Impact of chronic obstructive pulmonary disease (COPD) on attention functions. Respir Med 2010;104:52–60.
97. Dodd JW, Getov SV, Jones PW. Cognitive function in COPD. Eur Respir J 2010; 35:913–22.

98. Pereira ED, Viana CS, Taunay TC, et al. Improvement of cognitive function after a three-month pulmonary rehabilitation program for COPD patients. Lung 2011; 189:279–85.

99. Kinsman RA, Yaroush RA, Fernandez E, et al. Symptoms and experiences in chronic bronchitis and emphysema. Chest 1983;83:755–61.

100. Young T, Palta M, Dempsey J, et al. The occurrence of sleep-disordered breathing among middle-aged adults. N Engl J Med 1993;328:1230–5.

101. Simon-Tuval T, Scharf SM, Maimon N, et al. Determinants of elevated healthcare utilization in patients with COPD. Respir Res 2011;12:7.

102. Weitzenblum E, Chaouat A, Kessler R, et al. Overlap syndrome: obstructive sleep apnea in patients with chronic obstructive pulmonary disease. Proc Am Thorac Soc 2008;5:237–41.

103. Mermigkis C, Kopanakis A, Foldvary-Schaefer N, et al. Health-related quality of life in patients with obstructive sleep apnoea and chronic obstructive pulmonary disease (overlap syndrome). Int J Clin Pract 2007;61:207–11.

104. Criner GJ, Sternberg AL. National Emphysema Treatment Trial: the major outcomes of lung volume reduction surgery in severe emphysema. Proc Am Thorac Soc 2008;5:393–405.

105. Calverley PM, Rabe KF, Goehring UM, et al. Roflumilast in symptomatic chronic obstructive pulmonary disease: two randomised clinical trials. Lancet 2009;374: 685–94.

The Role and Potential of Imaging in COPD

George R. Washko, MD, MS

KEYWORDS

- COPD • Imaging • CT scan • MRI • PET • OCT

KEY POINTS

- New-generation computerized tomography with the visualization of lung parenchyma, airways, and vessels has helped clarify the association between radiological changes and clinical phenotypes.
- In chronic obstructive pulmonary disease (COPD), radiological phenotyping has been instrumental in the development of therapies, such as surgical and bronchoscopic lung volume reduction.
- The expansion of the knowledge of COPD using the integration of the data obtained through imaging and function will likely help plan therapeutic trials, such as regenerative therapy.
- The advent of radiological techniques capable of providing detailed information about lung structure and function is providing new insight into disease pathophysiology which may lead to improvements in clincial care.

INTRODUCTION

Chronic obstructive pulmonary disease (COPD) is a condition defined as incompletely reversible expiratory airflow obstruction caused by the exposure of noxious inhaled particulates.[1] Although the severity of the disease is assessed by the degree of lung function impairment, it is increasingly clear that COPD is a syndrome with numerous pulmonary and extrapulmonary manifestations, such as the emphysematous destruction of the lung parenchyma, lung cancer, remodeling of the airways and vasculature, cardiac impairment,[2] cachexia, and bone demineralization.[3] There is great interest in the clinical and research communities to refine our understanding of the potential association of these processes and it is thought that imaging may provide some of that insight.

The following article reviews the insights gained by imaging in smoking-related COPD. The unique contributions of various imaging modalities, such as computed

Dr Washko was supported by grant K23 HL089353 and an award from the Parker B. Francis Foundation.
Division of Pulmonary and Critical Care Medicine, Department of Medicine, Brigham and Women's Hospital, 75 Francis Street, Boston, MA 02115, USA
E-mail address: GWashko@Partners.org

tomography (CT), magnetic resonance imaging (MRI), optical coherence tomography (OCT), and positron emission tomography (PET), to a better understanding parenchymal, airway, and vascular disease is explored. Finally, the current and future contributions of imaging to clinical care are discussed.

CT
Parenchymal Disease

Smoking-related destruction of the lung parenchyma is typically thought to manifest as emphysema.[4] Defined by its appearance in the secondary pulmonary lobule (the most fundamental structural component of the lung containing airways, lymphatics, vasculature, and parenchyma encapsulated in connective tissue), emphysema is visually classified as being centrilobular, panlobular, and paraseptal disease.[5] Initial roentgenologic studies of the lungs of smokers identified several cardiac signs for the presence of emphysema, such as increased lucency of the lung fields, narrowing of the cardiac silhouette, and pruning of the peripheral vasculature (**Fig. 1**). Such findings are sensitive but lack the specificity required for large-scale clinical and research applications.[6,7]

With the introduction of CT into the medical sciences in the late 1970s, it became possible to visualize lung structure in vivo. One of the first applications of these imaging modalities was to develop subjective and objective methods for the assessment of emphysema.[8–11] Termed density mask analysis, Muller and colleagues[12] defined a Hounsfield unit threshold in the CT image that dichotomized the lung into emphysematous (density less than that Hounsfield unit threshold) and nonemphysematous (density greater than that Hounsfield unit threshold) tissue.[12] This type of densitometric analysis was found to be predictive of clinically significant metrics of disease, such as lung function, and correlated with histopathologic assessments of emphysema on explanted lung tissue.[12,13] With the caveat that the Hounsfield unit threshold used to delineate emphysematous from nonemphysematous tissue is subject to the image acquisition and reconstruction parameters, densitometric analysis of the lung parenchyma has become a cornerstone of radiologic characterization of lung disease

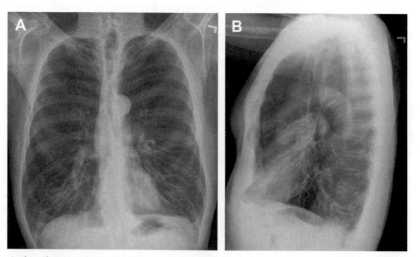

Fig. 1. (A, B) PA and Lateral chest radiograph of a patient with severe COPD and emphysema. Note the lucency of the lung fields, flattening of the diaphragms, narrowed cardiac silhouette, and paucity of peripheral vascular markings.

in smokers (**Fig. 2**).[14–18] Although densitometric analysis of the lung may provide global-, regional-, and lobar-specific measures of emphysema on the CT scan, when applied across a large region of lung, a major limitation is its relative inability to differentiate emphysema subtype (centrilobular, panlobular, and so forth). This limitation is most apparent when performing a head-to-head comparison of this technique with visual inspection of the lung parenchyma. Although the visual analysis of the lung parenchyma suffers from intraobserver and interobserver variability,[19] in several investigations it has been demonstrated to correlate with the pathologic condition, lung function, and predict the outcome in clinical investigations.[8–11,20,21] In an effort to address this, the community of radiological and computer scientists has focused on developing techniques that may objectively identify the emphysema type and distribution. These techniques are based largely on patterns of local features in the secondary pulmonary lobule and, for the purposes of this article, are collectively called textural analysis.

Texture analysis of the lung involves the selection of a discrete region of interest within the lung field and then assessing several parameters in this constrained region, such as density and the patterns of changes in density. Using such an approach,

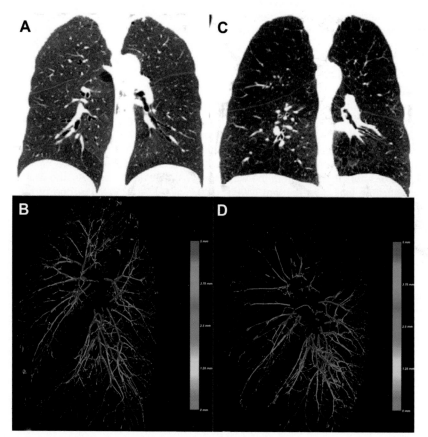

Fig. 2. (*A, C*) A coronal view of the lungs of a smoker with normal lung function (*A*) and one with moderate emphysema (*C*). (*B, D*) Volumetric reconstructions of the left lung pulmonary vasculature from a left midaxillary view. Vessels are color coded by diameter. Notice the loss of vasculature and thinning of the vessels in regions most affected by emphysema.

several groups of investigators have demonstrated that this technique could accurately identify disease type (using visual analysis as a gold standard) and provide more robust measures of lung disease for correlation in clinical investigations.[22–26] Indeed Xu and colleagues[27] demonstrated that such a technique could provide information that surpassed that provided by visual inspection. Although the sensitivity of textural analysis is potentially superior to visual inspection, it is computationally costly; until a more parsimonious approach to tissue classification is developed, it is limited to smaller-scale investigations.

Finally, it is increasingly clear that the manifestations of smoking-related parenchymal disease are not limited to low-attenuating tissue on the CT scan. Recently, Lederer and colleagues[28] demonstrated that a subset of smokers are more likely to have high-attenuating inflammatory, fibrotic, and atelectatic regions of the lung that are associated with a restrictive spirometric pattern of lung function. In a subsequent study, these lesions were found to be associated with reductions in lung volume and were inversely associated with emphysema.[29] Those smokers with such interstitial lung abnormalities (ILA) also tended to have pseudonormalization of their spirometry, likely from the mitigating effects of these abnormalities on reduced lung elastic recoil caused by emphysema. Further work is needed to determine the complete nature of ILA in smokers, but a subset of these patients may progress to clinically overt interstitial lung disease.[30] Also, given the common noxious exposure (tobacco smoke), a deeper understanding of the mechanisms that lead the lung down a fibrotic rather than emphysematous pathway of remodeling may offer insight into overall disease susceptibility.

Airway Disease

In obstructive lung disease, the site of expiratory airflow limitation is thought to be the small airways, those less than 2 mm in diameter.[31] Although this is beyond the resolution of clinical CT scanning, prior investigation suggests that radiological assessments of the central airways reflects remodeling in the lung periphery.[31] There are several metrics of central airway morphology in smokers. These metrics include the external or total bronchial area, the wall area (WA), the lumen area (Ai), the wall thickness, and the wall area percent (WA%; $100 \times$ [WA]/[Ai + WA]). In one of the first systematic analyses of airway morphology in smokers, Nakano and colleagues[32] assessed the apical segment of the right upper lobe (RB1) in 114 smokers. In their analysis, they found that those patients with the greatest WA% (increased ratio of WA to Ai) had the lowest forced expiratory volume in the first second of expiration expressed as a percent of the predicted. Based on this investigation, the WA% has become the most commonly used metric for clinical investigation largely because it has consistently provided the strongest correlation to spirometric measures of lung function. In a subsequent investigation, this same group demonstrated that central airway remodeling apparent on CT reflected distal histopathologic remodeling of the small airways, those with great central airway wall thickening had more small airway disease.[33] More recent work has suggested that the more peripheral the radiological assessments of airway structure in smokers (measures performed in airway generations closer to the small airways), the stronger the correlation with lung function.[34] Although this finding has compelled investigators to examine more and more distal airways, such measures are limited by the resolution of the CT images. For this reason, the most accurate measures of airway morphology are obtained from the third-generation segmental and possibly fourth-generation subsegmental airways.

Investigators have begun to look beyond airway wall thickening to assess airway disease in smokers. Included in these efforts are quantitative assessments of mural density or attenuation.[35] The premise behind these investigations is that as an airway wall thickens or remodels, both the shape and contents of the wall change. Normal bronchial cartilage may be gained or lost and normal connective tissue replaced by a scar. Preliminary investigation suggests that airway wall attenuation may provide additional information regarding airway disease in smokers.[35] Further work is needed to comprehensively understand the scanner-to-scanner variability and the influence of body habitus on these measures.

Recently, Hogg and colleagues[36] introduced a new paradigm for airway disease in smokers. Not only does airway remodeling lead to luminal obstruction and expiratory airflow obstruction but there also seems to be an outright loss of airways in advanced COPD. Using micro CT to examine the resected lung tissue, this group demonstrated that patients with advanced emphysema may have lost up to 90% of their terminal bronchioles. In addition to expiratory airway collapse caused by the loss of elastic recoil and fixed luminal obstruction of the small airways, a third potential mechanism for increased resistance to flow is the loss of parallel pathways.

Based on these findings, Diaz and colleagues[37] examined the chest CT scans of 50 smokers enrolled in the Lung Tissue Research Consortium and found that those patients with more advanced emphysema have pruning of the central airways on CT scan (loss of airways in generations 5–8). Further, even after the adjustment for densitometric measures of emphysema, the total airway count (sum of the airway generations visible in the third to eighth generation starting from the apical segment of the RB1) was an independent predictor of the Body mass index, Airflow obstruction, Dyspnea, and Exercise capacity (BODE) score, which is a validated multidimensional measure of mortality in COPD. Further histologic validation is needed to determine the extent to which airway loss manifests in the more proximal airway tree; however, airway dropout may be a marker of the extreme of airway disease.

As CT acquisition times have decreased, it is now feasible to perform more dynamic inspiratory/expiratory CT scanning of the chest. The addition of an expiratory image allows for the quantitative detection of the hallmark of a COPD, gas trapping. Visually, this may appear as mosaicism suggesting local gas trapping caused by an admixture of emphysema and airway disease. Using a Hounsfield unit threshold of -856 (attenuation value for normal), the expiratory image can also be quantitatively assessed whereby all tissue less than this value are designated as exhibiting gas trapping.[38] Although a current limitation of such an approach is the inability to differentiate the effects of emphysema and airway remodeling, new techniques are being developed that may allow for the subtraction of emphysema giving the user a clearer picture of the impact of small airway disease.

Vascular Remodeling

Pulmonary vascular disease is an independent predictor of morbidity and mortality in COPD. It is estimated that 305 to 70% of patients with COPD have clinically significant burdens of disease, and recent work has demonstrated that pathologic pulmonary vascular remodeling is found even in smokers with normal lung function.[39–45] The mechanisms for this process likely include inflammation, hypoxic vasoconstriction, and outright loss of parallel pathways caused by emphysematous destruction of the tissue. Although the standard visual assessment of pulmonary vascular remodeling includes measurements of the diameter of the main pulmonary artery, more recent investigations have capitalized on the ability of CT imaging to provide detailed measures of structure. These studies have demonstrated that remodeling of the distal intraparenchymal pulmonary vasculature yields compelling insights into the relation of vascular disease and emphysema, the effect of pulmonary vascular disease on pulmonary artery pressure, and a potential link between pulmonary vascular remodeling and atherosclerotic disease.[46–48]

More recently, Alford and colleagues[49] undertook an investigation of pulmonary vascular remodeling in the earliest stages of smoking-related lung disease. In a cohort of 43 patients (17 healthy, 12 smokers with no emphysema and normal lung function, 12 smokers with mild emphysema), using central venous boluses of iodinated contrast agent, this group was able to demonstrate that pulmonary vascular remodeling could be detected and quantitatively assessed at its earliest stages.[49] Although such an approach is not amenable to population-based studies, the findings of this study are consistent with the hypothesis that emphysema may begin as a vascular disease leading to a regional loss of tissue.

With the advances and large-scale application of CT scanning in clinical investigations, there have been several recent studies that have provided compelling insight into the clinical and functional impact of smoking-related lung disease. For example, using CT scans and epidemiologic and clinical data from the Multi Ethnic Study of Atherosclerosis, Barr and colleagues[2] clearly demonstrated that emphysema and its associated hyperinflation compromises cardiac function through reductions in left ventricular filling, possibly caused by occult pulmonary vascular remodeling. More recently, Han and colleagues depicted the complex relationship between radiological emphysema, airway disease, and acute exacerbations (AECOPD) of COPD.[50] The results of this investigation may allow clinicians and clinical investigators to identify who is at the greatest risk for an AECOPD to enrich both clinical studies and maximize preventive therapies in the outpatient setting. Lastly, to mention one of the most direct applications of CT imaging of the chest in therapeutic intervention, a trial of bronchoscopically placed one-way valves to achieve minimally invasive volume reduction demonstrated that those patients with incomplete interlobar fissures had the lowest chance of procedural benefit likely because of collateral ventilation.[51]

Possibly the greatest critique of CT imaging to date has been the lack of a clear vision of how quantitative assessments of parenchymal, airway, and vascular disease may guide the clinical care of patients with COPD. Although the quantitative CT scan is not yet integrated into clinical practice, the results of several recent investigations have provided a new understanding of the disease, and it is through this understanding that new therapies and therapeutic approaches to care will be discovered. These advances do not come without concern. The clinical and research community is increasingly aware of the risks associated with the radiation exposure necessary for CT acquisition. Although the estimates of the associations between the dose of radiation and the risk of cancer vary, this risk may be as high as 1/80 lifetime risk from a single CT.[52,53]

Finally, mention must be made of the overlap or co-occurrence of lung cancer and COPD. While it is unclear if the origins of cancer are found in airway or parenchymal remodeling it is thought that smokers with COPD who have emphysema on their CT are at the highest risk for developing cancer.[54–56] There are now several studies using screening CT scans of the chest to determine if early detection and presumably early intervention will reduce cancer-related mortality.[57–60] One of the largest and most recent studies, the National Lung Screening Trial, found a 20% relative reduction in mortality in patients undergoing annual screening CT scans.[61] Although these results are compelling, there are limitations to screening CT scans. Given the cost of each CT, it is impractical and impossible to screen the general population of smokers. Clearly, further refinements of who is at the greatest risk for the development of cancer need to be undertaken to develop a more focused screening algorithm. Also, screening CT scans of the chest of smokers leads to the detection of a large number of false-positive nodules that may require further evaluation.[62–64] In addition to the added cost of these procedures comes the morbidity associated with lung biopsy and fiber-optic bronchoscopic approaches to obtaining tissue for histopathology diagnosis.[64]

MRI

The basis for MRI is the perturbation of protons (hydrogen atoms) by a burst of radio waves. A strong magnetic field is applied to the tissue, which aligns the protons within. The brief application of a radio wave then forces these protons out of alignment. The energy emitted by the proton during this process and the process of returning to alignment is detected by the scanner and converted into the image displayed for clinical use. Unlike CT scanning, no ionizing radiation is used to generate the image. Given this obvious advantage, MRI has the potential to perform detailed real-time evaluations of tissue motion, which are then related to global and local tissue mechanics. A limiting factor for the application of MRI to the lung is, however, the lung architecture itself. The lung is primarily a gas-filled structure whose density (and therefore concentration of protons) is less than that of solid organs, such as the brain or liver. Because of this limitation, a good deal of research in lung imaging has been focused on the development and application of inhaled and intravenous contrast agents to enhance data collection.

Parenchyma

Although the strength of CT is its ability to accurately reflect details in tissue architecture, it is limited in its ability to detect function. Generally, tissue that seems normal on the CT scan is assumed to make full contribution to overall lung function. Several recent MRI studies using inhaled hyperpolarized noble gases, such as ^{3}helium (^{3}He) and ^{129}xenon (^{129}Xe), have offered new insight into lung structure and function and have great promise for demonstrating the falsity of this assumption.

The promise of hyperpolarized gases for imaging has been known for more than 25 years, and it was not until the late 1990s that their application in pulmonary research began to move toward its true potential.[65] To perform such experiments, a sample of helium or xenon is hyperpolarized using a laser and then on inhalation will initially distribute throughout the gas-containing regions of the lung. The initial diffusivity of the gas can then be assessed to provide quantitative information about lung structure, such as mean linear intercept, surface-to-volume ratio, airway radii, and number of alveoli.[66] ^{129}Xenon has the added advantage of being freely diffusible across the alveolar capillary membrane, and several investigators have demonstrated that this diffusion and washout in the capillary bed can be readily distinguishable. The integration of these steps, the diffusion of gas into the alveolus, the transfer across the alveolar-capillary membrane, and then removal by capillary blood flow, allows quantitative insight into one of the most basic functions of the lung: matching of ventilation and perfusion.[67–72]

Another interesting property of hyperpolarized noble gases is their increased rate of decay in the presence of oxygen. What may seem to be a limitation to pulmonary research has been demonstrated to offer additional information about function. Because of the regional heterogeneity in ventilation perfusion matching in the lung, oxygen tension is not uniform throughout the gas-containing regions of the parenchyma. The detection and quantification of this by measuring the differential rates of decay of ^{3}He or ^{129}Xe allows for an in-vivo assessment of the most fundamental aspect of lung function (**Fig. 3**).[73–75]

Airways

Unlike CT, MRI-based investigations of the airways do not tend to focus on the morphology of the more central tracheobronchial tree. Rather, MRI is more readily used to interrogate the flow of gas throughout the lung. The resulting flow of gas

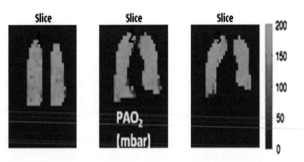

Fig. 3. Three-dimensional coronal maps of a healthy human patient depicting regional differences in oxygen tension using ^{3}He. At right is a color-coded bar of oxygen tension in millibars (1 mbar = 0.75 mm Hg). (*Courtesy of* Dr Samuel Patz.)

(diminished in more diseased areas of the lung) can be quantified and presented as a ventilation defect volume.[76–79] Such a measure may reflect regions afflicted by either emphysema or airway disease or potentially an admixture of the two. Again, unlike the CT scan, this assessment is not dependent on proximal airway structure reflecting distal remodeling, rather it is a direct measure of the properties of the distal lung parenchyma and small airways.

Vasculature

A strength of MRI is its ability to assess organ motion through the continuous or gated acquisition of data. As an example, electrocardiogram-gated MRI has become a standard for the calculation of cardiac function and offers more reproducible investigations of both right and left ventricular function than cardiac echo.[80–83] Given increasing interest in the interdependence of heart and lung in diseases, such as COPD, an in vivo tool to assess ventricular impairment is of great interest to clinical investigators. MRI also has been used to assess the distensibility of the central vessels.[84,85] Previous investigations in pulmonary hypertension suggest that such measures offer prognostic value for therapeutic intervention.[86] Finally, the true source of pulmonary vascular compromise in COPD is likely the distal small vessels. As mentioned previously, remodeling at these sites has been observed even in smokers with normal lung function.[43,44] Although direct morphologic assessment of the vascular at this level is beyond the resolution of clinical MRI, techniques, such as dynamic contrast-enhanced MRI perfusion, may offer a solution.[87–89] The premise to this technique is that after an intravenous contrast agent is introduced into the pulmonary arterial circulation, its local concentration will diminish proportionally to the ability of the lung to carry it away in the circulating blood volume. The more prolonged the decline in contrast concentration the lower the regional flow and, therefore, the greater relative regional pulmonary vascular resistance. Such a technique has been applied within pulmonary embolism or suspected pulmonary embolism.[87,90] Further work is needed to apply and validate this technique to pulmonary vascular disease associated with smoking.

There is great promise in the applications of MRI to investigations of smoking-related lung disease. This comes from both the novel applications of inhaled and intravenous contrast agents and the remarkable ability it provides for resolving lung structure. Recently Kirby and colleagues[91] demonstrated that in a longitudinal assessment of 20 patients (15 smokers, 5 healthy), ^{3}He proved to be a more sensitive measure of disease progression in the smokers over a 2-year period than standard spirometric and plethysmographic measures of lung function. Additional ongoing work at multiple institutions suggests that these techniques may improve our ability to monitor disease progression and the response to therapy. With time, MRI may play a significant role in both investigation and clinical care of patients with COPD.

PET

PET is a nuclear medicine technology based on the detection of regionalized concentrations of a positron emitting radionuclide. The localization of this tracer depends on the type of biologically active molecule that serves as its carrier. A commonly used molecule for clinical medicine is glucose, which is taken up by the most metabolically active tissues. Although PET has been widely used by clinicians for the detection and monitoring of malignancy, its applications in lung disease, such as COPD, have provided new insights into the disease pathology and potentially pathogenesis.

Recently, Vidal Melo and colleagues[92] demonstrated that there is significant heterogeneity of lung perfusion in mild and moderate COPD even after adjusting for regional changes in lung density and ventilation. Similar to work published by Alford and colleagues,[49] these changes in regional perfusion seem to precede visible changes to the lung structure, such as emphysema, suggesting that at least part of the progression of parenchymal disease in COPD is caused by vascular remodeling. Further work is needed to establish the relationship of longitudinal changes in regional lung perfusion and disease progression, but as the investigators suggest, assessments of vascular morphology and perfusion may indeed be a valuable biomarker for COPD.

OCT

OCT is an imaging method based on the refraction of light as it passes through tissues. A fiberoptic probe with a light source is introduced into the airways via a bronchoscope and the light patterns reflected by the tissue of interest are then reconstructed into an image. Unlike CT, MRI, or PET, OCT has the ability to resolve structures on the order of micrometers and can essentially provide in vivo images of tissue histology (**Fig. 4**). The

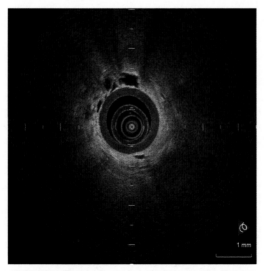

Fig. 4. A view using OCT. The fiberoptic probe can be seen at the center. Adjacent to the outer surface of the probe are alveolar ducts and alveoli. (*Courtesy of* Dr Anthony Lee of the British Columbia Cancer Research Center.)

primary strength of OCT is in examining airway morphology, which readily lends itself to airway disease in COPD. Recently, Coxson and colleagues[93] demonstrated in smokers that although CT measures of airway wall thickness correlate with lung function, it significantly overestimates airway size. OCT was a more sensitive measure of disease and simultaneously provided data on airway wall morphology and subepithelial remodeling and collagen deposition. Although OCT is not amenable to large-scale population-based studies, its ability to detect and monitor airway disease in smokers makes it a natural candidate for the investigation of pharmaceutical agents thought to reduce mural inflammation.[94]

Although there are definite niches and limitations to the imaging modalities presented in this article, each offers unique strengths and in aggregate has provided new and exciting insight into the potential pathogenesis and physiology of COPD. The greatest contribution to imaging has been its ability to facilitate in vivo investigations in both small cohorts and population-based investigations. It will be some time before MRI, PET, OCT, or even quantitative CT scanning becomes part of standard clinical practice, but they have already become the foundation for most clinical trials. It is clear that spirometric measures of lung function alone do not suffice for disease classification in smokers. They are too insensitive to disease heterogeneity and are only weakly correlated to both the symptoms and functional capacity experienced by patients with COPD. The future of investigation and clinical care lies in a combination of clinical characterization and image-based assessments of lung structure.

REFERENCES

1. Rabe KF, Hurd S, Anzueto A, et al. Global strategy for the diagnosis, management, and prevention of chronic obstructive pulmonary disease: gold executive summary. Am J Respir Crit Care Med 2007;176:532–55.
2. Barr RG, Bluemke DA, Ahmed FS, et al. Percent emphysema, airflow obstruction, and impaired left ventricular filling. N Engl J Med 2010;362:217–27.
3. Bon J, Fuhrman CR, Weissfeld JL, et al. Radiographic emphysema predicts low bone mineral density in a tobacco-exposed cohort. Am J Respir Crit Care Med 2011;183:885–90.
4. Snider GL. Emphysema: the first two centuries–and beyond. A historical overview, with suggestions for future research: part 1. Am Rev Respir Dis 1992; 146:1334–44.
5. Webb WR. Thin-section CT of the secondary pulmonary lobule: anatomy and the image–the 2004 Fleischer lecture. Radiology 2006;239:322–38.
6. Sutinen S, Christoforidis AJ, Klugh GA, et al. Roentgenologic criteria for the recognition of nonsymptomatic pulmonary emphysema. Correlation between roentgenologic findings and pulmonary pathology. Am Rev Respir Dis 1965;91: 69–76.
7. Nicklaus TM, Stowell DW, Christiansen WR, et al. The accuracy of the roentgenologic diagnosis of chronic pulmonary emphysema. Am Rev Respir Dis 1966;93: 889–99.
8. Foster WL Jr, Pratt PC, Roggli VL, et al. Centrilobular emphysema: CT-pathologic correlation. Radiology 1986;159:27–32.
9. Bergin C, Muller N, Nichols DM, et al. The diagnosis of emphysema. A computed tomographic-pathologic correlation. Am Rev Respir Dis 1986;133:541–6.
10. Hruban RH, Meziane MA, Zerhouni EA, et al. High resolution computed tomography of inflation-fixed lungs. Pathologic-radiologic correlation of centrilobular emphysema. Am Rev Respir Dis 1987;136:935–40.

11. Hayhurst MD, MacNee W, Flenley DC, et al. Diagnosis of pulmonary emphysema by computerised tomography. Lancet 1984;2:320–2.
12. Muller NL, Staples CA, Miller RR, et al. "Density mask". An objective method to quantitate emphysema using computed tomography. Chest 1988;94:782–7.
13. Kinsella M, Muller NL, Abboud RT, et al. Quantitation of emphysema by computed tomography using a "density mask" program and correlation with pulmonary function tests. Chest 1990;97:315–21.
14. Stern EJ, Frank MS. CT of the lung in patients with pulmonary emphysema: diagnosis, quantification, and correlation with pathologic and physiologic findings. AJR Am J Roentgenol 1994;162:791–8.
15. Heremans A, Verschakelen JA, Van fraeyenhoven L, et al. Measurement of lung density by means of quantitative CT scanning. A study of correlations with pulmonary function tests. Chest 1992;102:805–11.
16. Gould GA, Redpath AT, Ryan M, et al. Lung CT density correlates with measurements of airflow limitation and the diffusing capacity. Eur Respir J 1991;4:141–6.
17. Gevenois PA, de Maertelaer V, De Vuyst P, et al. Comparison of computed density and macroscopic morphometry in pulmonary emphysema. Am J Respir Crit Care Med 1995;152:653–7.
18. Gevenois PA, De Vuyst P, de Maertelaer V, et al. Comparison of computed density and microscopic morphometry in pulmonary emphysema. Am J Respir Crit Care Med 1996;154:187–92.
19. Hersh CP, Washko GR, Jacobson FL, et al. Interobserver variability in the determination of upper lobe-predominant emphysema. Chest 2007;131:424–31.
20. Washko GR, Criner GJ, Mohsenifar Z, et al. Computed tomographic-based quantification of emphysema and correlation to pulmonary function and mechanics. COPD 2008;5:177–86.
21. Fishman A, Martinez F, Naunheim K, et al. A randomized trial comparing lung-volume-reduction surgery with medical therapy for severe emphysema. N Engl J Med 2003;348:2059–73.
22. Uppaluri R, Mitsa T, Sonka M, et al. Quantification of pulmonary emphysema from lung computed tomography images. Am J Respir Crit Care Med 1997;156:248–54.
23. Uppaluri R, Hoffman EA, Sonka M, et al. Computer recognition of regional lung disease patterns. Am J Respir Crit Care Med 1999;160:648–54.
24. Chabat F, Yang GZ, Hansell DM. Obstructive lung diseases: texture classification for differentiation at ct. Radiology 2003;228:871–7.
25. Sluimer IC, van Waes PF, Viergever MA, et al. Computer-aided diagnosis in high resolution CT of the lungs. Med Phys 2003;30:3081–90.
26. Sorensen L, Shaker SB, de Bruijne M. Quantitative analysis of pulmonary emphysema using local binary patterns. IEEE Trans Med Imaging 2010;29:559–69.
27. Xu Y, Sonka M, McLennan G, et al. MDCT-based 3-d texture classification of emphysema and early smoking related lung pathologies. IEEE Trans Med Imaging 2006;25:464–75.
28. Lederer DJ, Enright PL, Kawut SM, et al. Cigarette smoking is associated with subclinical parenchymal lung disease: the multi-ethnic study of atherosclerosis (mesa)-lung study. Am J Respir Crit Care Med 2009;180:407–14.
29. Washko GR, Hunninghake GM, Fernandez IE, et al. Lung volumes and emphysema in smokers with interstitial lung abnormalities. N Engl J Med 2011;364:897–906.
30. Tsushima K, Sone S, Yoshikawa S, et al. The radiological patterns of interstitial change at an early phase: over a 4-year follow-up. Respir Med 2010;104:1712–21.

31. Hogg JC, Macklem PT, Thurlbeck WM. Site and nature of airway obstruction in chronic obstructive lung disease. N Engl J Med 1968;278:1355–60.

32. Nakano Y, Muro S, Sakai H, et al. Computed tomographic measurements of airway dimensions and emphysema in smokers. Correlation with lung function. Am J Respir Crit Care Med 2000;162:1102–8.

33. Nakano Y, Wong JC, de Jong PA, et al. The prediction of small airway dimensions using computed tomography. Am J Respir Crit Care Med 2005;171:142–6.

34. Hasegawa M, Nasuhara Y, Onodera Y, et al. Airflow limitation and airway dimensions in chronic obstructive pulmonary disease. Am J Respir Crit Care Med 2006; 173:1309–15.

35. Washko GR, Dransfield MT, Estepar RS, et al. Airway wall attenuation: a biomarker of airway disease in subjects with COPD. J Appl Physiol 2009;107:185–91.

36. Hogg JC, McDonough JE, Sanchez PG, et al. Micro-computed tomography measurements of peripheral lung pathology in chronic obstructive pulmonary disease. Proc Am Thorac Soc 2009;6:546–9.

37. Diaz AA, Valim C, Yamashiro T, et al. Airway count and emphysema assessed by chest CT imaging predicts clinical outcome in smokers. Chest 2010;138:880–7.

38. Coxson HO, Rogers RM, Whittall KP, et al. A quantification of the lung surface area in emphysema using computed tomography. Am J Respir Crit Care Med 1999;159:851–6.

39. Chatila WM, Thomashow BM, Minai OA, et al. Comorbidities in chronic obstructive pulmonary disease. Proc Am Thorac Soc 2008;5:549–55.

40. Falk JA, Kadiev S, Criner GJ, et al. Cardiac disease in chronic obstructive pulmonary disease. Proc Am Thorac Soc 2008;5:543–8.

41. Chaouat A, Naeije R, Weitzenblum E. Pulmonary hypertension in COPD. Eur Respir J 2008;32:1371–85.

42. Hasleton PS, Heath D, Brewer DB. Hypertensive pulmonary vascular disease in states of chronic hypoxia. J Pathol Bacteriol 1968;95:431–40.

43. Barbera JA, Riverola A, Roca J, et al. Pulmonary vascular abnormalities and ventilation-perfusion relationships in mild chronic obstructive pulmonary disease. Am J Respir Crit Care Med 1994;149:423–9.

44. Peinado VI, Barbera JA, Ramirez J, et al. Endothelial dysfunction in pulmonary arteries of patients with mild COPD. Am J Physiol 1998;274:L908–13.

45. Hale KA, Niewoehner DE, Cosio MG. Morphologic changes in the muscular pulmonary arteries: relationship to cigarette smoking, airway disease, and emphysema. Am Rev Respir Dis 1980;122:273–8.

46. Matsuoka S, Washko GR, Dransfield MT, et al. Quantitative CT measurement of cross-sectional area of small pulmonary vessel in COPD: correlations with emphysema and airflow limitation. Acad Radiol 2010;17:93–9.

47. Matsuoka S, Washko GR, Yamashiro T, et al. Pulmonary hypertension and computed tomography measurement of small pulmonary vessels in severe emphysema. Am J Respir Crit Care Med 2010;181:218–25.

48. Matsuoka S, Yamashiro T, Diaz A, et al. The relationship between small pulmonary vascular alteration and aortic atherosclerosis in chronic obstructive pulmonary disease: quantitative CT analysis. Acad Radiol 2011;18:40–6.

49. Alford SK, van Beek EJ, McLennan G, et al. Heterogeneity of pulmonary perfusion as a mechanistic image-based phenotype in emphysema susceptible smokers. Proc Natl Acad Sci U S A 2010;107:7485–90.

50. Han MK, Kazerooni EA, Lynch DA, et al. Chronic obstructive pulmonary disease exacerbations in the COPD gene study: associated radiologic phenotypes. Radiology 2011;261(1):274–82.

51. Sciurba FC, Ernst A, Herth FJ, et al. A randomized study of endobronchial valves for advanced emphysema. N Engl J Med 2010;363:1233–44.
52. Smith-Bindman R. Is computed tomography safe? N Engl J Med 2010;363:1–4.
53. Smith-Bindman R, Lipson J, Marcus R, et al. Radiation dose associated with common computed tomography examinations and the associated lifetime attributable risk of cancer. Arch Intern Med 2009;169:2078–86.
54. Petty TL. Are COPD and lung cancer two manifestations of the same disease? Chest 2005;128:1895–7.
55. Wilson DO, Weissfeld JL, Balkan A, et al. Association of radiographic emphysema and airflow obstruction with lung cancer. Am J Respir Crit Care Med 2008;178:738–44.
56. de Torres JP, Bastarrika G, Wisnivesky JP, et al. Assessing the relationship between lung cancer risk and emphysema detected on low-dose CT of the chest. Chest 2007;132:1932–8.
57. International Early Lung Cancer Action Program Investigators, Henschke CI, Yankelevitz DF, et al. Survival of patients with stage I lung cancer detected on CT screening. N Engl J Med 2006;355:1763–71.
58. Infante M, Cavuto S, Lutman FR, et al. A randomized study of lung cancer screening with spiral computed tomography: three-year results from the Dante trial. Am J Respir Crit Care Med 2009;180:445–53.
59. Gohagan JK, Marcus PM, Fagerstrom RM, et al. Final results of the lung screening study, a randomized feasibility study of spiral CT versus chest x-ray screening for lung cancer. Lung Cancer 2005;47:9–15.
60. Marcus PM, Bergstralh EJ, Fagerstrom RM, et al. Lung cancer mortality in the mayo lung project: impact of extended follow-up. J Natl Cancer Inst 2000;92:1308–16.
61. National Lung Screening Trial Research Team, Aberle DR, Adams AM, et al. Reduced lung-cancer mortality with low-dose computed tomographic screening. N Engl J Med 2011;365:395–409.
62. Henschke CI, McCauley DI, Yankelevitz DF, et al. Early lung cancer action project: overall design and findings from baseline screening. Lancet 1999;354:99–105.
63. Sone S, Takashima S, Li F, et al. Mass screening for lung cancer with mobile spiral computed tomography scanner. Lancet 1998;351:1242–5.
64. Wilson DO, Weissfeld JL, Fuhrman CR, et al. The Pittsburgh lung screening study (PLUSS): outcomes within 3 years of a first computed tomography scan. Am J Respir Crit Care Med 2008;178:956–61.
65. Happer W. Spin exchange, past, present and future. Ann Phys Fr 1985;10:645–57.
66. Yablonskiy DA, Sukstanskii AL, Woods JC, et al. Quantification of lung microstructure with hyperpolarized 3he diffusion MRI. J Appl Physiol 2009;107:1258–65.
67. Patz SMI, Hrovat MI, Dabaghyan M, et al. Diffusion of hyperpolarized 129xe in the lung: a simplified model of 129xe septal uptake and experimental results. New J Phys 2011;13:2–18.
68. Driehuys B, Cofer GP, Pollaro J, et al. Imaging alveolar-capillary gas transfer using hyperpolarized 129xe MRI. Proc Natl Acad Sci U S A 2006;103:18278–83.
69. Patz S, Hersman FW, Muradian I, et al. Hyperpolarized (129)xe MRI: a viable functional lung imaging modality? Eur J Radiol 2007;64:335–44.
70. Patz S, Muradian I, Hrovat MI, et al. Human pulmonary imaging and spectroscopy with hyperpolarized 129xe at 0.2t. Acad Radiol 2008;15:713–27.
71. Ruppert K, Mata JF, Brookeman JR, et al. Exploring lung function with hyperpolarized (129)xe nuclear magnetic resonance. Magn Reson Med 2004;51:676–87.

72. Mansson S, Wolber J, Driehuys B, et al. Characterization of diffusing capacity and perfusion of the rat lung in a lipopolysaccharide disease model using hyperpolarized 129xe. Magn Reson Med 2003;50:1170–9.
73. Deninger AJ, Eberle B, Bermuth J, et al. Assessment of a single-acquisition imaging sequence for oxygen-sensitive (3)He-MRI. Magn Reson Med 2002;47:105–14.
74. Deninger AJ, Mansson S, Petersson JS, et al. Quantitative measurement of regional lung ventilation using 3He MRI. Magn Reson Med 2002;48:223–32.
75. Mansson S, Deninger AJ, Magnusson P, et al. 3He MRI-based assessment of posture-dependent regional ventilation gradients in rats. J Appl Physiol 2005;98:2259–67.
76. de Lange EE, Mugler JP 3rd, Brookeman JR, et al. Lung air spaces: MR imaging evaluation with hyperpolarized 3He gas. Radiology 1999;210:851–7.
77. Kauczor HU, Hofmann D, Kreitner KF, et al. Normal and abnormal pulmonary ventilation: visualization at hyperpolarized He-3 MR imaging. Radiology 1996;201:564–8.
78. MacFall JR, Charles HC, Black RD, et al. Human lung air spaces: potential for MR imaging with hyperpolarized He-3. Radiology 1996;200:553–8.
79. Woodhouse N, Wild JM, Paley MN, et al. Combined helium-3/proton magnetic resonance imaging measurement of ventilated lung volumes in smokers compared to never-smokers. J Magn Reson Imaging 2005;21:365–9.
80. McLure LE, Peacock AJ. Cardiac magnetic resonance imaging for the assessment of the heart and pulmonary circulation in pulmonary hypertension. Eur Respir J 2009;33:1454–66.
81. Bottini PB, Carr AA, Prisant LM, et al. Magnetic resonance imaging compared to echocardiography to assess left ventricular mass in the hypertensive patient. Am J Hypertens 1995;8:221–8.
82. Grothues F, Smith GC, Moon JC, et al. Comparison of interstudy reproducibility of cardiovascular magnetic resonance with two-dimensional echocardiography in normal subjects and in patients with heart failure or left ventricular hypertrophy. Am J Cardiol 2002;90:29–34.
83. Benza R, Biederman R, Murali S, et al. Role of cardiac magnetic resonance imaging in the management of patients with pulmonary arterial hypertension. J Am Coll Cardiol 2008;52:1683–92.
84. Bogren HG, Klipstein RH, Mohiaddin RH, et al. Pulmonary artery distensibility and blood flow patterns: a magnetic resonance study of normal subjects and of patients with pulmonary arterial hypertension. Am Heart J 1989;118:990–9.
85. Gan CT, Lankhaar JW, Westerhof N, et al. Noninvasively assessed pulmonary artery stiffness predicts mortality in pulmonary arterial hypertension. Chest 2007;132:1906–12.
86. Jardim C, Rochitte CE, Humbert M, et al. Pulmonary artery distensibility in pulmonary arterial hypertension: an MRI pilot study. Eur Respir J 2007;29:476–81.
87. Amundsen T, Kvaerness J, Jones RA, et al. Pulmonary embolism: detection with MR perfusion imaging of lung–a feasibility study. Radiology 1997;203:181–5.
88. Hatabu H, Gaa J, Kim D, et al. Pulmonary perfusion: qualitative assessment with dynamic contrast-enhanced MRI using ultra-short TE and inversion recovery turbo flash. Magn Reson Med 1996;36:503–8.
89. Hatabu H, Gaa J, Kim D, et al. Pulmonary perfusion and angiography: evaluation with breath-hold enhanced three-dimensional fast imaging steady-state precession MR imaging with short TR and TE. AJR Am J Roentgenol 1996;167:653–5.

90. Berthezene Y, Croisille P, Wiart M, et al. Prospective comparison of MR lung perfusion and lung scintigraphy. J Magn Reson Imaging 1999;9:61–8.
91. Kirby M, Mathew L, Wheatley A, et al. Chronic obstructive pulmonary disease: longitudinal hyperpolarized (3)He MR imaging. Radiology 2010;256:280–9.
92. Vidal Melo MF, Winkler T, Harris RS, et al. Spatial heterogeneity of lung perfusion assessed with (13)N PET as a vascular biomarker in chronic obstructive pulmonary disease. J Nucl Med 2010;51:57–65.
93. Coxson HO, Quiney B, Sin DD, et al. Airway wall thickness assessed using computed tomography and optical coherence tomography. Am J Respir Crit Care Med 2008;177:1201–6.
94. Coxson HO, Mayo J, Lam S, et al. New and current clinical imaging techniques to study chronic obstructive pulmonary disease. Am J Respir Crit Care Med 2009; 180:588–97.

The Importance of the Assessment of Pulmonary Function in COPD

Kristina L. Bailey, MD

KEYWORDS

- Chronic obstructive pulmonary disease • Spirometry • Lung volumes
- Diffusing capacity of the lung for carbon monoxide

KEY POINTS

- Spirometry should be performed in every case of suspected chronic obstructive pulmonary disease.
- Pulmonary function testing can also aid in assessing the severity of disease and in managing the disease after the diagnosis is made.

INTRODUCTION

Chronic obstructive pulmonary disease (COPD) is defined by airflow limitation caused by chronic bronchitis or emphysema. Spirometry is an essential step in the diagnosis and staging of COPD. Guidelines advise spirometry as the gold standard for COPD diagnosis.[1,2] Spirometry is also an important part of monitoring COPD. Despite this, many patients are treated for presumed COPD without ever undergoing pulmonary function testing. This article reviews pulmonary function testing and the abnormalities seen in COPD. Discussed is the role spirometry plays in the diagnosis and management of COPD, and in quantifying the severity of COPD.

ROLE OF SPIROMETRY IN THE DIAGNOSIS OF COPD

Spirometry is the gold standard for the diagnosis of COPD. In symptomatic patients, spirometry can help determine whether the patient's symptoms are caused by respiratory disease or other conditions. Unfortunately, a large proportion of patients with COPD go undiagnosed.[3] Frequently the disease is not diagnosed until it is quite advanced. Targeted screening of symptomatic patients with risk factors for COPD results in better diagnosis rates and more appropriate therapy.[4]

Spirometry is often underused in COPD diagnosis. More than a third of patients with a new COPD diagnosis have never had pulmonary function testing, but are given a clinical diagnosis.[5] It is important to confirm a clinical diagnosis of COPD with spirometry.

Pulmonary, Critical Care, Sleep and Allergy Division, Department of Internal Medicine, University of Nebraska Medical Center, 985910 Nebraska Medical Center, Omaha, NE 68198–5910, USA
E-mail address: kbailey@unmc.edu

Med Clin N Am 96 (2012) 745–752
doi:10.1016/j.mcna.2012.04.011
0025-7125/12/$ – see front matter © 2012 Elsevier Inc. All rights reserved.

Epidemiologic data show that when spirometry is not used, COPD is often underdiagnosed for those with the disease and overdiagnosed for those without the disease.[6] If the diagnosis is missed in a patient with COPD, they will not have the benefit of treatment. If the patient is given an incorrect diagnosis of COPD, this also has deleterious consequences. Not only will the patient not be treated for the true cause of their symptom, but they also will likely be given treatment for COPD, which could give them unnecessary side effects. To ensure appropriate diagnosis and treatment, spirometry must be performed.

INTRODUCTION TO PULMONARY FUNCTION TESTING

Pulmonary function testing has three basic components: (1) spirometry, (2) lung volumes, and (3) diffusing capacity of the lung for carbon monoxide (DLCO). Each of these components can be affected by COPD. However, only spirometry is necessary to make the diagnosis of COPD.

Spirometry

Spirometry consists of (1) forced vital capacity (FVC), (2) forced expiratory volume in 1 second (FEV_1), and (3) FEV_1/FVC ratio. To perform spirometry, the patient takes the biggest breath possible and blows it out as fast as they can. This is called a "forced exhalation maneuver." During this procedure, the total volume of air that the patient can exhale in one breath is measured; this is the FVC. The amount of air that the patient can exhale in the first second is also measured; this is the FEV_1. Each is measured in liters and is reported as percent of predicted for that patient. The percent predicted is based on reference values that take into account the age, gender, and race of the patient. The FVC is a measure of the amount of air the lungs hold. The FEV_1 is a measure of how easily air flows through the lungs. Patients with COPD often have narrowing or inflammation of the airways. This hinders how fast air can leave the lungs. This leads to a decrease in the FEV_1. If the FEV_1 is decreased disproportionately to the FVC, a diagnosis of COPD is made. To determine if the decrease is disproportionate, the FEV_1/FVC ratio is calculated. An FEV_1/FVC ratio of less than 0.70 after bronchodilator is typically considered diagnostic of COPD. However, the use of a fixed cut-off has created some controversy, which is described later in this article.

Along with spirometry, a flow-volume loop is also typically generated. The flow-volume loop plots flow on the y axis and volume on the x axis. A normal flow-volume loop (**Fig. 1**A) has a characteristic shape. In obstructive lung disease, such as COPD, the expiratory limb takes on a coved shape (see **Fig. 1**B).

Lung Volumes

In addition to spirometry, lung volumes can also be measured. Lung volumes consist of total lung capacity (TLC), residual volume (RV), and functional residual capacity. TLC is the volume of air contained in the lung after a full inhalation. RV is the volume of air left in the lung after a full exhalation. Functional residual capacity is the volume of gas left in the lungs after a tidal breath.

Lung volumes are measured by helium dilution, nitrogen washout, or body plethysmography. Body plethysmography has come to be the gold standard in COPD, because helium dilution and nitrogen washout can underestimate TLC in COPD. Helium dilution and nitrogen washout can only measure air that communicates with the airways. Bullae, which are common in COPD, are not measured by these methods.

Emphysema destroys lung tissue, leading to loss of elastic recoil. Loss of elastic recoil allows the lungs to be stretched to abnormally large volumes, resulting in an

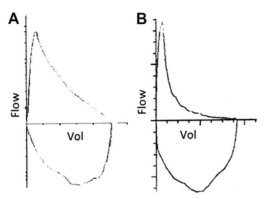

Fig. 1. (A) Normal flow-volume loop. (B) Flow-volume loop of a patient with COPD showing coving of the expiratory limb.

increased TLC. RV can also be increased in COPD when disease progression destroys the elastic tethers that help hold small airways open during exhalation. This leads to premature closing of the airways, which causes abnormal amounts of air to be trapped in the lung. In some patients, there is also inflammation of the small airways, which causes narrowing, further contributing to air trapping and the increase in RV.

Air trapping can lead to hyperinflation. There is a static and dynamic component of hyperinflation. Static hyperinflation refers to the baseline level of air trapping seen at rest. This is caused by the loss of elastic recoil properties of the lung and fixed airway obstruction. Dynamic hyperinflation occurs during exercise or times of rapid respiratory rate. In these situations, the patient is unable to finish exhaling before the next breath starts. With each breath, the patient becomes progressively more hyperinflated. This puts the respiratory muscles at a disadvantage, and increases the work of breathing.

Diffusing Capacity of the Lung for Carbon Monoxide

DLCO is a measure of how easily carbon monoxide (CO) molecules transfer from the alveolar gas to the hemoglobin of red cells in the pulmonary circulation. To measure DLCO, the patient inhales a single breath containing a minute amount of CO and holds it for 10 seconds. The breath is then exhaled and the exhaled breath is analyzed for CO. The change in the concentration of CO is then multiplied by the single breath TLC to calculate DLCO. Some patients with severe COPD may have difficulty performing the breath hold required to measure DLCO.

In COPD, DLCO decreases with increasing severity of disease. This is because in emphysema, the lung has lost alveoli, resulting in a lower surface area available for diffusion. In addition, there is also a loss of capillary bed, which can also decrease DLCO. When DLCO falls below 55% of predicted, the patient should undergo oximetry during exercise to determine if oxygen is required.[7]

DIAGNOSIS OF COPD BASED ON SPIROMETRY

A diagnosis of COPD is confirmed by spirometry when the FEV_1/FVC ratio is less than 0.70. Although there is some controversy about what the cutoff should be, the Global Initiative for Chronic Obstructive Lung Disease (GOLD) guidelines[2] and the combined American College of Physicians, American College of Chest Physicians, American

Thoracic Society, and the European Respiratory Society COPD guidelines[8] recommend using the fixed cutoff of less than 0.70. This criterion is set regardless of age and gender to simplify the diagnosis of COPD. However, the fixed ratio cutoff is not perfect. The FEV_1/FVC ratio is known to decline with normal aging. Using this cutoff may lead to an overdiagnosis of COPD in the elderly[9,10] and an underdiagnosis in young adults.[11] This is caused by age-related changes in FEV_1/FVC ratio.

Because of these imperfections in the FEV_1/FVC ratio, there have been several alternate methods proposed to diagnose obstruction. One proposal is to use the lower limit of normal (LLN) for the cutoff of FEV_1/FVC ratio. LLN takes into consideration age, height, and gender for each individual. This minimizes the age-related changes in the FEV_1/FVC ratio, and may reduce the misclassification of airway obstruction.[10] However, it also may be more difficult for primary care providers to perform and interpret. In addition, using this cutoff may not improve clinical care. Despite the proposed overdiagnosis in the elderly, the FEV_1/FVC ratio still correlates better with COPD exacerbations and mortality than using LLN.[12]

It may be difficult for some patients to perform a forced exhalation maneuver for several reasons, including poor mental status and coughing. Proposed alternatives include using slow vital capacity or FEV in 6 seconds (FEV_6) instead of FVC. Slow vital capacity measures the vital capacity while breathing in and out in a slow and steady manner rather than the forced maneuver used to measure the FVC. Slow vital capacity was found to be useful in elderly patients who are unable to perform an FVC maneuver without coughing.[13] However, it was not easier for patients with poor mental status to perform.[13] Another option is the FEV_1/FEV_6 ratio. The FEV_1/FEV_6 ratio has been shown to be an acceptable surrogate for the FEV_1/FVC ratio.[14] It is also thought to be an easier test for patients to perform than the FVC maneuver.

DIFFERENTIATING COPD FROM ASTHMA WITH BRONCHODILATOR REVERSIBILITY TESTING

Asthma and COPD have many features in common, including symptoms of shortness of breath. Bronchodilator reversibility testing can be used to help differentiate asthma from COPD. In both diseases, spirometry can show an obstructive pattern. However, the airway obstruction caused by asthma is typically completely reversed (FEV_1/FVC ratio is normal) with bronchodilator therapy. In contrast, in patients with COPD the obstruction remains after bronchodilator treatment (FEV_1/FVC ratio remains <0.7). Although the airway obstruction remains in COPD, there may be improvement in the FEV_1 after bronchodilator therapy. Significant improvement in FEV_1 after bronchodilator is defined as an increase in FEV_1 by 12% and 200 mL.

Although bronchodilator reversibility testing can be helpful in distinguishing between COPD and asthma, it is not a perfect test. Some patients with COPD have significant reversibility of their FEV_1 after bronchodilator. Likewise, some patients with severe, long-standing asthma may not have complete reversibility after bronchodilator. The test must be interpreted along with the clinical context.

QUANTIFYING COPD SEVERITY WITH SPIROMETRY

Spirometry can be used to quantify COPD severity. Several scales have been used in the past and COPD staging guidelines have been criticized because they do not accurately reflect severity of disease. Data are emerging that indicate that COPD stage correlates with other important measures of severity. For instance, COPD stage correlates well with patient reports of dyspnea.[15] In addition, COPD severity is associated with a higher rate of severe exacerbations requiring hospitalization.

Table 1
GOLD guidelines

GOLD 2001	GOLD 2011	FEV$_1$/FVC ratio	FEV$_1$ (% predicted)
0: "At risk"	Not applicable		
I: Mild	I: Mild	≤0.7	≥80
II: Moderate	II: Moderate	≤0.7	50–79
III: Severe	III: Severe	≤0.7	30–49
IV: Very severe	IV: Very severe	≤0.7	<30

The GOLD guidelines ratings of severity have gone through several changes. The initial guidelines in 2001 included a stage 0 ("at risk"), which included people with normal spirometry who had a history of smoking, exposure to pollutants, respiratory symptoms, or a family history of respiratory disease. The current GOLD guidelines have removed stage 0.[2] These changes are summarized in **Table 1**. The percent predicted FEV$_1$ is used to grade the severity of COPD. It should be noted that the post-bronchodilator FEV$_1$ should be used to determine severity stage. It is more reproducible than the prebronchodilator FEV$_1$.[16] Stage I or "mild" COPD is defined as a FEV$_1$/FVC ratio of less than 0.7 and an FEV$_1$ greater than 80% predicted, stage II is an FEV$_1$ of 50% to 79% predicted, stage III is 30% to 49% predicted, and stage IV is less than 30% predicted.

ROLE OF SPIROMETRY IN THE MANAGEMENT OF COPD

Spirometry plays an essential role in not only the diagnosis, but also the management of COPD. Spirometry can guide therapy for COPD, enable monitoring of disease progression, help determine prognosis, and estimate long-term survival.

Spirometry has been shown to prompt changes in therapy for patients with COPD.[17] Several guidelines make recommendations for treatment based on severity as measured by FEV$_1$. The American College of Physicians, American College of Chest Physicians, American Thoracic Society, and European Respiratory Society guidelines recommend treatment with inhaled bronchodilators for those with an FEV$_1$ of less than 60% predicted, and pulmonary rehabilitation for those with an FEV$_1$ of less than 50% predicted. The 2011 GOLD guidelines take this one step further, using more than just the patient's FEV$_1$ to help guide treatment.[2] Spirometry alone cannot give an accurate picture of the severity of an individual patient's disease. Symptoms and number of exacerbations must also be considered. The 2011 GOLD guidelines propose a method

Table 2
Modified Medical Research Council questionnaire for assessing the severity of breathlessness

Grade 0	I only get breathless with strenuous exercise
Grade 1	I get short of breath when hurrying on the level or walking up a slight hill
Grade 2	I walk slower than people of the same age on the level because of breathlessness, or I have to stop for breath when walking on my own pace on the level
Grade 3	I stop for breath after walking about 100 m or after a few minutes on the level
Grade 4	I am too breathless to leave the house or I am breathless when dressing or undressing

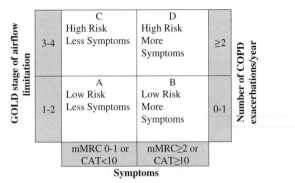

Fig. 2. The combined COPD assessment. Patients are assigned lettered groups A through D based on spirometry, symptoms, and number of exacerbations per year. If there is a discrepancy between which group the patient would fall into, always choose the higher-risk group. For example, a patient who is GOLD stage II, with a CAT of 22, and two COPD exacerbations a year falls into group D rather than group B. CAT, COPD assessment test; mMRC, Modified British Medical Research Council. (*Modified from* The global strategy for the diagnosis, management and prevention of COPD. 2011. Available at: http://www.goldcopd.org/. Accessed April 1, 2012.)

to combine spirometry, symptoms, and numbers of exacerbations to produce a more comprehensive picture. In this classification, patients are placed into groups A through D, with group A having the lowest severity and group D having the highest severity. To calculate the patient's group, one must have (1) spirometry, (2) a measurement of symptoms, and (3) the number of COPD exacerbations the patient has per year. The patient's symptoms can be quantified using either the COPD assessment test (www.catestonline.org) or the Modified British Medical Research Council questionnaire (**Table 2**). One can then use **Fig. 2** to determine into which category the patient falls. The GOLD guidelines also make recommendations for initial therapy based on the patient's group. Group A should be treated with a short-acting β-agonist or a short-acting anticholinergic. Group B should be treated with a long-acting β-agonist or anticholinergic. Groups C and D should be treated with an inhaled corticosteroid and a long-acting β-agonist or long-acting anticholinergic. These recommendations are summarized in **Fig. 3**.

Spirometry also is an objective way of monitoring for disease progression. It is often helpful to determine whether an increase of shortness of breath is caused by worsening COPD or other etiologies, such as heart disease. This is especially important because many patients with COPD also have concomitant heart disease.

	Initial pharmacologic therapy		Non-pharmacologic therapy	
A	**Short-acting** beta-agonist or anticholinergic prn		Smoking cessation	Consider pulmonary rehabilitation
B				
C	**Long-acting** beta-agonist or anti-cholinergic	**Plus** inhaled corticosteroid		
D				

Fig. 3. COPD therapy based on GOLD stage. (*Adapted from* The global strategy for the diagnosis, management and prevention of COPD. 2011. Available at: http://www.goldcopd.org/. Accessed April 1, 2012.)

Spirometry can also be used to help determine the long-term survival and prognosis of a patient with COPD. Classically, the FEV_1 has been used to determine prognosis.[18] With decreasing FEV_1, mortality increases. However, the FEV_1 alone does not give the entire picture of the patient's status. Other combinations of criteria that include the FEV_1 are being studied, such as the BODE index.[19]

SUMMARY

Spirometry is the gold standard for making the diagnosis of COPD. It should be performed in every case of suspected COPD. Other pulmonary functions, such as lung volumes, can give insight into physiologic consequences of COPD, such as hyperinflation. Pulmonary function testing can also aid in assessing the severity of disease and in managing the disease after diagnosis is made.

REFERENCES

1. Rabe KF, Hurd S, Anzueto A, et al. Global strategy for the diagnosis, management, and prevention of chronic obstructive pulmonary disease: GOLD executive summary. Am J Respir Crit Care Med 2007;176(6):532–55.
2. From the global strategy for the diagnosis, management and prevention of COPD. 2011. Available at: http://www.goldcopd.org/. Accessed April 1, 2012.
3. Mannino DM, Gagnon RC, Petty TL, et al. Obstructive lung disease and low lung function in adults in the United States: data from the National Health and Nutrition Examination Survey, 1988-1994. Arch Intern Med 2000;160(11):1683–9.
4. Walker PP, Mitchell P, Diamantea F, et al. Effect of primary-care spirometry on the diagnosis and management of COPD. Eur Respir J 2006;28(5):945–52.
5. Han MK, Kim MG, Mardon R, et al. Spirometry utilization for COPD: how do we measure up? Chest 2007;132(2):403–9.
6. Joo MJ, Au DH, Lee TA. Use of spirometry in the diagnosis of chronic obstructive pulmonary disease and efforts to improve quality of care. Transl Res 2009;154(3): 103–10.
7. Owens GR, Rogers RM, Pennock BE, et al. The diffusing capacity as a predictor of arterial oxygen desaturation during exercise in patients with chronic obstructive pulmonary disease. N Engl J Med 1984;310(19):1218–21.
8. Qaseem A, Wilt TJ, Weinberger SE, et al. Diagnosis and management of stable chronic obstructive pulmonary disease: a clinical practice guideline update from the American College of Physicians, American College of Chest Physicians, American Thoracic Society, and European Respiratory Society. Ann Intern Med 2011;155(3):179–91.
9. Hardie JA, Buist AS, Vollmer WM, et al. Risk of over-diagnosis of COPD in asymptomatic elderly never-smokers. Eur Respir J 2002;20(5):1117–22.
10. Swanney MP, Ruppel G, Enright PL, et al. Using the lower limit of normal for the FEV1/FVC ratio reduces the misclassification of airway obstruction. Thorax 2008; 63(12):1046–51.
11. Cerveri I, Corsico AG, Accordini S, et al. Underestimation of airflow obstruction among young adults using FEV1/FVC <70% as a fixed cut-off: a longitudinal evaluation of clinical and functional outcomes. Thorax 2008;63(12):1040–5.
12. Mannino DM, Sonia Buist A, Vollmer WM. Chronic obstructive pulmonary disease in the older adult: what defines abnormal lung function? Thorax 2007;62(3):237–41.
13. Allen SC, Charlton C, Backen W, et al. Performing slow vital capacity in older people with and without cognitive impairment–is it useful? Age Ageing 2010; 39(5):588–91.

14. Jing JY, Huang TC, Cui W, et al. Should FEV1/FEV6 replace FEV1/FVC ratio to detect airway obstruction? a metaanalysis. Chest 2009;135(4):991–8.
15. Mahler DA, Ward J, Waterman LA, et al. Patient-reported dyspnea in COPD reliability and association with stage of disease. Chest 2009;136(6):1473–9.
16. Lin SH, Kuo PH, Kuo SH, et al. Severity staging of chronic obstructive pulmonary disease: differences in pre- and post-bronchodilator spirometry. Yonsei Med J 2009;50(5):672–6.
17. Chavannes N, Schermer T, Akkermans R, et al. Impact of spirometry on GPs' diagnostic differentiation and decision-making. Respir Med 2004;98(11):1124–30.
18. Anthonisen NR, Wright EC, Hodgkin JE. Prognosis in chronic obstructive pulmonary disease. Am Rev Respir Dis 1986;133(1):14–20.
19. Cote CG, Pinto-Plata VM, Marin JM, et al. The modified BODE index: validation with mortality in COPD. Eur Respir J 2008;32(5):1269–74.

Role of Exercise in Testing and in Therapy of COPD

Miguel Divo, MD, Victor Pinto-Plata, MD*

KEYWORDS

- Six-minute walk test • Cardiopulmonary exercise test • Stair-climbing test
- Shuttle walk test • Hyperinflation • Oxygen consumption

KEY POINTS

- Patients with chronic obstructive pulmonary disease (COPD) frequently complain of exercise limitation that when associated with severe dyspnea leads to further deconditioning and worse health status.
- The determination of functional capacity using exercise testing is of use to clinicians, as it helps provide a prognosis and to plan for therapeutic interventions.
- Several field exercise tests, such as the 6-minute walk distance and stair climbing are within the reach of most health care providers. The more comprehensive shuttle walk distance and cardiopulmonary exercise test provide complementary information and are available at many medical centers.
- Exercise training, the cornerstone of pulmonary rehabilitation, has been shown to improve dyspnea and health-related quality of life and decrease health care use. It is indicated in any patients with COPD who are limited in their exercise capacity.

INTRODUCTION

A clinical exercise test is performed to assess an organ or system reserve capacity. Most organs have a large physiologic reserve that allows it to adapt to increasing demands. In chronic diseases, this reserve may decrease gradually and patients usually remain largely asymptomatic because they limit their exercise until the reserve is greatly reduced to a degree where minimal activity results in dyspnea. The lack of regular exercise in many patients with chronic conditions also contributes to the delay in symptoms but adds a deconditioning factor that by itself worsens dyspnea and further reduces functional capacity.

Exercise capacity tests are helpful in measuring the physiologic reserve of the respiratory, cardiovascular, hematologic and osteomuscular systems, which are difficult to ascertain by test performed at rest. The test results could be used to assess clinical status, offer prognosis, and assist in the management of patients complaining of

Pulmonary and Critical Care Medicine Division, Brigham and Women's Hospital, Harvard Medical School, 75 Francis Street, Boston MA 02115, USA
* Corresponding author.
E-mail address: vpinto-plata@partners.org

Med Clin N Am 96 (2012) 753–766
doi:10.1016/j.mcna.2012.05.004
0025-7125/12/$ – see front matter © 2012 Elsevier Inc. All rights reserved.

dyspnea, arguably, the major complaint and most disabling symptom in patients with chronic obstructive pulmonary disease (COPD).

Several factors, including skeletal muscle dysfunction, hyperinflation, deconditioning, anxiety, and depression, usually play a role in the etiology of dyspnea[1] and could be present even in patients with relatively mild disease.[2] Patients usually become dyspneic with physical activities but as the disease progresses, it is present with minimal activities or even at rest. An exercise test should be obtained in symptomatic patients with COPD to determine their pulmonary physiologic reserve, identifying the presence of other organ systems as the etiology of exercise limitation, and detection and treatment of exercise-induced hypoxemia. An exercise test is also helpful to detect changes in exercise capacity or respiratory parameters over time, usually after a therapeutic intervention.

The forced expiratory volume in the first second (FEV_1) is the traditional measurement that characterizes disease severity. The Global Initiative for Chronic Obstructive Lung Disease (GOLD) and other international societies, such as the American Thoracic Society (ATS) and European Respiratory Society, use the ratio of FEV_1 to the forced vital capacity (FVC) less than 70 to define obstruction, and the FEV_1 expressed as percent of predicted to categorized disease severity.[3,4] Based on the GOLD criteria,[3] the disease severity is divided into 4 categories: stage I or mild COPD (FEV_1 $\geq$80%), stage II or moderate (50% $\leq$ FEV_1 <80%), stage III or severe (30% $\leq$ FEV_1 <50%), and stage IV or very severe (FEV_1 <30%). This staging is important to categorize disease severity; however, COPD also has systemic involvement, not captured by spirometry. In fact, several other attributes or important clinical characteristics of the disease are not well captured by the FEV_1. Among them are body mass index,[5] the level of dyspnea,[6] exacerbations,[7] quality of life,[8] and exercise capacity, even when measured with a simple test, such as the distance walked over 6 minutes (6MWT).[9,10] All of these variables provide independent additional information to the measurement of lung function in the prediction of survival. Some of these characteristics have become important elements to classify patients with COPD[11,12] into phenotypic subgroups of the disease[13] (see the article by Martinez and Han elsewhere in this issue).

The measurement of the exercise capacity and other disease outcomes are paramount to better define a patient's health status, predict health care use, measure response to intervention, and prognosticate survival. In the past few years, several multidimensional score systems have been created using a combination of several of these variables.[11,12,14,15] Among them, the BODE index, which integrates the body mass index (weight in kilograms divided by height in m^2), degree of airflow obstruction, measured with the FEV_1, severity of dyspnea using the modified Medical Research Council Dyspnea scale, and exercise endurance (measured by the 6MWT) has become the most widely accepted. Each one of the variables have a scaled cutoff score value and the sum of them provide the BODE score, with values ranging from 0 to 10. Higher scores correlate with an increase risk for death, and its prediction value is superior than the FEV_1 alone.[11] The BODE score has also demonstrated to be a useful tool for the evaluation of possible candidate with COPD for lung transplantation,[16] and longitudinal changes correlates with outcomes after interventions such as pulmonary rehabilitation,[17] lung transplantation[18] and lung volume reduction surgery.[19] The most important contributor to the ultimate performance of the BODE index is the inclusion exercise performance, supporting its use in the practical assessment and management of patients with COPD.

MODALITIES OF EXERCISE TESTING

There are several modalities of exercise tests for patients with COPD. They are used according to the clinical scenario, the patient's ability to perform a particular test, the information required, and the technical capacity and infrastructure of the institution or setting (medical office or tertiary care institution) where the test is completed. They may be classified according to the technical requirement and cost, level of exercise intensity, and intrinsic characteristics (standardization and reproducibility). More important, the indication and the information expected from a test is critical to order the appropriate exercise modality.

These modalities include the 6MWT, stair-climbing test, shuttle test (incremental and endurance), cardiopulmonary exercise test (CPET), and cardiac stress test. **Table 1** shows a summary of the characteristics of each test. In this monograph, we discuss the first 4 modalities.

Six-Minute Walk Test

The 6MWT was first introduced in 1963 as a field test for fitness assessment by McGavin and colleagues,[20] who used it to determine disability in patients with chronic bronchitis. The test is currently performed in 6 minutes, since Butland and colleagues[21] determined a high correlation coefficient between a 6- and a 12-minute walk (r = 0.955). It is a simple test to perform, does not require special training of personnel, and is easy to administer, well tolerated, and reflects the functional exercise level for activities of daily living (ADLs). It evaluates the global and integrative response of all the systems involved during exercise, including cardiovascular, pulmonary, and muscular. A guideline document from the ATS[4] suggests a standardized method to perform the test. The suggested location is a 100-ft (30-m) corridor, although different lengths are acceptable (50–150 ft or 20–50 m). The corridor should have marked distances that allow the proper measurement of the distance walked. Two cones on each end of the corridor will mark the turning point. The patient should wear comfortable clothing and shoes. The equipment required includes a stopwatch,

Table 1
Characteristics of different exercise modalities

Modality of Test	Technical Requirement	Intensity	Indication	Standardization
Stair Climbing	Minimal	Submaximal to maximal	Postoperative risk Functional capacity	Minimal
Six-Minute Walk Test (6MWT)	Moderate Timer Corridor Oximeter	Submaximal to maximal	Functional capacity	Guidelines available
Shuttle Test	Complex Timer Hall CD and CD player	Maximal	Functional capacity	Instructions available
Cardiopulmonary Exercise Test (CPET)	Complex Needs a specialized laboratory with medical supervision	Maximal	Functional capacity Comprehensive cardiopulmonary status	Comprehensive guidelines available

Data from Zeballos RJ, Weisman IM. Modalities of clinical exercise testing. In: Weisman IM, Zeballos RJ. Clinical Exercise Testing. Prog Respir Res. Basel: Karger, 2002, Vol 32, pp 30-42; and Casaburi R, ZuWallack R. Pulmonary rehabilitation for management of chronic obstructive pulmonary disease. N Engl J Med 2009;360:1329–35.

a lap counter, and a source of oxygen, sphygmomanometer and oximeter. We believe the oxygen saturation monitoring should be a routine measurement during this test because in patients with COPD, this test is more likely to detect exercise hypoxemia than any other test including treadmill or cycle ergometry.

The 6MWT can be performed by a respiratory therapist, nurse, or trained medical personnel in a primary care office. Before the start of the test, pulse, respiratory rate, dyspnea level, oxygen saturation, and blood pressure are measured. The patient is instructed to walk as far as possible for 6 minutes but may slow down or stop during the test and resume it within the 6-minute period. The patient should not talk during the test and at the end, the same set of vital signs, dyspnea level, and oxygen saturation should be recorded to document any changes and determine the need for intervention/therapy (supplemental oxygen, pulmonary rehabilitation, or bronchodilators). There is a Current Procedural Terminology code for simple pulmonary stress testing (94620). The indication and interpretation should accompany this report.[22]

Different equations have been published to determine the predicted value in a healthy population.[23–25] Enright and Sherrill[23] evaluated 173 healthy men and women aged 40 to 80 who participated in the Tucson Epidemiologic Study of Airways Obstructive Disease. The median distance walked for men was 576 m and 494 for women. One equation for each gender was determined and these reference equations explained 40% of the variance. Troosters and colleagues[24] studied 51 healthy controls aged 50 to 85 years in Leuven, Belgium. The average distance was 631 (±93) meters and the distance walked was 84 m longer in men than in women. Their equation included the same factors as the one from Enright and Sherrill[23]: height, weight, age, and gender and explained 66% of the variability. Subsequent work by Casanova and colleagues[26] better defined the distance walked by a healthy population when they studied a larger set (444 subjects) in a multicenter study in 7 countries (10 centers). The mean distance walked was 571 (±90) meters and men walked 30 m more than women. The maximal heart rate during the walk was also included in the equation (besides the previously mentioned factors) but there was a large variability among countries and the routine use of the equation was not recommended.

The total distance walked during the 6MWT and the predicted value using any of the previously mentioned equations, should be reported along with the level of dyspnea (before and after the test) and the oxygen saturation. By convention, the distance is usually reported in meters. It is important to notice, however, that the predicted value in some instances is not so critical, as a threshold value of 350 m in patients with COPD has demonstrated clinical relevance, independent of the observed predicted value.[9] Indeed, Cote and colleagues[9] followed 1379 patients with COPD from the BODE cohort study for more than 2 years (55 ± 30 months). They used a receiver operating characteristics curve to determine the threshold values with the best specificity and sensitivity to predict mortality. The study compared a walked distance of 350 m with 3 other threshold values calculated with the predictive equations of Troosters and colleagues,[24] Enright and Sherrill,[23] and 6MWT work. The investigators found no difference in the Kaplan-Meier survival analyses among these methods. A distance of 350 m had a sensitivity of 68%, a specificity of 70%, and an area under the curve (AUC) of 0.754 to predict mortality. These findings have been validated in the ECLIPSE (Evaluation of COPD Longitudinally to Identify Predictive Surrogate Endpoints) study, a large, multicenter cohort of 2110 patients followed for 3 years.[27] In this study, a distance of 334 m had the best-predicted value for increased risk of death (AUC: 0.67) and 357 m for exacerbation-related hospitalization (AUC 0.60). This study also determined a different decline in the walk distance per year according to the disease severity: GOLD stage II, 1.6 (+/−1.2) m; GOLD stage III, 9.8 (+/−1.3) m; and GOLD stage IV, 8.5 (+/−2.4) m.

Physical activity is reduced, particularly in patients with moderate and severe disease. Measuring physical activity and functional status of patients with COPD is particularly important, as both correlate with exacerbations, hospital admissions, and mortality.[28] The level of physical activity could be measured using different tools, including questionnaires to estimate it or direct measurement using pedometers or accelerometers. The use of these tools in a regular patient with COPD in the office may be impractical; however, daily physical activity of patients with COPD is highly correlated with the 6MWT and less so with more intense exercise testing.[29] In fact, Garcia-Rio and coworkers[30] studied 110 patients with moderate and severe COPD and measured their daily physical activity over a 5-day period using a triaxial accelerometer, a device that records patients' movements as a marker of physical activity. The investigators found a good correlation between the level of physical activity and the 6MWT (r = 0.72, P = .001), better than the correlation with maximal exercise on a stationary bike (r = 0.63). A multiple regression analysis showed that the level of hyperinflation during the exercise and the distance walked in 6 minutes were the best predictors of physical activity. Therefore, the walk test is a simple tool to measure the level of functional capacity in patients with COPD, an important factor in health care use and survival.

Although the ATS guidelines support the measurement of oxygen saturation (SpO2) as an optional test,[4] a subsequent study demonstrated the importance of such monitoring.[31] In a multicenter study, 576 outpatients with different levels of COPD severity were followed for 60 months (range 12 to 94 months) and the value of the oxygen saturation during the walk test as a predictor of survival was compared with age, gender, spirometry values, the distance walked, comorbidities, and baseline PaO_2. The presence of oxygen desaturation, even on those patients with a baseline partial pressure of oxygen in arterial blood (PaO_2) higher than 60 mm Hg at rest, was an independent predictor of mortality (relative risk 2.63; 95% confidence interval 1.53 to 4.51, $P<.001$). Measurement of the oxygen saturation during the walk test can also help determine which patients benefit from supplemental oxygen during ambulation (oxygen saturation 88% or less).

The test is indicated for all symptomatic patients with COPD, particularly those with dyspnea or reduced physical activity despite pharmacologic intervention, patients with severe disease (FEV_1 <50%), patients with recent or frequent admissions to the hospital for respiratory or nonrespiratory conditions, and patients considered candidates for pulmonary rehabilitation.

Although labeled as a submaximal exercise test, it has been shown to have a similar oxygen uptake at minute 6 compared with peak exercise in a cycle ergometer in patients with severe COPD.[32] Furthermore, it has a better discriminative power to predict mortality compared with the maximal oxygen consumption obtained during a CPET.[33]

In summary, the 6MWT is an exercise field test that is easy to perform and that provides additional and critical information for the care of patients with COPD. It should be considered an essential piece in the evaluation and management of symptomatic patients with this condition.

Stair Climbing

One of the ADLs that is impaired in patients with COPD is that of climbing stairs. It is a highly prevalent complaint, particularly in patients with moderate and severe disease. In a large study of 890 patients with COPD referred for pulmonary rehabilitation, the most prevalent limited activities were walking (68%), stair climbing (35%), and cycling (30%).[34] Therefore, an evaluation of this activity may be warranted in a subgroup of patients who are required to use stairways.

Stair climbing has been traditionally used to determine the fitness of lung surgery candidates and to estimate the risk of postoperative complications in those patients.[35] It also has been used to determine the level of hypoxemia in patients who complain of dyspnea during stair climbing. Although less sophisticated than a cardiopulmonary exercise test to estimate surgical suitability before lung resection, it is in some instances the only available tool to make such determination, because a CPET is not widely available. It is still used in several clinical centers for preoperative assessment because it is practical, does not require technical support, and patients can be tested the same day of an office visit without any special preparation. It may be used as a screening test to determine those patients who require cardiopulmonary exercise testing.[36] In that study, more than half of the patients who were unable to climb more than 14 m had an oxygen consumption of less than 15 mL/kg, but 98% of the patients who climbed more than 22 m had a normal oxygen uptake. Therefore, patients undergoing lung resection for lung cancer (many will also have COPD) who are unable to climb 22 m should be referred for a CPET before lung surgery.

The physiologic demand of a stair-climbing test is higher than the one imposed by a 6MWT.[37] In this study, 16 patients with severe COPD performed a 44-step climbing test and a 6MWT in a randomized, crossover fashion. The level of oxygen desaturation was similar in both tests but the stair-climbing test caused more dyspnea, lung hyperinflation, a higher median blood lactate (1.1 vs 0.3 mmol/L, $P<.001$), a more pronounced drop in mean pH (-0.05 ± 0.02 vs -0.03 ± -0.03, $P = .02$) and a higher increase in mean systolic blood pressure (27 ± 11 vs 13 ± 16 mm Hg; $P = .009$).

Unfortunately, there is no standardized procedure for the stair-climbing test as there is for the 6MWT. Usually, patients climb as many stairs as possible until they are limited by symptoms (dyspnea, leg fatigue, chest pain, dizziness). Subjects may or may not grab the rail during the climbing. Some researchers consider the end of the test when the patient stops for the first time but others allow patients to continue until the patient is unable to climb any longer. The results are reported as flights of stairs or floors reached, but the definition of a flight of stairs is also not uniform (11–25 steps). The number of steps climbed is probably the best report, as this number could be multiplied by the height of the step and converted to a distance (usually meters). It is not necessary but probably advisable to use an oximetry and document the oxygen saturation and heart rate at the beginning and end of the test.

The difference in the report of the results may bring some limitation when results from different groups are compared (**Table 2**). The lack of standardization includes the speed of climbing (subject's own pace or brisk walk), use of the handrail for balance, inclination of the stairway, and height of the stair's steps but could be diminished by reporting the distance climbed (explained previously).

Several studies have measured the oxygen consumption of stair climbing and the correlation with the 6MWT and CPET.[38] The number of steps climbed correlated well linearly with the maximal oxygen consumption (VO_2 max) on a cycle ergometer ($r = 0.72$) in 31 men with COPD. The VO_2 max also correlated, but weakly, with the distance walk in meters ($r^2 = 0.27$) and the number of steps in stair climbing ($r^2 = 0.33$) in another study with 50 patients with COPD.[39] All in all, stair climbing is a good field test with applicability in the area of preoperative evaluation. It lacks the standard qualities of the 6MWT and other tests but it does resemble a maximal exercise test in terms of the physiologic response.

Shuttle Walk Test and the Endurance Shuttle Walk Test

The shuttle walk test (SWT) is a walk test that uses an audio signal to direct the walking pace of a subject back and forth on a 10-m course.[40] The walking speed is increased

Table 2
Reports on stair-climbing test and postoperative complications by different authors

Author	Year	Type of Surgery	Stairs Climbed	Outcome
Van Nostrand et al[53]	1968	Pneumonectomy	<2 flights (~36 steps)	Higher mortality (50%)
Olsen et al[54]	1991	Wedge, lobectomy, pneumonectomy	<3 flights (75 steps)	Higher postoperative complication, longer intubation and length of stay
Holden et al[55]	1992	Wedge, lobectomy pneumonectomy	44 steps	Worse 90-d survival
Girish et al[35]	2001	Wedge, lobectomy pneumonectomy upper abdominal	<2 flights (<36 steps)	Higher mortality and increased postoperative respiratory insufficiency
Brunelli et al[36]	2010	Lobectomy	More than 19.6 (4.4) m or 126 (28) steps	No Complications

Abbreviation: Year, year of publication.

every minute, and the test ends when the subject cannot reach the turnaround point within the required time. It correlates well with the 6MWT (r = O.68) and the exercise performed is similar to a symptom-limited, maximal, incremental treadmill test. When compared with CPET results expressed in maximal watts,[41] the incremental SWT distance has a relative better correlation (R = 0.75, $P<.001$) than the 6MWT distance (r = 0.63 P = .002).

The requirements to perform a shuttle test include a flat surface at least 10 m long, timed signal played on a compact disk player, a measuring tape to establish a 10-m surface, and 2 cones placed 0.5 m from each end. The subject should walk from one cone to the opposite one and reach it before the next beep. Every minute, the speed is increased and each speed of walking is referred to as a level, with 12 levels in total. As the level increases, there is an increment in the number of shuttles in each level. For example, in levels 1, 2, and 3, the subject must complete 3, 4, and 5 shuttles respectively. The test is terminated when the subject is more than 0.5 m away from the cone at the moment of the beep. The test is scored as the total number of shuttles and is converted and reported in meters by multiplying the number of shuttles by 10 (distance in meters in each shuttle).

A variation of this test, the endurance shuttle walk test (ESWT), uses an externally controlled, constant paced walking speed. It is used to measure endurance. The rationale for this test is that most ADLs represent a sustained submaximal level of exercise. First, an incremental SWT is performed to determine the highest level or speed. Then, a timed signal recorded with a speed between 75% and 95% predicted of the maximum is selected. The subject is then instructed to walk for as long as possible and the time spent at a certain speed or the distance walked is recorded (endurance). This test has been used to determine improvement after pulmonary rehabilitation[42] and response to bronchodilator treatment.[43,44] These 2 tests are more popular in Europe than in the United States.

Cardiopulmonary Exercise Test

The CPET is a more sophisticated test modality that integrates the measurement of exercise output with all the physiologic components of the exercise machinery, including gas exchange, as well as the ventilatory and cardiovascular parameters. It is the preferred test when assessing physiologic response to exercise and partitioning the elements participating in that response. Compared with the previously described modalities, CPET not only provides a quantification of exercise capacity, but it can also point to the locus of exercise limitation, which is especially useful when competing causes could explain the symptoms reported by patients. Another added benefit of this modality is the possibility of obtaining key physiologic parameters that could help to tailor an exercise program and ensure the safety of the subject. CPET is an integral component of the pulmonary function laboratory and requires supervision by a trained technician and a physician. The most common indication for CPET are listed in **Box 1**. Within the CPET modality there are several variants of the test, each aimed to address a particular clinical question with different degrees of invasiveness or complexity, as described in **Table 3**.

The extent of exercise limitation in COPD is associated with the degree of airway obstruction.[45] However, factors responsible for an abnormal exercise response are multiple and interdependent, and include ventilatory limitation, gas exchange abnormalities, dynamic hyperinflation, abnormal O_2 delivery (anemia, cardiac dysfunction), and peripheral muscle dysfunction.[46–49] The individual contribution of each factor varies between individuals and resting pulmonary or cardiac function tests do not predict a particular exercise response. Furthermore, patients with COPD may have other comorbidities and the CPET may indentify potential confounding factors amenable to targeted therapeutic intervention.

Exercise in the Therapy of Patients with COPD

As we have discussed, COPD is an insidious and progressive disease that affects a patient's ability to perform physical activities because of the limitation imposed by early and disproportionate dyspnea, which creates a vicious circle that ends up disabling individuals. This in turn leads to a worse health-related quality of life,[2] anxiety, and social isolation.[47,48] Relieving dyspnea and regaining the ability of performing those important ADLs using exercise as a therapeutic intervention is an essential focus of the treatment of this disease. Promoting healthy lifestyle, including exercise, is an integral component of the therapeutic armamentarium of clinicians. Therefore, it is important that health care providers understand the principle of exercise prescription to provide clear and specific instructions to their patients. In the

---

Box 1
Most common indications for a CPET in patients with COPD

Indications

1. Unexplained dyspnea, or dyspnea out of proportion with the degree of airflow obstruction.

2. Presence of multiple comorbidities that could influence a patient's symptoms.

3. To quantify and prescribe objectively the level of exercise intensity before the initiation of a pulmonary rehabilitation or exercise program, in addition to ruling out exercise-induced cardiac ischemia or arrhythmias.

4. Assessment of increased perioperative risk in a patient undergoing thoracic surgery.

5. Objective quantification of response to a particular therapy (eg, pre-post rehabilitation, lung volume reduction).

6. Assessment and quantification of dynamic hyperinflation.

7. Research in COPD.

Table 3
Cardiopulmonary exercise test modalities

CPET Category	Description	Aim
Simple	Either stationary bike or treadmill exercise, gas exchange assessed noninvasively by pulse oximeter	
CPET with ABG	Performance of resting and peak exercise ABG, or serial measurement if an arterial line is placed	More precise measurement of exercise induced hypoxemia, determination of A-a gradient, Vd/Vt, lactic acid levels, baseline carboxy or metahemoglobinemia
CEPT with measurement of pulmonary artery pressures and right heart function	Placement of pulmonary artery catheter in addition to arterial line	Provides data for determination of oxygen extraction (mixed venous O_2 saturation) and diagnosis of exercise-induced pulmonary hypertension
CPET with assessment of dynamic hyperinflation	Measurement of baseline and serial inspiratory capacity	Determination if the degree of airflow limitation produces dynamic hyperinflation
Assessment of exercise-induced bronchospasm	Measurement of baseline and serial postexercise FEV_1	Less used in COPD, useful in the diagnosis of exercise-induced asthma

Abbreviations: A-a gradient, alveolar-arterial gradient; ABG, arterial blood gases; COPD, chronic obstructive pulmonary disease; CPET, cardiopulmonary exercise test; FEV_1, forced expiratory volume in the first second; Vd/Vt, ratio of physiologic dead space over tidal volume.

end, it is the clinician who decides between a simple home exercise routine or more intense highly supervised hospital (center)-based programs. To effectively achieve this goal, it is important not only to know how to prescribe exercise as a therapy but also to know which resources are available in the area.

Programs: Simple Home Based Versus Formal Pulmonary Rehabilitation

Although exercise training can be achieved at home with simple programs, for patients with more severe obstruction, as defined by the GOLD stages II to IV, a more structured pulmonary rehabilitation program is recommended.[1,3] The selection of patients for the program is commonly dictated by third party payers. In the United States, it has classically depended on policies drafted by Centers for Medicare and Medicaid Services (CMS) mandates. For CMS, besides a diagnosis of COPD GOLD stage II or higher, there must be evidence of potential improvement or maintenance of health status. It is important to highlight that airflow limitation correlates poorly with the degree of breathlessness or walking distance (6MWT), as evidenced by the considerable overlap between GOLD stages.[2] Therefore, the evaluation of breathlessness and walking distance should be integrated in the evaluation of patients with COPD to determine the level of impairment and the potential for a beneficial response to rehabilitation.

Pulmonary rehabilitation programs are either inpatient or more commonly outpatient, usually including 2 to 3 sessions per week for 6 to 8 weeks. Programs based on variations of this basic structure have demonstrated benefits in several patient-centered outcomes, including quality of life, exercise capacity, symptom perception, hospital readmissions, and survival while marginally affecting the degree of airway obstruction.[17,28] The benefits of rehabilitation are by-products of multiple interventions from structured programs, including exercise training, optimization of pharmacotherapy, education, supervision, group support, and nutritional support.

Program Components

The prescription of an exercise plan should be tailored to each patient. An ideal starting point is the objective assessment of pulmonary function, exercise limitation, degree of breathlessness, response to physical load, and consideration of comorbidities that could contribute to the exercise limitation.[50] Depending on available resources, spirometry, lung volume measurement and diffusing capacity, CPET, and dyspnea perception at rest (Medical Research Council dyspnea scale) and during exercise (Borg dyspnea scale) provide the needed parameters to prescribe an exercise program and ensure safety during exertion.

The most important component of pulmonary rehabilitation is exercise training. This is governed by principles that have to be considered when designing an individualized exercise program or when giving general advice to your patient:

1. Training specificity; which means that exercising a certain body part primarily will develops the muscles of that body part. For COPD, lower extremity exercise (walking and biking) are strongly recommended and complemented with strength exercise to shoulder girdle muscle using upper extremity exercise.
2. Frequency; the exact frequency has never been determined but most programs include a minimum of 3 sessions per week and at least 1 or 2 days to rest.
3. Duration of the exercise session; which is usually built in incremental fashion as the individual endurance improves. It is possible to consider that the total duration does not require a continuous session; therefore, it could be divided into shorter series interposed by resting periods.
4. Intensity of exercise; usually measured by targeting a heart rate with or without dyspnea level. The benefit target is in the range of 65% to 85% of maximal heart rate. For the optimal prescription of exercise, a CPET is an excellent tool that provides a guide to plan the intensity of exercise to dyspnea and heart rate. With the results from the laboratory, it is usually to target a maximal oxygen uptake work rate aimed to reach 60% to 80% of the peak oxygen uptake (VO2 max), which is usually close to the anaerobic threshold.
5. Exercise modality (endurance or resistance training); most patients with COPD will benefit from endurance training (aerobic), which is the principal component in pulmonary rehabilitation programs. Resistive training is complementary, especially when the patient reaches a plateau, or to strengthen the accessory muscles of breathing.
6. Reversal of training effect (use it or loose it). Maintenance and motivation are essential to keep a sustained effect, plus maintenance reflects that the patient has committed to a healthy lifestyle consistently. Emphasizing this point is of importance for patients so they incorporate the gains into their daily routine.
7. Safety. Starting an exercise plan for a patient with COPD should consider safety first. This requires evaluating patients to see if they can exercise on their own or if a more structured program is required, as in the case of formal pulmonary rehabilitation.

Techniques to Improve Training

Dyspnea is considered as "the pain of breathing" and limiting dyspnea could potentially enhance the patient's capacity to train. Techniques, such as supplemental oxygen during exercise, have been shown to facilitate training and increasing the time that patients can perform exercise. In patients with very severe dyspnea with exercise, single-limb training may help decrease the level of symptoms and allow similar end-result training.[51] The use of a mixture of oxygen and helium and noninvasive positive pressure ventilation helps decrease the work of breathing during the training. This probably decreases the oxygen cost of breathing, thus allowing more oxygen to be delivered to the systemic circulation, thereby improving exercise performance.[52] All of these techniques have proven to be of value in many different settings and some, such as oxygen supplementation during training, are easy to implement. More validation of the value of these techniques on patient-centered outcomes is needed before any of them is routinely recommended.

SUMMARY

The stair-climbing test, 6MWT, and shuttle test are exercise tests that requires less technical support than the CPET and are more available to any physician. The 6MWT is the simplest and most likely to be cost effective, as it provides useful information regarding prognosis, ADLs, and health care use at a very low cost. In addition, the 6MWT can be used to evaluate response to several interventions, including physical rehabilitation, medications, lung volume reduction interventions, and transplantation. The 6MWT has also been useful in and has become an integral part of the evaluation and response to treatment in other medical conditions, including congestive heart failure, pulmonary hypertension, and pulmonary fibrosis. The stair-climbing test seems to be most useful for preoperative evaluations when a CPET is not available. We have also used it on patients unable to perform a good CPET because of lack of familiarity with bicycle pedaling. The shuttle walk test may be used to better determine a maximal exercise capacity when a CPET is not available and to measure the effects of pulmonary rehabilitation in patients unfamiliar with a CPET. The role of exercise as a therapeutic tool is central to the concept of pulmonary rehabilitation. Exercise training improves not only functional dyspnea and health-related quality of life, but also has been shown to decrease health care resource use. As part of a comprehensive pulmonary rehabilitation initiated after a hospitalization for exacerbation, it has been shown to decrease readmission rates.

REFERENCES

1. Casaburi R, ZuWallack R. Pulmonary rehabilitation for management of chronic obstructive pulmonary disease. N Engl J Med 2009;360:1329–35.
2. Agusti A, Calverley PM, Celli B, et al. Characterisation of COPD heterogeneity in the ECLIPSE cohort. Respir Res 2010;11:122.
3. Global Initiative for Chronic Obstructive Lung Disease. Global strategy for the diagnosis, management and prevention of COPD: update 2010. Available at: http://wwwgoldcopd.com/. Accessed August 13, 2011.
4. ATS statement: guidelines for the six-minute walk test. Am J Respir Crit Care Med 2002;166:111–7.
5. Schols AM, Slangen J, Volovics L, et al. Weight loss is a reversible factor in the prognosis of chronic obstructive pulmonary disease. Am J Respir Crit Care Med 1998;157:1791–7.
6. Nishimura K, Izumi T, Tsukino M, et al. Dyspnea is a better predictor of 5-year survival than airway obstruction in patients with COPD. Chest 2002;121:1434–40.
7. Soler-Cataluna JJ, Martinez-Garcia MA, Roman Sanchez P, et al. Severe acute exacerbations and mortality in patients with chronic obstructive pulmonary disease. Thorax 2005;60:925–31.

8. Jones PW, Quirk FH, Baveystock CM. The St George's respiratory questionnaire. Respir Med 1991;85(Suppl B):25–31 [discussion: 3–7].
9. Cote CG, Casanova C, Marin JM, et al. Validation and comparison of reference equations for the 6-min walk distance test. Eur Respir J 2008;31:571–8.
10. Pinto-Plata VM, Cote C, Cabral H, et al. The 6-min walk distance: change over time and value as a predictor of survival in severe COPD. Eur Respir J 2004; 23:28–33.
11. Celli BR, Cote CG, Marin JM, et al. The body-mass index, airflow obstruction, dyspnea, and exercise capacity index in chronic obstructive pulmonary disease. N Engl J Med 2004;350:1005–12.
12. Puhan MA, Garcia-Aymerich J, Frey M, et al. Expansion of the prognostic assessment of patients with chronic obstructive pulmonary disease: the updated BODE index and the ADO index. Lancet 2009;374:704–11.
13. Han MK, Agusti A, Calverley PM, et al. Chronic obstructive pulmonary disease phenotypes: the future of COPD. Am J Respir Crit Care Med 2010;182:598–604.
14. Jones RC, Donaldson GC, Chavannes NH, et al. Derivation and validation of a composite index of severity in chronic obstructive pulmonary disease: the DOSE Index. Am J Respir Crit Care Med 2009;180:1189–95.
15. Esteban C, Quintana JM, Moraza J, et al. BODE-index vs HADO-score in chronic obstructive pulmonary disease: which one to use in general practice? BMC Med 2010;8:28.
16. Kotloff RM, Thabut G. Lung transplantation. Am J Respir Crit Care Med 2011;184: 159–71.
17. Cote CG, Celli BR. Pulmonary rehabilitation and the BODE index in COPD. Eur Respir J 2005;26:630–6.
18. Lahzami S, Bridevaux PO, Soccal PM, et al. Survival impact of lung transplantation for COPD. Eur Respir J 2010;36:74–80.
19. Martinez FJ, Foster G, Curtis JL, et al. Predictors of mortality in patients with emphysema and severe airflow obstruction. Am J Respir Crit Care Med 2006; 173:1326–34.
20. McGavin CR, Gupta SP, McHardy GJ. Twelve-minute walking test for assessing disability in chronic bronchitis. Br Med J 1976;1:822–3.
21. Butland RJ, Pang J, Gross ER, et al. Two-, six-, and 12-minute walking tests in respiratory disease. Br Med J (Clin Res Ed) 1982;284:1607–8.
22. Salzman SH. The 6-min walk test: clinical and research role, technique, coding, and reimbursement. Chest 2009;135:1345–52.
23. Enright PL, Sherrill DL. Reference equations for the six-minute walk in healthy adults. Am J Respir Crit Care Med 1998;158:1384–7.
24. Troosters T, Gosselink R, Decramer M. Six minute walking distance in healthy elderly subjects. Eur Respir J 1999;14:270–4.
25. Gibbons WJ, Fruchter N, Sloan S, et al. Reference values for a multiple repetition 6-minute walk test in healthy adults older than 20 years. J Cardiopulm Rehabil 2001;21:87–93.
26. Casanova C, Celli BR, Barria P, et al. The 6-min walk distance in healthy subjects: reference standards from seven countries. Eur Respir J 2011;37:150–6.
27. Spruit MA, Polkey MI, Celli B, et al. Predicting outcomes from 6-minute walk distance in chronic obstructive pulmonary disease. J Am Med Dir Assoc 2012; 13(3):291–7.
28. Garcia-Aymerich J, Lange P, Benet M, et al. Regular physical activity reduces hospital admission and mortality in chronic obstructive pulmonary disease: a population based cohort study. Thorax 2006;61:772–8.

29. Pitta F, Troosters T, Spruit MA, et al. Characteristics of physical activities in daily life in chronic obstructive pulmonary disease. Am J Respir Crit Care Med 2005; 171:972–7.
30. Garcia-Rio F, Lores V, Mediano O, et al. Daily physical activity in patients with chronic obstructive pulmonary disease is mainly associated with dynamic hyper-inflation. Am J Respir Crit Care Med 2009;180:506–12.
31. Casanova C, Cote C, Marin JM, et al. Distance and oxygen desaturation during the 6-min walk test as predictors of long-term mortality in patients with COPD. Chest 2008;134:746–52.
32. Troosters T, Vilaro J, Rabinovich R, et al. Physiological responses to the 6-min walk test in patients with chronic obstructive pulmonary disease. Eur Respir J 2002;20:564–9.
33. Cote CG, Pinto-Plata VM, Marin JM, et al. The modified BODE index: validation with mortality in COPD. Eur Respir J 2008;32:1269–74.
34. Annegarn J, Meijer K, Passos VL, et al. Problematic activities of daily life are weakly associated with clinical characteristics in COPD. J Am Med Dir Assoc 2012;13(3):284–90.
35. Girish M, Trayner E Jr, Dammann O, et al. Symptom-limited stair climbing as a predictor of postoperative cardiopulmonary complications after high-risk surgery. Chest 2001;120:1147–51.
36. Brunelli A, Xiume F, Refai M, et al. Peak oxygen consumption measured during the stair-climbing test in lung resection candidates. Respiration 2010; 80:207–11.
37. Dreher M, Walterspacher S, Sonntag F, et al. Exercise in severe COPD: is walking different from stair-climbing? Respir Med 2008;102:912–8.
38. Pollock M, Roa J, Benditt J, et al. Estimation of ventilatory reserve by stair climbing. A study in patients with chronic airflow obstruction. Chest 1993;104: 1378–83.
39. Montes de Oca M, Ortega Balza M, Lezama J, et al. [Chronic obstructive pulmo-nary disease: evaluation of exercise tolerance using three different exercise tests]. Arch Bronconeumol 2001;37:69–74 [in Spanish].
40. Singh SJ, Morgan MD, Scott S, et al. Development of a shuttle walking test of disability in patients with chronic airways obstruction. Thorax 1992;47:1019–24.
41. Luxton N, Alison JA, Wu J, et al. Relationship between field walking tests and incremental cycle ergometry in COPD. Respirology 2008;13:856–62.
42. Pepin V, Laviolette L, Brouillard C, et al. Significance of changes in endurance shuttle walking performance. Thorax 2011;66:115–20.
43. Brouillard C, Pepin V, Milot J, et al. Endurance shuttle walking test: responsive-ness to salmeterol in COPD. Eur Respir J 2008;31:579–84.
44. Bedard ME, Brouillard C, Pepin V, et al. Tiotropium improves walking endurance in chronic obstructive pulmonary disease. Eur Respir J 2012;39(2):265–71.
45. Pinto-Plata VM, Celli-Cruz RA, Vassaux C, et al. Differences in cardiopulmonary exercise test results by American Thoracic Society/European Respiratory Society-Global Initiative for Chronic Obstructive Lung Disease stage categories and gender. Chest 2007;132:1204–11.
46. Cortopassi F, Divo M, Pinto-Plata V, et al. Resting handgrip force and impaired cardiac function at rest and during exercise in COPD patients. Respir Med 2011;105:748–54.
47. Montes de Oca M, Rassulo J, Celli BR. Respiratory muscle and cardiopulmonary function during exercise in very severe COPD. Am J Respir Crit Care Med 1996; 154:1284–9.

48. O'Donnell DE, Revill SM, Webb KA. Dynamic hyperinflation and exercise intolerance in chronic obstructive pulmonary disease. Am J Respir Crit Care Med 2001; 164:770–7.

49. Vassaux C, Torre-Bouscoulet L, Zeineldine S, et al. Effects of hyperinflation on the oxygen pulse as a marker of cardiac performance in COPD. Eur Respir J 2008; 32:1275–82.

50. Crisafulli E, Costi S, Luppi F, et al. Role of comorbidities in a cohort of patients with COPD undergoing pulmonary rehabilitation. Thorax 2008;63:487–92.

51. Dolmage TE, Goldstein RS. Effects of one-legged exercise training of patients with COPD. Chest 2008;133:370–6.

52. Johnson JE, Gavin DJ, Adams-Dramiga S. Effects of training with heliox and noninvasive positive pressure ventilation on exercise ability in patients with severe COPD. Chest 2002;122:464–72.

53. Van Nostrand D, Kjelsberg MO, Humphrey EW. Preresectional evaluation of risk from pneumonectomy. Surg Gynecol Obstet 1968;127:306–12.

54. Olsen GN, Bolton JW, Weiman DS, et al. Stair climbing as an exercise test to predict the postoperative complications of lung resection. Two years' experience. Chest 1991;99:587–90.

55. Holden DA, Rice TW, Stelmach K, et al. Exercise testing, 6-min walk, and stair climb in the evaluation of patients at high risk for pulmonary resection. Chest 1992;102:1774–9.

Defining Patient-Reported Outcomes in Chronic Obstructive Pulmonary Disease
The Patient-Centered Experience

Jonathan P. Singer, MD, MS[a],*, Roger D. Yusen, MD, MPH[b]

KEYWORDS

- Chronic obstructive pulmonary disease • Health-related quality of life • Utility
- Disability • Patient-reported outcomes

KEY POINTS

- Patients with chronic obstructive pulmonary disease (COPD) have reduced health-related quality of life (HRQOL), and HRQOL worsens as COPD progresses.
- Measures of HRQOL can serve as measures of disease severity and predict outcomes.
- These measures are sensitive to change following interventions, and can thus be used as measures of intervention effect.

INTRODUCTION

The impact of chronic obstructive pulmonary disease (COPD) on global morbidity and mortality makes it one of the most important diseases in the world.[1] COPD has now become the third most frequent cause of death in the United States.[2]

COPD progresses with or without therapy. Research has only identified a few therapies that slow disease progression or reduce mortality, and these include smoking cessation,[3] oxygen therapy for hypoxemia,[4] and lung volume reduction therapy or lung transplantation for select cases.[5] A cure for COPD remains elusive. Thus, important goals for disease management consist of improving quality of life (QOL) through symptom relief, optimization of functioning, and avoidance of adverse consequences of therapies.[6]

Patients, clinicians, and investigators alike recognize the primacy of improving QOL. Regulatory agencies have begun to demand that clinical trials of therapies for patients

[a] Division of Pulmonary, Critical Care, Allergy and Sleep Medicine and Cardiovascular Research Institute, University of California, San Francisco, 350 Parnassus, Suite 609, San Francisco, CA 94117, USA; [b] Divisions of Pulmonary and Critical Care Medicine and General Medical Sciences, Washington University, St Louis, MO, USA
* Corresponding author.
E-mail address: jon.singer@ucsf.edu

Med Clin N Am 96 (2012) 767–787
doi:10.1016/j.mcna.2012.05.005
0025-7125/12/$ – see front matter © 2012 Elsevier Inc. All rights reserved.

with COPD incorporate patient-centered outcomes as end points.[7] Despite the widespread recognition of the importance of QOL, defining the patient experience and the impact of COPD on QOL remains challenging.[8] Various ways exist to define, assess, and interpret the patient experience and QOL. This review defines measures of the patient experience (eg, QOL), discusses characteristics of instruments used in research and clinical trials to measure QOL, and reports findings of studies that assessed QOL of patients with COPD.

DEFINING THE PATIENT EXPERIENCE AND PATIENT-REPORTED OUTCOMES

Experts have coined the phrase patient-reported outcomes (PRO) to describe a measure of a patient's health status directly elicited from the patient.[9] Multiple instruments that measure PROs exist. Classification of PROs range from unidimensional symptom scales, which include the Baseline Dyspnea Index[10] (BDI), the Modified Medical Research Council (MMRC) Dyspnea Scale,[11] and the University of California, San Diego, Shortness of Breath Questionnaire (UCSD SOBQ),[12] as well as multidimensional health-related QOL (HRQOL) instruments. HRQOL instruments are further classified as generic (or general), such as the Medical Outcome Study 36-item Short-Form Health Survey[13] (SF-36) and the Sickness Impact Profile (SIP),[14] or disease specific, such as the St George's Respiratory Questionnaire (SGRQ).[15]

DEFINING AND MEASURING HRQOL

QOL has multiple conceptual dimensions; factors that affect it include financial status, social support, physical environment, health, spirituality, and access to basic needs such as food, water, and housing.[16] The World Health Organization (WHO) conceptualizes QOL as an "individuals' perception of their position in life in the context of the culture and value systems in which they live and in relation to their goals, expectations, standards, and concerns."[17] The medical field concentrates on a more restrictive concept of health-related QOL, which focuses specifically on the effects of health, illness, and consequent medical therapy on QOL. Similar to QOL, HRQOL has multiple dimensions that encompass domains that include symptoms, physical functioning, cognitive performance, psychosocial conditions, emotional status, and adaptation to disease.[16]

Theoretic constructs of HRQOL drive much of the development of instruments used to measure HRQOL.[18] Because of the multidimensionality of HRQOL, researchers typically select items (ie, questions) for HRQOL measurement instruments to test the impact of health and illness on different dimensions. For example, in the SGRQ, an HRQOL instrument designed for patients with asthma or COPD, items include questions on symptoms (eg, cough, dyspnea), activity (eg, capacity for walking), and the subjective impact of COPD on a patient's physical and emotional status.[15]

Clinical trials that have HRQOL as an outcome should use reliable, valid, responsive, and discriminative HRQOL instruments (**Table 1**).[18] Among other things, a reliable instrument repeatedly yields the same results when administered in similar settings (eg, stable clinical status and same interviewer). A valid instrument measures what it purports to measure. Multiples types of validity exist, and the overall body of evidence supports the degree of validity of an instrument. A responsive instrument has the ability to detect small but clinically relevant changes that follow a change in clinical status or therapy over time. The discriminative ability of an HRQOL instrument refers to the ability of the instrument to separate individuals with differing degrees of impairment. Psychometrics is a specialized field concerned with the development and assessment of PROs, including HRQOL instruments, and psychometric properties of instruments determine their quality.

Table 1
Important measurement properties of patient-reported outcome assessment tools

Measurement Property	Method of Assessment	Description	Considerations
Reliability	Test-retest reproducibility	Stability of scores when the person undergoing testing has not experienced a change in the concept of interest	Most important type of reliability for instruments used in clinical trials
	Internal consistency	Extent to which the different items (ie, questions) consistently measure the same underlying construct (eg, Cronbach coefficient α)	Internal consistency alone is not sufficient evidence of reliability
	Interinterviewer agreement	Agreement between responses when an instrument is administered to the same person by different interviewers	Only relevant to instruments administered by an interviewer
Validity	Content, face validity / Construct validity	Completeness, relevance, and comprehensibility of items in assessing the concept of interest	Difficult to answer quantitatively; requires the use of qualitative methods
	Convergent validity	Correlation with other measures of related constructs in the hypothesized manner, consistent with the proposed conceptual framework	Referent measures may be previously validated PROs or non-PRO measures
	Divergent, discriminant validity	Lack of correlation with measures that are intend to be different or conceptually distinct	—
	Predictive validity	Ability to accurately predict future health status or other relevant outcomes	—
Responsiveness (longitudinal validity)	Calculation of responsiveness statistic (eg, effect size)	Ability to detect changes in the measured concept over time, usually in response to a specific intervention or known change in health	Responsiveness of an instrument may depend on the time interval
Interpretability	MID or MCID	Smallest difference in score that is considered meaningful to patients and clinically relevant	MID may be determined by different methods; may vary for different subpopulations

Abbreviations: MCID, minimal clinically important difference; MID, minimum important difference.
Adapted from Chen H, Taichman DB, Doyle RL. Health-related quality of life and patient-reported outcomes in pulmonary arterial hypertension. Proc Am Thorac Soc 2008;5:623–30.

Researchers classify instruments for measuring HRQOL as generic or specific for a particular disease. Both generic and disease-specific HRQOL instruments have advantages and limitations. Developers of generic instruments for measuring HRQOL, such as the SF-36 and the SIP, designed them to have broad applicability across different diseases, which allows comparisons of the impact of different diseases on HRQOL across the multiple conceptual dimensions of HRQOL. Some instruments (eg, SF-36) have established population norms for healthy persons. Because treatments may cause systemic effects, generic HRQOL instruments may also better detect the overall impact of treatment side effects than organ/disease-specific HRQOL instruments. The breadth of generic instruments also creates the disadvantage of decreasing sensitivity for detecting changes in HRQOL in diseases in which certain conceptual dimensions dominate the impact on QOL. For example, although persons with COPD often have the particularly troubling symptoms of dyspnea and cough, few items in generic HRQOL instruments focus on these symptoms. Thus, generic HRQOL instruments may not detect small but clinically significant improvements related to such disease-specific symptoms.

Disease-specific HRQOL measures focus on that specific disease, and its treatments affect QOL. Disease-specific HRQOL measurement may involve the assessment of symptoms, functioning, and the impact of symptoms and functioning on social and role function and emotional status. Disease-specific measures complement the advantages and disadvantages of generic measures in that they may have greater responsiveness to change and ability to discriminate among individuals with differing degrees of impairment for a specific disease. By definition, disease-specific instruments do not broadly apply to other diseases; they have a lower responsiveness to the systemic effects of a disease or treatment on changes in HRQOL.[18]

ACCOUNTING FOR PATIENT PREFERENCES

Utility assessment involves the quantitative measurement of how patients feel about health outcomes. Utilities, which can capture degree of impairment, degree of bother, and willingness to undergo risk to reduce bother, offer an important means for measuring QOL and the effects of interventions.

Similar to other HRQOL instruments, generic and disease-specific utility instruments exist, but they also have unique advantages. Utility scores typically range on a continuum from 0 (eg, death or worst health state) to 1 (ideal health). Because utility measures account for death, studies that use utility measurement to evaluate HRQOL do not have the selection bias of only including living patients in the analyses. In addition, utility data support the estimation of quality-adjusted life-years (QALYs), which take into consideration quantity as well as QOL consequences of illnesses and their treatments.[19,20] For example, the QALYs of a person living 2 years with a health state of 0.3 are considered equivalent to those of another person living 1 year with a health state of 0.6 and then dying ($2 \times 0.3 = [1 \times 0.6] + [1 \times 0]$). Preference-based utility measurement may play an important role in the evaluation of high-risk interventions such as lung volume reduction surgery or lung transplantation.[21–23] By determining QALYs, researchers can use utilities to determine the cost-effectiveness or cost-utility of interventions.[24]

Researchers can measure preferences for a health state directly from the subject or indirectly from a population sample's preferences. Examples of direct utility assessment include Standard Gamble,[25] Visual Analog Scale, Time-Trade-Off, and Willingness to Pay. Examples of indirect utility assessment include the Quality of Well-Being (QWB) Scale,[26] EuroQol 5D (EQ-5D),[27] and Health Utility Index (HUI).[28] Other publications have summarized the relative merits of using direct or indirect measures of subject preferences (**Table 2**).[29–31]

Table 2
Characteristics of commonly used patient-reported outcome assessment tools for patients with COPD

Instrument	Items (n)	Administration and Estimated Completion Time (min)	Domains/ Dimensions/ Attributes Assessed	Domains Scored; Possible Range (Worst to Best); MID
Generic				
Medical Outcomes Study SF Health Survey	12, 20 or 36 (eg, SF-36)	Self or interviewer; 5–15	Physical functioning Role limitations caused by physical health Bodily pain General health Vitality Social functioning Role limitations caused by mental health Mental health	PCS: 0–100 MCS: 0–100 Individual domains: 0–100 MID: 5–15 (varies per domain)
Nottingham Health Profile	38	Self; 5–10	Physical mobility Pain Social isolation Emotional reactions Energy Sleep	Individual domains 100–0, no overall score MID: unknown
Sickness Impact Profile	136	Self or interviewer; 20–30	Ambulation Mobility Body care/ movement Communication Alertness behavior Emotional behavior Social interaction Sleep and rest Eating Work Home management Recreation and pastimes	Physical dimension Psychosocial dimensions Individual categories Overall score, range 0–100 MID: unknown
COPD specific				
SGRQ	50	Self; 10–15	Symptoms Activities Impact	Individual domains, overall score 100–0 MID: 4
CRQ	20	Interviewer, 20	Dyspnea Fatigue Emotional function Mastery	Individual domains 1–7 Summary score 1–7 MID: 0.5
UCSD SOBQ	24	Self or interviewer, 5–10	Dyspnea Fear	120–0

(continued on next page)

Table 2
(continued)

Instrument	Items (n)	Administration and Estimated Completion Time (min)	Domains/ Dimensions/ Attributes Assessed	Domains Scored; Possible Range (Worst to Best); MID
Modified Medical Research Council Dyspnea Scale	1	Self, 1	Dyspnea	4–0
BDI/TDI		Self, interviewer, or computerized,	Functional impairment Magnitude of task needed to evoke dyspnea Magnitude of effort needed to evoke dyspnea	0–12 for BDI −9 to 9 for TDI
Multiattribute or Preference-Based Utility				
Indirect				
EQ-5D	5	Self or interviewer, 2	Mobility Self-care Usual activities Pain/discomfort Anxiety/ depression	0–1; 0, death or worst possible health state, 1, best possible health state
QWB	18	Interviewer, 7–10	Mobility and confinement Physical activity Social activity	0–1 0, death or worst possible health state, 1, best possible health state
HUI Mark 3	31	Self or interviewer, 2–5	Vision Hearing Speech Ambulation Dexterity Emotion Cognition Pain	0–1 0, death or worst possible health state, 1, best possible health state
Direct				
Standard Gamble	NA	Interviewer	Disease specific or general	0–1 0, death or worst possible health state, 1, best possible health state
Other				
Visual Analog Scale	1	Self	Disease specific or general	0–100

Abbreviations: BDI/TDI, Baseline Dyspnea Index; CRQ, Chronic Respiratory Disease Questionnaire; EQ-5D, EuroQol 5D; HUI, Health Utility Index; MCS, mental component summary; MID, minimum important difference; PCS, physical component summary; QWB, Quality of Well Being Scale; SF, short form; SGRQ, St George's Respiratory Questionnaire; TDI, Transitional Dyspnea Index; UCSD SOBQ, UC San Diego Shortness of Breath Questionnaire.

INTERPRETING HRQOL MEASURES

The interpretation of HRQOL outcomes should include the determination of statistical and clinical significance. Some HRQOL instruments have undergone study to define the smallest clinically relevant or meaningful change for a patient (ie, minimum important difference [MID]). However, studies may show changes in HRQOL scores that exceed the MID but fail to achieve statistical significance. In some cases, the non–statistically significant outcome may have resulted because of inadequate statistical power to detect differences. If a larger sample size had been studied, the negative (not statistically significant) result may have turned out to be positive (statistically significant).

Some controversy exists around the interpretation of HRQOL summary scores. In addition to summary scores, many multidimensional instruments have profile or dimension scores that represent specific health concepts. For example, in addition to physical and mental summary scores, the SF-36 has profile scores for each of the 8 health concepts evaluated: physical functioning, role physical, bodily pain, general health, vitality, social functioning, role emotional, and mental health. Studies therefore can present HRQOL data in a summary score or in multiple profile scores. Some proponents of separately presenting scores of the different dimensions base their argument on the multidimensional nature of HRQOL.[18] They argue that innumerable combinations of profile scores to produce a summary score does not provide interpretable information. Although proponents of the summary score approach acknowledge this limitation, they argue that making real-life decisions often requires comparing single scores.[18] Thus, clinical trials evaluating medical technologies commonly use summary scores.

Interventional studies in patients with COPD commonly show significant changes in physiologic outcomes (eg, forced expiratory volume in 1 second [FEV_1]) without showing changes in HRQOL, and vice versa. Interventions that effect positive changes in subjective dyspnea, cough, exercise capacity, or depression/anxiety may not necessarily affect physiologic measures of lung function. Thus, HRQOL end points complement physiologic end points, and they allow the assessment of outcomes that matter most to patients. They also increase the ability to detect positive, clinically meaningful outcomes in clinical trials.

Many methods for estimating the effects of treatment on HRQOL fail to formally account for subjects who die or drop out of a study. If those who die or drop out had worse HRQOL than those who remained alive and continued follow-up in the study, then this limitation introduces bias that can lead to erroneously favorable estimates of HRQOL. The risk of bias increases with higher dropout or death rates (eg, interventions that carry significant mortality risk, such as lung transplantation). Statistical imputation techniques address this bias by substituting estimates for missing data.[32] The worst-case scenario or extreme case analysis imputation method assigns study participants who die or drop out the poorest possible HRQOL score. As an alternative, studies can use the previously described utility measures that account for both survival and subject preference for health states to estimate HRQOL. In doing so, the HRQOL estimates include scores for the patients who died (typically assigned a subject preference score of 0). As with non–utility-based HRQOL assessment, studies using utility assessment should also address how to deal with missing data not caused by death.

PREDICTIVE MODELS

Researchers have developed important multidimensional predictive models that incorporate PROs for patients with COPD. Three predictive models, the Body-Mass Index,

Degree of Airflow Obstruction and Dyspnea, and Exercise Capacity (BODE),[33] the modified BODE (mBODE),[34] and the Age, Dyspnea, Obstruction (ADO)[35] indices incorporate a combination of physiologic measures and symptom scores. The BODE index uses a 10-point scale that incorporates body mass index (B), airflow obstruction as measured by FEV_1 percent predicted (O), dyspnea as measured by the MMRC Dyspnea Scale (D), and exercise capacity as measured by the 6-minute walk test (E). Higher BODE scores predict risk of death.[33] The mBODE replaces the MMRC Dyspnea Scale with the UCSD SOBQ as the dyspnea (D) measure.[34] Recognizing that predictors may have differential impacts on risk of mortality, investigators developed the weighted ADO index, which incorporates age (A), dyspnea as measured by either the German Chronic Respiratory Questionnaire or the Spanish translation of the MMRC Dyspnea Scale (D), and airflow obstruction as measured by FEV_1 (O).[35] The ADO index uses a 10-point scale. When developing the index, each predictor was found to have a different quantitative impact on risk of death. To account for the finding that each predictor had a different quantitative impact on risk of death, the ADO index weights each predictor based on regression coefficients. In addition to predicting risk of death relative to a referent group, the ADO index can calculate an absolute risk of death for an individual patient. Researchers who conduct large epidemiologic studies of lung disease do not routinely have measures of lung function and exercise capacity uniformly available. Developers of the COPD Severity Score[36] instrument addressed this problem. The COPD Severity Score measures 5 aspects of COPD severity that include respiratory symptoms, systemic corticosteroid use, other COPD medication use, previous hospitalization or intubation, and use of home oxygen to produce a multidimensional 35-point index. It accounts for current symptoms and the therapy needed to achieve the current symptom status. Because the COPD Severity Score does not use measures of lung function or exercise capacity, researchers may administer it by telephone survey. Examples of the predictive abilities of these instruments are presented later.

HRQOL IN COPD

Most studies evaluating PROs in patients with COPD are in 1 of 3 general categories: (1) cross-sectional studies that correlate PROs with physiologic measures, (2) studies that evaluate the impact of COPD on PROs, and (3) interventional trials that use PROs as outcome measures to evaluate the impact of pharmacologic and nonpharmacologic therapies.[16]

ASSOCIATIONS OF PROs WITH PHYSIOLOGIC MEASURES

The negative effects of COPD on HRQOL become more pronounced as COPD severity worsens.[37,38] Disease-specific HRQOL instruments discriminate more than generic HRQOL instruments among different levels of COPD severity. However, multiple studies have shown that correlations between HRQOL and FEV_1 only range from modest[39] to poor.[40] For example, in a study of 120 participants with different Global Obstructive Lung Disease (GOLD) stages (GOLD I has best lung function and GOLD IV has worst) of COPD, Pickard and colleagues[37] showed that SGRQ scores (range 0–100, with higher scores representing poorer HRQOL) were markedly worse in GOLD stage III (52.2 ± 19.6) and IV (54.1 ± 13.5) compared with GOLD stage I (28.8 ± 15.0) and II (37.2 ± 18.6). Exercise capacity, as measured by the 6-minute walk distance (6MWD), often shows a stronger correlated with HRQOL than FEV_1[15] or oxygenation.[41]

COPD has systemic consequences that affect functioning.[42] Because HRQOL has multiple dimensions, extrapulmonary factors should also correlate with HRQOL in patients with COPD. Subjects with COPD at the extremes of weight and those with low lean body mass have all shown poorer HRQOL that those with less extreme weight.[43] Low lean body mass may reflect sarcopenia and frailty, both of which affect exercise capacity. Poorer leg strength, a reflection of both deconditioning and sarcopenia, negatively affects exercise capacity as measured by 6MWD.[44] Exercise capacity modestly correlates with HRQOL.[45,46] Beyond muscle impairments, patients with COPD often have extrapulmonary comorbidities that include cardiovascular disease, diabetes, and insomnia. Of those comorbidities, insomnia and musculoskeletal disorders most strongly correlate with HRQOL.[47,48] Although the effects of individual comorbidities other than insomnia and musculoskeletal disorders do not noticeably affect HRQOL, the effect of multiple comorbidities in subjects with COPD modestly to weakly correlate with poorer HRQOL.[47–49]

Patients with COPD frequently suffer from anxiety and depression, and these conditions have undergone much investigation. Studies have found a prevalence of anxiety or depression in patients with COPD that ranges from 6% to 50%.[50] More recent studies report a higher prevalence of 42% to 57% of depressive symptoms.[51,52] In a cohort of stable Veterans Affairs outpatients with chronic breathing problems including COPD, 80% of 1334 subjects were positive on a brief telephone screen for anxiety, depression, or both.[53] Of those, 80% were ultimately found to have anxiety, depression, or both during formal evaluation. In addition, depressed patients with COPD are more likely to be ongoing smokers[54] and are less likely to quit after completing smoking cessation programs.[55] Compared with nondepressed patients with COPD, depressed patients with COPD spend more days admitted to the hospital,[56] have worse HRQOL,[57] and may have higher mortality.[58] Depression and anxiety have strong independent and combined associations with poorer HRQOL in patients with COPD.

THE IMPACT OF COPD ON PROs

Acute exacerbations of COPD, manifest as increased cough, sputum production, and dyspnea, have immediate negative effects on HRQOL. Studies consistently reported poor HRQOL SGRQ domain scores ranging from 41 to 80 during acute exacerbations.[59–61] During acute COPD exacerbations, patients also show poor scores in certain SF-36 that include physical component, general health, vitality, and role emotional domain scores.[59] The number of acute exacerbations in the prior year has a strong association with poorer HRQOL during any subsequent acute exacerbations. For example, Doll and colleagues[62] reported on 162 subjects tested during an acute exacerbation. Those with 0 to 1 exacerbations in the prior year had SGRQ total scores of 40.1 ± 21.0 compared with scores of 58.5 ± 18.6 in those subjects who had experienced 5 or more exacerbations. SGRQ scores increased (ie, worsened) linearly for those who had 2, 3, or 4 exacerbations in the prior year. Further, poorer SGRQ scores have a significant association with subsequent readmission to the hospital.[63] As patients recover from the exacerbation, HRQOL scores improve. Doll and colleagues[62] reported that, in the 162 subjects tested during acute exacerbation, SGRQ total scores improved by nearly 7 points as patients recovered (6.92 ± 19.23, $P<.001$).

HRQOL also predicts important health outcomes. Poorer HRQOL predicts subsequent hospitalizations for COPD, independent of age, lung function, and gender. For 266 middle-aged to older aged adults with COPD in the United Kingdom, for each 5-point decrement in SGRQ score, subjects had an approximately 15% increased risk of hospitalization in the ensuing 12 months[63] Similarly, in a United States longitudinal cohort study of 1202 middle-aged adults with COPD, each 1 standard deviation worsening in baseline disease-specific HRQOL was associated with a 40% increased risk of subsequent hospitalization for COPD; a similar decrement in generic HRQOL conferred a 60% increased risk.[64] Additionally, Domingo-Salvany and colleagues[65] reported that poorer HRQOL independently predicts mortality after controlling for age, FEV_1, and body mass index. In a cohort of 312 men with COPD, the investigators showed that a 1 standard deviation worsening in SGRQ total score or SF-36 Physical Component Summary score conferred a 30% increase in overall mortality. Further, a 4-point increase in the SGRQ, a minimally important difference change, resulted in a 5.1% increase in overall mortality (95% confidence interval [CI] 0.97–9.4%). Marin and colleagues[66] showed that subjects with COPD and poor baseline HRQOL have markedly poorer survival than those with a higher baseline HRQOL. After 10 years of follow-up, persons in the poorest quartile of baseline SGRQ scores had an overall mortality of approximately 70%, compared with a mortality of approximately 30% for those in the highest quartile.

Regarding the prognostic models for patients with COPD, in the landmark study that defined the BODE index, Celli and colleagues[33] showed that each 1 point increase in baseline BODE score was associated with a 34% increase in the risk of death within 2 years (hazard ratio [HR] 1.34, 95% CI 1.26–1.42; $P<.0001$). The BODE score better predicts death than FEV_1 alone.[67] However, in cohorts of Swiss and Spanish subjects with COPD, the BODE index underestimated 3-year mortality in older patients (age >70 years) with severe COPD (GOLD stage IV) and overestimated 3-year mortality in older patients with at least moderate COPD ($\geq$GOLD stage II) with a first hospital admission for a COPD exacerbation.[35] The mBODE also predicts mortality. Investigators from the National Emphysema Treatment Trial (NETT) showed that subjects experiencing a greater than 1-point increase in mBODE score 6 months after randomization (lung volume reduction surgery [LVRS] vs medical management) had a 2-fold higher risk of mortality over the 2-year follow-up period (HR 2.35; 95% CI 1.71–3.23; $P<.001$). Subjects experiencing a greater than 1-point decrease (improvement) in mBODE score 6 months after randomization had a 40% lower risk of mortality over the 2 year follow-up period (HR 0.57; 95% CI 0.41–0.78; $P<.001$).[68] Higher baseline ADO scores (range 0–10) predict subsequent mortality. For each 1-point increase in ADO score, the odds of death within 3 years increase by 42% (odds ratio 1.42; 95% CI 1.19–1.69; $P<.05$).[35] The COPD Severity Score correlates with other measures of general and disease-specific HRQOL, and it predicts acute exacerbations and hospitalizations for COPD (**Table 3**).[69]

INTERVENTIONS THAT AFFECT HRQOL
Pharmacologic

Recognizing the importance of HRQOL as trial end points, many large pharmacologic and surgical interventional trials have included HRQOL measures as secondary outcomes and a few have used them as primary outcomes. Studies typically do not have adequate power to detect significant differences in secondary outcomes. However, lack of evidence does not necessarily imply lack of benefit. A full review of the impact of medications on HRQOL is beyond the scope of this article, so it focuses on reviewing some of the large multicenter randomized controlled trials (RCTs).

Several large interventional trials have evaluated the impact of inhaled medications on disease-specific HRQOL in patients with COPD. The Inhaled Steroids in Obstructive Lung Disease in Europe (ISOLDE) trial was the first long-term multicenter randomized controlled study of inhaled corticosteroids in patients with COPD. The study randomized 751 participants to either inhaled fluticasone propionate or placebo.

Table 3
Characteristics of multidimensional COPD severity grading instruments

Instrument	Components	Points Assigned for Given Value	Range (Best to Worst)
BODE	Body mass index (kg/m^2)	>21 = 0 points; ≤21 = 1	0–10
	FEV$_1$ % predicted	≥65 = 0 points; 50–64 = 1; 36–49 = 2; ≤35 = 3	
	MMRC dyspnea scale	0–1 = 0 points; 2 = 1; 3 =2; 4 = 3	
	6MWD (m)	≥350 = 0; 250–349 = 1; 150–249 = 2; ≤149 = 3	
mBODE	Body-mass index (kg/m^2)	>21 = 0 points; ≤21 = 1	0–10
	FEV$_1$ % predicted	≥65 = 0 points; 50–64 = 1; 36–49 = 2; ≤35 = 3	
	UCSD SOBQ	≤52 = 0 points; 53–63 = 1; 64–77 =2; ≥78 = 3	
	6MWD (m)	≥350 = 0; 250–349 = 1; 150–249 = 2; ≤149 = 3	
ADO	Age (y)	40–49 = 0 points; 50–59 = 1; 60–69 = 2; 70–79 = 3	0–10
	MMRC dyspnea scale	0–1 = 0 points; 2 = 1; 3 =2; 4 = 3	
	FEV$_1$ % predicted	≥65 = 0 points; 50–64 = 1; 36–49 = 2; ≤35 = 3	
COPD Severity Score	Respiratory symptoms (maximum 7 points)	Dyspnea on exertion, current • None = 0; hurrying on level ground or walking uphill = 1; walking with peers on level ground = 2; walking at own pace on level ground = 2 Dyspnea during past 14 d or nights • None = 1; 1–2 d or nights = 1; 3–6 = 2; 7–13 = 3; every day or night = 4	0–35
	Systemic corticosteroid use (maximum 5 points)	Ever used = 1; ≥3 times a week for ≥3 mo during last year = 3; used in the past 2 wk = 1	
	Other medication use (maximum 10 points)	Metered-dose inhaler use, past 2 wk • Short-acting β-agonists = 1; long-acting β-agonists = 1; inhaled corticosteroids = 1; ipratropium bromide =1 Nebulizer use, past 2 wk • Short-acting β-agonists = 1; ipratropium bromide = 1 Oral medications, past 2 wk • β-agonists = 1; theophylline = 1 Oral antibiotics for lung condition, past 12 mo • 1–2 courses = 1; ≥3 courses = 2	
	Hospitalization/intubation/oxygen use (maximum 13 points)	Hospitalized for COPD, past 5 y = 3 Intubated for COPD, past 5 y = 5 Home oxygen, current day or nighttime use = 5	

Although the study used the rate of decline in FEV_1 over 3 years 3as its primary outcome, it included acute exacerbations and SGRQ scores as secondary outcomes; a 4-point change in SGRQ was considered clinically important. Fluticasone did not affect the rate of decline in FEV_1, although it did reduce rate of acute exacerbations by 25% ($P = .026$). Although HRQOL declined in both randomized treatment groups, the fluticasone group took longer to deteriorate (SGRQ of ≥ 4 points) than did the placebo group ($P = .004$). The withdrawal rates over the 3-year study of 43% in the fluticasone group and 53% in the placebo group raise questions about bias when interpreting these outcome data.[70] Poor reporting of deaths over the study period may also have introduced selection bias.

Several modest-sized studies showed that tiotroprium, a long-acting antimuscarinic agent, improved exacerbation rates, dyspnea, and HRQOL.[71–73] The Understanding the Potential Long-Term Impacts on Function with Tiotropium (UPLIFT) 4-year, double-blind, multicenter, international interventional trial randomized 5593 subjects with COPD to either once-daily tiotropium or placebo.[74] UPLIFT used end points similar to those used in ISOLDE The tiotropium group maintained a modest, statistically significant improvement in FEV_1 compared with the placebo group (87–103 mL before bronchodilator use and 47 to 65 mL after bronchodilator use) over the course of the trial. The 2 randomized treatment groups showed a similar rates of decline in HRQOL as measured by the SGRQ. The tiotropium group overall had a significant improvement in SGRQ compared with placebo of between 2.2 to 3.3 points in each of the 4 years analyzed that did not meet the clinically important difference (all P-values <0.001). Analyzing change in a dichotomous fashion, a greater proportion of subjects in the tiotropium group had a clinically meaningful improvement of 4 points or more in the SGRQ in each of the 4 years of follow-up (all P-values <0.001). Analyses used random-effects modeling and included patients with at least 2 postrandomization SGRQ measures (every 6 months after randomization); imputation was not performed. The impact of death on HRQOL was not considered. Compared with the placebo group, the tiotropium group showed a delay in time to first exacerbation, mean number of exacerbations, and time to hospitalization for exacerbation, and these may have accounted for some of the observed improvement in HRQOL.

Many studies have evaluated combination therapy. In a randomized, double-blind, placebo-controlled trial of 1465 patients studied repeatedly over 12 months, Calverley and colleagues[75] showed that combined therapy with salmeterol and fluticasone propionate reduced exacerbations and improved HRQOL by a clinically meaningful difference (≥ 4-point improvement in SGRQ) compared with placebo. Although repeated-measures analyses were used, the impact of death on HRQOL was not considered. The Toward a Revolution in COPD Health (TORCH) multiarm, double-blind, placebo-controlled, randomized multinational trial compared combined salmeterol and fluticasone propionate with each component alone and with placebo over a 3-year period. The study used all-cause mortality as the primary end point; secondary end points included exacerbation frequency and HRQOL as measured by the SGRQ. Of the 6184 subjects randomized to each of the 4 groups, between 851 and 1011 subjects in each group completed the study. The study came close to showing a reduction in mortality in the combination treatment group compared with placebo (HR 0.825; 95% CI 0.681–1.002; $P = .052$). Subjects on combination therapy had fewer COPD exacerbations and hospitalizations. Subjects experienced an improvement in the SGRQ score (3.1 points averaged over 3 years) that was statistically significant but not clinically meaningful (defined by at least a 4.0-point change). Subjects in each treatment arm manifested the greatest magnitude of improvement in the SGRQ within the first 6 months of the trial. Thereafter, the SGRQ scores worsened.

At the end of 3 years, subjects receiving combination therapy had an improvement in SGRQ of approximately 1.7 points compared with baseline versus a worsening of approximately 2.3 points in the placebo group. Those excluded from the HRQOL analyses included 25% of subjects who received placebo, and 19% of subjects who received combination therapy did not complete the HRQOL questionnaires. It is unlikely that the data were missing at random, and the impact of the data being missing remains unknown. As in other studies, death rates and missing data likely affected HRQOL results in ways that are difficult to predict. Therefore, data from these trials should undergo cautious interpretation because they reflect only those subjects alive and well enough to complete the survey instruments.

As discussed earlier, acute exacerbations are associated with poorer HRQOL. In addition to modest improvements in FEV_1, the pharmacologic trials such as UPLIFT,[74] TORCH,[76] and MACRO (Macrolide Azithromycin to Prevent Rapid Worsening of Symptoms Associated With Chronic Obstructive Pulmonary Disease; azithromycin vs placebo)[77] all reduced the number of acute exacerbations in patients with COPD. Although difficult to predict, the reduction in acute exacerbations observed in these trials may explain some of the improved HRQOL observed in these trials.

Supplemental Oxygen

The landmark Nocturnal Oxygen Therapy Trial (NOTT) showed a mortality benefit of long-term oxygen therapy for hypoxemic patients with COPD.[4] The study randomized 203 subjects with COPD and resting oxygen tension on arterial blood gas (PaO_2) less than or equal to 55 mm Hg or less than or equal to 59 mm Hg and features of pulmonary hypertension to either continuous or nocturnal oxygen therapy. The study measured generic HRQOL with the SIP. The group randomized to supplemental oxygen had improved HRQOL compared with the group not randomized to supplemental oxygen, although the manuscript did not show the magnitude of difference.

Ambulatory oxygen may improve HRQOL in persons who have exertional oxyhemoglobin desaturation.[78] The double-blind, crossover study over 12 weeks randomized 50 patients who did not fulfill criteria for long-term oxygen therapy (LTOT), based on a resting oxygen tension on arterial blood gas less than or equal to 55 mm Hg or exertional desaturation to SaO_2 less than or equal to 88%, to either supplemental oxygen at 4 L/min or no supplemental oxygen (tank with room air inspired oxygen concentration) after completion of a formal pulmonary rehabilitation program. For 6 weeks, study participants used a flow rate of 4 L/min for any activity during which they would normally experience dyspnea; after 6 weeks, they crossed over to using either oxygen or air. The study used the Chronic Respiratory Questionnaire (CRQ) (disease-specific) and the SF-36 to assess HRQOL. Use of oxygen affected statistical improvements in each CRQ domain, although the study failed to achieve the prespecified MIDs. The study showed significant improvements associated with oxygen therapy in SF-36 domains of role physical, general health, social functioning, and role emotional.

Pulmonary Rehabilitation

Beyond declines in lung function that manifest as dyspnea and limited exercise capacity, COPD results in systemic functional limitations that lead to physical deconditioning. This physical deconditioning further increases dyspnea on exertion. Recognizing this complex interplay, pulmonary rehabilitation (PR) is designed to reduce symptoms, decrease disability, and improve HRQOL. The multifaceted PR incorporates education, exercise training, and psychosocial/behavioral interventions. In the second update of a Cochrane Review, Lacasse and colleagues[79] performed a meta-analysis of 31 RCTs that convincingly showed that formal PR achieves its goals of reducing patient-reported dyspnea, fatigue, perceived control over their disease, improved exercise capacity, and both disease-specific and generic HRQOL. The review included RCTs with formal exercise programs lasting at least 4 weeks. Of 31 RCTs, 11 measured HRQOL with validated disease-specific HRQOL instruments. These 11 studies used either the CRQ or the SGRQ. PR led to a change in each domain of the CRQ tested (fatigue, emotional function, mastery, and dyspnea) that exceeded the MID of 0.5 points. Similarly, PR achieved a 6-point improvement in SGRQ total score, exceeding the 4-point MID (95% CI -8.98 to -3.24, lower scores represent improved HRQOL). The benefits of a single course of PR eventually wane.[80]

Disease Management Programs

Clinicians developed disease management programs because of the recognition that the daily responsibilities of COPD care lays with the patients and their families. Such programs are designed to improve patient outcomes through intensive education and frequent communication with COPD-trained health care providers. Patients or health care providers may manage such programs. In general, management programs include an emphasis on adherence to guidelines and use nurses with specialized training in COPD and central coordination that maintains records of communication between patients and nurse managers.[81] Disease management programs have had varied results on HRQOL. In a 1-year multicenter trial, Bourbeau and colleagues[82] randomized 96 patients to a case-management program and 95 patients to usual care. Study eligibility required participants to have had a hospitalization for an acute COPD exacerbation in the year preceding study entry. At 4 months after randomization, the disease management group had significantly better (4-point difference in SGRQ) SGRQ activity and impact domain and overall scores than the usual care group, although a significant difference in the symptom domain did not occur. At 1 year after randomization, only the disease management group showed a significantly better HRQOL (SRGQ impact domain only) compared with baseline. A separate trial of 248 patients randomized to a self-management intervention or usual care failed to show significant differences in HRQOL as measured by SGRQ.[83] In a Cochrane Review of 2239 patients in 15 group comparisons derived from 14 interventional trials, self-management programs resulted in statistically significant improvements in HRQOL at 12 months after randomization, but the interventions did not show clinically important differences in HRQOL (eg, SGRQ total score difference -2.58; 95% CI -5.14 to -0.02).[84] More recently, Chavannes and colleagues[85] randomized 152 subjects with mild to moderate COPD from primary care clinics to either usual care or an intensive case-management program. After 1 year, SGRQ scores improved in the intervention group (SGRQ -4.61; 95% CI -7.2 to -2.0; P = .001) compared with no change in the control group (SGRQ -0.7; 95% CI -3.0 to 1.6; P = .6). Those with an FEV_1/forced vital capacity ratio less than 0.7 and symptoms of dyspnea (Modified Medical Research Council Dyspnea Scale >2) had the greatest improvements (SGRQ -13.42; 95% CI -20.8 to -6.1; P = .002) compared with no change in the usual care group (SGRQ -0.3; 95% CI -5.5 to 4.9; P = .9).

Surgical Interventions: LVRS

The NETT[5] was designed to determine how LVRS affected mortality and exercise capacity compared with maximum medical therapy (MT). Secondary outcomes included disease-specific (UCSD SOBQ and SGRQ) and general (QWB) HRQOL. The investigators chose an 8-point change in SGRQ as the minimal clinically important difference, a change twice as big as that normally used in studies, in recognition of the high mortality risk associated with the intervention. After an interim analysis showed patients with the most advanced emphysema (FEV$_1$ $\leq$20% predicted and either a diffusing capacity of carbon monoxide $\leq$20% predicted or a radiographically determined homogeneous distribution of emphysema) had an unacceptably high risk of death, the NETT excluded such patients from further enrollment. The NETT chose several factors, including baseline exercise capacity and heterogeneity of emphysema distribution on computed tomography (CT) scan, a priori for subgroup analysis. The study randomized a total of 1218 patients to LVRS (608) or MT (610). As expected, patients in the LVRS group had a significantly higher 90-day mortality (7.9%, 95% CI 5.9–10.3) than the MT group (1.3%, 95% CI 0.6–2.6; P<.001). At the end of the study (median follow-up duration of 29.2 months), the 2 randomized treatment groups had similar overall mortality. Although the surgical and medical groups both showed declines in QOL during follow-up, the medical group declined more rapidly. Even in the subgroup of NETT high-risk patients, in which the LVRS group had a markedly higher death rate than the medical group, the 2 treatment groups had similar quality-adjusted survival during follow-up, showing that the higher mortality associated with LVRS was offset with gains in QOL.[86] Post hoc analyses found varying outcomes in 4 main subgroups based on exercise capacity (high vs low; low baseline exercise capacity defined as 25 W for women and 40 W for men) and distribution of emphysema on CT scan (predominantly upper lobe vs other). Only the upper lobe–predominant emphysema and low exercise capacity subgroup showed a survival benefit associated with LVRS (P<.005).The overall mortality in the LVRS group was either similar to MT or higher in the other subgroups. Thus, the investigators suggested that LVRS should be reserved for patients with upper lobe–predominant emphysema and low baseline exercise capacity. However, the information provided by HRQOL instruments suggested an alternative interpretation. First, those patients randomized to LVRS had a 5-fold higher risk of deriving improved HRQOL measured by the QWB than those randomized to MT. Further, 3 of the 4 subgroups described earlier (the exception being the group that was not upper lobe predominant/high exercise capacity) showed marked improvements in HRQOL (ORs 5.7–8.4). Variation of the imputation method chosen to address missing QOL data significantly affected the findings.[32]

The NETT investigators also evaluated QALYs gained by LVRS compared with MT alone. As previously described, QALYs incorporate both survival and HRQOL into a composite measure. After 3 years, the LVRS group experienced higher mean QALYs than the MT group (1.46 vs 1.27; P<.001).[87] The NETT investigators later reported on the same outcomes after a longer median follow-up period of 4.3 years.[88] With the longer follow-up, the non–high-risk LVRS group had a lower mortality (relative risk 0.85; P = .02); improved exercise capacity (>10 W) at 1, 2, and 3 years (all P-values <0.001); and improved disease-specific HRQOL (SGRQ $\geq$8-point improvement) up to 4 years after randomization (P-values $\leq$0.005). The proportion of patients having LVRS and achieving improved HRQOL ($\geq$8-point change in SGRQ) were 40%, 32%, 20%, and 10% after years 1, 2, 3, 4 compared with the MT improvements of 9%, 8%, 8%, and 4%. Patients who died or were missing data at each time point were considered not improved. Although the upper lobe–predominant/low exercise capacity subgroup had the largest impact of LVRS on HRQOL, even those in the upper lobe–predominant/high exercise capacity group had a 4.6-fold to 7.0-fold higher risk of improved HRQOL over 4 years of follow-up compared with the MT group (all P-values $\leq$0.003). LVRS failed to improve HRQOL only in the group that was not upper lobe predominant/low exercise capacity.

As another method to determine the impact of LVRS on both survival and HRQOL in a post hoc analysis, the NETT investigators created a composite end point of death or a clinically meaningful decline in HRQOL (8 points on SGRQ).[89] Using this composite end point, the NETT investigators showed that LVRS improved the composite survival/HRQOL end point in most patients; patients who did not derive a composite survival/HRQOL benefit were those with emphysema that was not upper lobe predominant and high perioperative mortality.

Surgical Interventions: Lung Transplantation

The primary indications for lung transplantation consist of poor HRQOL and low estimated short-term survival.[90] Several studies have shown improvements in energy and mobility, decreased anxiety and depression, and improvements in HRQOL following lung transplantation.[91–93] However, few studies have focused exclusively on the impact of lung transplantation on HRQOL in patients with COPD.[21–23] Washington University (St Louis, MO, USA) and University of Toronto (Toronto, Canada) researchers have conducted QOL cohort studies of patients with COPD undergoing lung transplantation.[94–96] The Washington University group found low pretransplant HRQOL (utility assessment via the Standard Gamble) in a cohort of 99 patients with COPD who underwent lung transplantation in the pre–lung allocation score (LAS) time-dependent donor lung allocation system. Lung transplantation conferred a large improvement in HRQOL approximately 6 months after transplantation.[96] More recently, the investigators conducted a similar study of a cohort of 114 patients with COPD in the LAS system, and observed similar findings.[95] These utility-based studies included all deaths in the analyses and used imputation to estimate the small amount of missing data. The Toronto group analyzed a convenience sample of 112 subjects with COPD in which 66 underwent lung transplantation and 55 of these completed posttransplant HRQOL assessments.[94] Those who did not complete posttransplantation HRQOL assessments were assigned the worse possible score. The patients showed poor HRQOL before transplantation, and they had significantly improved disease-specific HRQOL (assessed by the SGRQ) at approximately 4 months after lung transplantation. These short-term reports show findings consistent with a small long-term study that had significant selection bias.[97]

SUMMARY

Patients with COPD have reduced HRQOL, and HRQOL worsens as COPD progresses. Although long-term interventions such as smoking cessation, supplemental oxygen therapy for hypoxemia, LVRS, and lung transplantation may save lives, these and other therapies have variable but important effects on PROs. Measures of HRQOL can serve as measures of disease severity and predict outcome. Moreover, these measures are sensitive to change following interventions, and can thus be used as measures of intervention effect. Future research will provide a better understanding of the effects of COPD on HRQOL and the impact of various interventions.

REFERENCES

1. World Health Report. Geneva (Switzerland): World Health Organization; 2000.
2. Murphy SL, Xu J, Kochanek K. Deaths: preliminary data for 2010. National vital statistics reports. Hyattsville (MD): National Center for Health Statistics; 2012.
3. Anthonisen NR, Connett JE, Kiley JP, et al. Effects of smoking intervention and the use of an inhaled anticholinergic bronchodilator on the rate of decline of FEV1. The Lung Health Study. JAMA 1994;272:1497–505.

4. Continuous or nocturnal oxygen therapy in hypoxemic chronic obstructive lung disease: a clinical trial. Nocturnal Oxygen Therapy Trial Group. Ann Intern Med 1980;93:391–8.

5. Fishman A, Martinez F, Naunheim K, et al. A randomized trial comparing lung-volume-reduction surgery with medical therapy for severe emphysema. N Engl J Med 2003;348:2059–73.

6. Rabe KF, Hurd S, Anzueto A, et al. Global strategy for the diagnosis, management, and prevention of chronic obstructive pulmonary disease: GOLD executive summary. Am J Respir Crit Care Med 2007;176:532–55.

7. Guidance for industry: patient-reported outcome measures: use in medical product development to support labeling claims: draft guidance. Health Qual Life Outcomes 2006;4:79.

8. Yusen R. What outcomes should be measured in patients with COPD? Chest 2001;119:327–8.

9. Doward LC, McKenna SP. Defining patient-reported outcomes. Value Health 2004;7(Suppl 1):S4–8.

10. Fletcher CM, Elmes PC, Fairbairn AS, et al. The significance of respiratory symptoms and the diagnosis of chronic bronchitis in a working population. Br Med J 1959;2:257–66.

11. Mahler DA, Weinberg DH, Wells CK, et al. The measurement of dyspnea. Contents, interobserver agreement, and physiologic correlates of two new clinical indexes. Chest 1984;85:751–8.

12. Eakin EG, Resnikoff PM, Prewitt LM, et al. Validation of a new dyspnea measure: the UCSD Shortness of Breath Questionnaire. University of California, San Diego. Chest 1998;113:619–24.

13. Ware JE Jr, Sherbourne CD. The MOS 36-item short-form health survey (SF-36). I. Conceptual framework and item selection. Med Care 1992;30:473–83.

14. Bergner M, Bobbitt RA, Carter WB, et al. The Sickness Impact Profile: development and final revision of a health status measure. Med Care 1981;19:787–805.

15. Jones PW, Quirk FH, Baveystock CM, et al. A self-complete measure of health status for chronic airflow limitation. The St. George's respiratory questionnaire. Am Rev Respir Dis 1992;145:1321–7.

16. Curtis JR, Martin DP, Martin TR. Patient-assessed health outcomes in chronic lung disease: what are they, how do they help us, and where do we go from here? Am J Respir Crit Care Med 1997;156:1032–9.

17. Measuring quality of life, 1997. Available at: http://www.who.int/mental_health/media/68.pdf. Accessed May 9, 2012.

18. McDowell I. Measuring health: a guide to rating scales and questionnaires. 3rd edition. New York: Oxford University Press; 2006.

19. Weinstein MC, Fineber HV, Elstein AS, et al. Clinical decision analysis. Philadelphia: WB Saunders; 1980.

20. Sox HC, Blatt MA, Higgins MC, et al. Medical decision making. Boston: Butterworth; 1988.

21. Yusen RD. Technology and outcomes assessment in lung transplantation. Proc Am Thorac Soc 2009;6:128–36.

22. Yusen RD. Lung transplantation outcomes: the importance and inadequacies of assessing survival. Am J Transplant 2009;9:1493–4.

23. Yusen RD. Survival and quality of life of patients undergoing lung transplant. Clin Chest Med 2011;32:253–64.

24. Weinstein MC, Pliskin JS, Stason WB. Coronary artery bypass surgery. Decision and policy analysis. In: Bunker JP, Barnes BA, Mosteller F, editors. Costs, risks, and benefits of surgery. New York: Oxford University Press; 1977. p. 342–71.

25. Gafni A. The Standard Gamble method: what is being measured and how it is interpreted. Health Serv Res 1994;29:207–24.

26. Anderson JP, Kaplan RM, Berry CC, et al. Interday reliability of function assessment for a health status measure. The quality of well-being scale. Med Care 1989; 27:1076–83.

27. EuroQol–a new facility for the measurement of health-related quality of life. The EuroQol Group. Health Policy 1990;16:199–208.

28. Furlong WJ, Feeny DH, Torrance GW, et al. The Health Utilities Index (HUI) system for assessing health-related quality of life in clinical studies. Ann Med 2001;33:375–84.

29. Dolan P. Whose preferences count? Med Decis Making 1999;19:482–6.

30. Nord E, Pinto JL, Richardson J, et al. Incorporating societal concerns for fairness in numerical valuations of health programmes. Health Econ 1999;8:25–39.

31. Weinstein MC, Siegel JE, Gold MR, et al. Recommendations of the Panel on Cost-effectiveness in Health and Medicine. JAMA 1996;276:1253–8.

32. Blough DK, Ramsey S, Sullivan SD, et al. The impact of using different imputation methods for missing quality of life scores on the estimation of the cost-effectiveness of lung-volume-reduction surgery. Health Econ 2009;18:91–101.

33. Celli BR, Cote CG, Marin JM, et al. The body-mass index, airflow obstruction, dyspnea, and exercise capacity index in chronic obstructive pulmonary disease. N Engl J Med 2004;350:1005–12.

34. Martinez FJ, Foster G, Curtis JL, et al. Predictors of mortality in patients with emphysema and severe airflow obstruction. Am J Respir Crit Care Med 2006;173:1326–34.

35. Puhan MA, Garcia-Aymerich J, Frey M, et al. Expansion of the prognostic assessment of patients with chronic obstructive pulmonary disease: the updated BODE index and the ADO index. Lancet 2009;374:704–11.

36. Eisner MD, Trupin L, Katz PP, et al. Development and validation of a survey-based COPD Severity Score. Chest 2005;127:1890–7.

37. Pickard AS, Yang Y, Lee TA. Comparison of health-related quality of life measures in chronic obstructive pulmonary disease. Health Qual Life Outcomes 2011;9:26.

38. Stahl E, Lindberg A, Jansson SA, et al. Health-related quality of life is related to COPD disease severity. Health Qual Life Outcomes 2005;3:56.

39. Hajiro T, Nishimura K, Tsukino M, et al. A comparison of the level of dyspnea vs disease severity in indicating the health-related quality of life of patients with COPD. Chest 1999;116:1632–7.

40. van Schayck CP, Rutten-van Molken MP, van Doorslaer EK, et al. Two-year bronchodilator treatment in patients with mild airflow obstruction. Contradictory effects on lung function and quality of life. Chest 1992;102:1384–91.

41. Prigatano GP, Wright EC, Levin D. Quality of life and its predictors in patients with mild hypoxemia and chronic obstructive pulmonary disease. Arch Intern Med 1984;144:1613–9.

42. Eisner MD, Blanc PD, Yelin EH, et al. COPD as a systemic disease: impact on physical functional limitations. Am J Med 2008;121:789–96.

43. Shoup R, Dalsky G, Warner S, et al. Body composition and health-related quality of life in patients with obstructive airways disease. Eur Respir J 1997;10:1576–80.

44. Singer J, Yelin EH, Katz PP, et al. Respiratory and skeletal muscle strength in chronic obstructive pulmonary disease: impact on exercise capacity and lower extremity function. J Cardiopulm Rehabil Prev 2011;31:111–9.

45. Gonzalez E, Herrejon A, Inchaurraga I, et al. Determinants of health-related quality of life in patients with pulmonary emphysema. Respir Med 2005;99:638–44.
46. Katsura H, Yamada K, Wakabayashi R, et al. The impact of dyspnoea and leg fatigue during exercise on health-related quality of life in patients with COPD. Respirology 2005;10:485–90.
47. van Manen JG, Bindels PJ, Dekker EW, et al. Added value of co-morbidity in predicting health-related quality of life in COPD patients. Respir Med 2001;95:496–504.
48. Wijnhoven HA, Kriegsman DM, Hesselink AE, et al. The influence of co-morbidity on health-related quality of life in asthma and COPD patients. Respir Med 2003;97:468–75.
49. van Manen JG, Bindels PJ, Dekker FW, et al. The influence of COPD on health-related quality of life independent of the influence of comorbidity. J Clin Epidemiol 2003;56:1177–84.
50. van Ede L, Yzermans CJ, Brouwer HJ. Prevalence of depression in patients with chronic obstructive pulmonary disease: a systematic review. Thorax 1999;54:688–92.
51. Lacasse Y, Rousseau L, Maltais F. Prevalence of depressive symptoms and depression in patients with severe oxygen-dependent chronic obstructive pulmonary disease. J Cardiopulm Rehabil 2001;21:80–6.
52. Yohannes AM, Baldwin RC, Connolly MJ. Depression and anxiety in elderly outpatients with chronic obstructive pulmonary disease: prevalence, and validation of the BASDEC screening questionnaire. Int J Geriatr Psychiatry 2000;15:1090–6.
53. Kunik ME, Roundy K, Veazey C, et al. Surprisingly high prevalence of anxiety and depression in chronic breathing disorders. Chest 2005;127:1205–11.
54. Wagena EJ, Kant I, Huibers MJ, et al. Psychological distress and depressed mood in employees with asthma, chronic bronchitis or emphysema: a population-based observational study on prevalence and the relationship with smoking cigarettes. Eur J Epidemiol 2004;19:147–53.
55. Cinciripini PM, Wetter DW, Fouladi RT, et al. The effects of depressed mood on smoking cessation: mediation by postcessation self-efficacy. J Consult Clin Psychol 2003;71:292–301.
56. Yellowlees PM, Alpers JH, Bowden JJ, et al. Psychiatric morbidity in patients with chronic airflow obstruction. Med J Aust 1987;146:305–7.
57. Clary GL, Palmer SM, Doraiswamy PM. Mood disorders and chronic obstructive pulmonary disease: current research and future needs. Curr Psychiatry Rep 2002;4:213–21.
58. Almagro P, Calbo E, Ochoa de Echaguen A, et al. Mortality after hospitalization for COPD. Chest 2002;121:1441–8.
59. Andersson I, Johansson K, Larsson S, et al. Long-term oxygen therapy and quality of life in elderly patients hospitalised due to severe exacerbation of COPD. A 1 year follow-up study. Respir Med 2002;96:944–9.
60. Davies L, Wilkinson M, Bonner S, et al. "Hospital at home" versus hospital care in patients with exacerbations of chronic obstructive pulmonary disease: prospective randomised controlled trial. BMJ 2000;321:1265–8.
61. Spencer S, Jones PW. Time course of recovery of health status following an infective exacerbation of chronic bronchitis. Thorax 2003;58:589–93.
62. Doll H, Grey-Amante P, Duprat-Lomon I, et al. Quality of life in acute exacerbation of chronic bronchitis: results from a German population study. Respir Med 2002;96:39–51.

63. Osman IM, Godden DJ, Friend JA, et al. Quality of life and hospital re-admission in patients with chronic obstructive pulmonary disease. Thorax 1997;52:67–71.

64. Singer JP, Blanc PD, Iribarren C, et al. Health-related quality of life predicts severe exacerbations of COPD. Am J Respir Crit Care Med 2009;179:A1519.

65. Domingo-Salvany A, Lamarca R, Ferrer M, et al. Health-related quality of life and mortality in male patients with chronic obstructive pulmonary disease. Am J Respir Crit Care Med 2002;166:680–5.

66. Marin JM, Cote CG, Diaz O, et al. Prognostic assessment in COPD: health related quality of life and the BODE index. Respir Med 2011;105:916–21.

67. Ong KC, Earnest A, Lu SJ. A multidimensional grading system (BODE index) as predictor of hospitalization for COPD. Chest 2005;128:3810–6.

68. Martinez FJ, Han MK, Andrei AC, et al. Longitudinal change in the BODE index predicts mortality in severe emphysema. Am J Respir Crit Care Med 2008;178: 491–9.

69. Omachi TA, Yelin EH, Katz PP, et al. The COPD Severity Score: a dynamic prediction tool for health-care utilization. COPD 2008;5:339–46.

70. Burge PS, Calverley PM, Jones PW, et al. Randomised, double blind, placebo controlled study of fluticasone propionate in patients with moderate to severe chronic obstructive pulmonary disease: the ISOLDE trial. BMJ 2000;320: 1297–303.

71. Brusasco V, Hodder R, Miravitlles M, et al. Health outcomes following treatment for six months with once daily tiotropium compared with twice daily salmeterol in patients with COPD. Thorax 2003;58:399–404.

72. Donohue JF, van Noord JA, Bateman ED, et al. A 6-month, placebo-controlled study comparing lung function and health status changes in COPD patients treated with tiotropium or salmeterol. Chest 2002;122:47–55.

73. Vincken W, van Noord JA, Greefhorst AP, et al. Improved health outcomes in patients with COPD during 1 yr's treatment with tiotropium. Eur Respir J 2002; 19:209–16.

74. Tashkin DP, Celli B, Senn S, et al. A 4-year trial of tiotropium in chronic obstructive pulmonary disease. N Engl J Med 2008;359:1543–54.

75. Calverley P, Pauwels R, Vestbo J, et al. Combined salmeterol and fluticasone in the treatment of chronic obstructive pulmonary disease: a randomised controlled trial. Lancet 2003;361:449–56.

76. Calverley PM, Anderson JA, Celli B, et al. Salmeterol and fluticasone propionate and survival in chronic obstructive pulmonary disease. N Engl J Med 2007;356: 775–89.

77. Albert RK, Connett J, Bailey WC, et al. Azithromycin for prevention of exacerbations of COPD. N Engl J Med 2011;365:689–98.

78. Eaton T, Garrett JE, Young P, et al. Ambulatory oxygen improves quality of life of COPD patients: a randomised controlled study. Eur Respir J 2002;20:306–12.

79. Lacasse Y, Goldstein R, Lasserson TJ, et al. Pulmonary rehabilitation for chronic obstructive pulmonary disease. Cochrane Database Syst Rev 2006;3:CD003793.

80. Nishiyama O, Taniguchi H, Kondoh Y, et al. Factors in maintaining long-term improvements in health-related quality of life after pulmonary rehabilitation for COPD. Qual Life Res 2005;14:2315–21.

81. Seemungal TA, Wedzicha JA. Integrated care: a new model for COPD management? Eur Respir J 2006;28:4–6.

82. Bourbeau J, Julien M, Maltais F, et al. Reduction of hospital utilization in patients with chronic obstructive pulmonary disease: a disease-specific self-management intervention. Arch Intern Med 2003;163:585–91.

83. Monninkhof E, van der Valk P, van der Palen J, et al. Effects of a comprehensive self-management programme in patients with chronic obstructive pulmonary disease. Eur Respir J 2003;22:815–20.
84. Effing T, Monninkhof EM, van der Valk PD, et al. Self-management education for patients with chronic obstructive pulmonary disease. Cochrane Database Syst Rev 2007;4:CD002990.
85. Chavannes NH, Grijsen M, van den Akker M, et al. Integrated disease management improves one-year quality of life in primary care COPD patients: a controlled clinical trial. Prim Care Respir J 2009;18:171–6.
86. Yusen RD, Littenberg B. Integrating survival and quality of life data in clinical trials of lung disease: the case of lung volume reduction surgery. Chest 2005;127:1094–6.
87. Ramsey SD, Berry K, Etzioni R, et al. Cost effectiveness of lung-volume-reduction surgery for patients with severe emphysema. N Engl J Med 2003;348:2092–102.
88. Naunheim KS, Wood DE, Mohsenifar Z, et al. Long-term follow-up of patients receiving lung-volume-reduction surgery versus medical therapy for severe emphysema by the National Emphysema Treatment Trial Research Group. Ann Thorac Surg 2006;82:431–43.
89. Benzo R, Farrell MH, Chang CC, et al. Integrating health status and survival data: the palliative effect of lung volume reduction surgery. Am J Respir Crit Care Med 2009;180:239–46.
90. Orens JB, Estenne M, Arcasoy S, et al. International guidelines for the selection of lung transplant candidates: 2006 update–a consensus report from the Pulmonary Scientific Council of the International Society for Heart and Lung Transplantation. J Heart Lung Transplant 2006;25:745–55.
91. Limbos MM, Joyce DP, Chan CK, et al. Psychological functioning and quality of life in lung transplant candidates and recipients. Chest 2000;118:408–16.
92. Rodrigue JR, Baz MA, Kanasky WF Jr, et al. Does lung transplantation improve health-related quality of life? The University of Florida experience. J Heart Lung Transplant 2005;24:755–63.
93. Smeritschnig B, Jaksch P, Kocher A, et al. Quality of life after lung transplantation: a cross-sectional study. J Heart Lung Transplant 2005;24:474–80.
94. Eskander A, Waddell TK, Faughnan ME, et al. BODE index and quality of life in advanced chronic obstructive pulmonary disease before and after lung transplantation. J Heart Lung Transplant 2011;30:1334–41.
95. Mittler B, Brown K, Yusen RD. Impact of lung transplantation in the U.S. Lung Allocation Score system on quality of life in patients with chronic obstructive pulmonary disease. J Heart Lung Transplant 2012;31:S27.
96. Yusen RD, Brown KL, Habrock TE, et al. The impact of lung transplantation on quality of life in patients with COPD. J Heart Lung Transplant 2005;24:S156–7.
97. Gerbase MW, Spiliopoulos A, Rochat T, et al. Health-related quality of life following single or bilateral lung transplantation: a 7-year comparison to functional outcome. Chest 2005;128:1371–8.

COPD Exacerbations
Causes, Prevention, and Treatment

Alex J. Mackay, MBBS, BSc (Hons), MRCP*, John R. Hurst, PhD, FRCP

KEYWORDS

- Chronic obstructive pulmonary disease • Exacerbation • Respiratory viruses
- Bacteria

KEY POINTS

- Respiratory viruses (in particular rhinovirus) and bacteria both play a major role in the etiology of exacerbate COPD.
- A distinct group of patients appears susceptible to frequent exacerbations, irrespective of disease severity and this phenotype is stable over time.
- Many current therapeutic strategies help reduce exacerbation frequency.

Chronic obstructive pulmonary disease (COPD) is associated with episodes of acute deterioration in respiratory health termed "exacerbations." Exacerbations are characterized by a worsening of symptoms from the usual stable state, especially dyspnea, increased sputum volume, and purulence. When diagnosing COPD exacerbations, clinicians must also exclude other causes for respiratory deterioration, such as pneumothoraces, pulmonary emboli, and pneumonia, using clinical examination and appropriate investigations if required. Exacerbations are among the most common causes of emergency medical hospital admission in the United Kingdom[1] (and elsewhere) and the rate at which they occur seems to reflect an independent susceptibility phenotype.[2] Exacerbations are important events in the natural history of COPD that help drive lung function decline,[3,4] increase the risk of cardiovascular events,[5] and are responsible for much of the morbidity[6] and mortality[7] associated with this highly prevalent condition.

FREQUENT EXACERBATOR PHENOTYPE

Patients with a history of frequent exacerbations exhibit faster decline in lung function,[3] have worse quality of life,[6] have increased risk of hospitalization,[8] and have greater mortality (**Fig. 1**).[7] Therefore, it is important to identify patients at risk of

Financial Disclosures: Dr Hurst has received support to attend meetings or speaker and advisory fees from AstraZeneca, Bayer, Boehringer Ingelheim, Chiesi, GlaxoSmithKline, and Pfizer.
Academic Unit of Respiratory Medicine, Royal Free Campus, UCL Medical School, Rowland Hill Street, London NW3 2PF, UK
* Corresponding author.
E-mail address: alexander.mackay@ucl.ac.uk

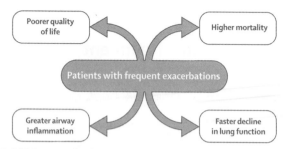

Fig. 1. Effect of COPD exacerbations in the group with frequent exacerbations. (*From* Wedzicha JA, Seemungal TA. COPD exacerbations: defining their cause and prevention. Lancet 2007;370(9589):786–96; with permission.)

frequent exacerbations. Exacerbations become more frequent and severe as COPD severity increases.[9] However, a distinct group of patients seems to be susceptible to exacerbations, irrespective of disease severity, and the major determinant of exacerbation frequency is a history of prior exacerbations.[2] This phenotype of susceptibility to exacerbations is stable over time and is seen across all severity of airflow obstruction,[2] suggesting that patients with the frequent exacerbator phenotype are prone to exacerbations as a result of intrinsic susceptibility, and develop exacerbations when exposed to particular triggers, such as respiratory infections.

Exacerbations are associated with increased systemic and airway inflammation and may be triggered by bacterial and respiratory viral infections. They may also be precipitated by environmental factors (**Fig. 2**).

VIRAL INFECTIONS
Rhinovirus

Rhinovirus is responsible for the common cold and initial evidence that respiratory viral infections were important triggers of COPD exacerbations came from the association of coryzal symptoms with exacerbations. Seemungal and colleagues[10] found that up to 64% of exacerbations were associated with a symptomatic cold occurring up to 18 days before exacerbation onset. Additionally, exacerbations associated with dyspnea and coryza at onset are associated with larger falls in peak flow, prolonged recovery times, and higher levels of airway inflammatory markers (interleukin [IL]-6).[11,12]

Studies using molecular biology polymerase chain reaction techniques have provided further evidence of the role of rhinovirus in the cause of COPD exacerbations. In studies from the London COPD cohort, up to 40% of exacerbations were associated with respiratory viral infections. Rhinovirus was the most common respiratory virus detected and found in 58% of viral exacerbations.[10] Rohde and colleagues[13] corroborated these findings in a separate study of hospitalized patients, detecting respiratory viruses in 56% of exacerbations. Rhinovirus was again the most prevalent virus, being detected in 36% of virus-associated exacerbations.

Experimental Rhinovirus Infection Models

Mallia and colleagues[14] have used experimental rhinovirus infection to provide evidence of a direct causal relationship between respiratory virus infection and acute exacerbations of COPD. In that study, 13 subjects with COPD and 13 control subjects with a similar smoking history but normal lung function were closely observed after infection with rhinovirus serotype 16. Daily upper and lower respiratory symptom scores were increased significantly above baseline levels and were significantly

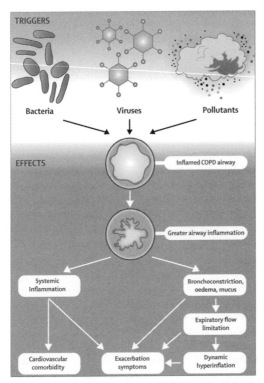

Fig. 2. Triggers of COPD exacerbations and associated pathophysiologic changes leading to increased respiratory symptoms. (*From* Wedzicha JA, Seemungal TA. COPD exacerbations: defining their cause and prevention. Lancet 2007;370(9589):786–96; with permission.)

greater in the COPD group compared with control subjects. Postbronchodilator peak expiratory flow fell and in blood and airway inflammatory markers increased significantly from baseline in patients with COPD but not control subjects. Nasal lavage virus load was significantly higher in the COPD group compared with control subjects and peak sputum virus load in subjects with COPD correlated positively with peak serum C-reactive protein concentration and sputum inflammatory markers (neutrophils, IL-6, IL-8, neutrophil elastase, and tumor necrosis factor-α). Furthermore, there was a temporal relationship between virus detection in the respiratory tract and the onset of symptoms and airflow obstruction, and virus clearance was followed by clinical recovery. Thus, Mallia and colleagues[14] provide direct evidence that the symptomatic and physiologic changes seen at acute exacerbations of COPD can be precipitated by rhinovirus infection.

Susceptibility to Virus-Induced Exacerbations

Defective immunity may lead to increased susceptibility to virus-induced exacerbations. Interferon-β is an essential component of antirhinoviral immunity and Mallia and colleagues[14] have reported impaired interferon-β response to rhinovirus infection in COPD. Furthermore, cells from patients with COPD manifest increased viral titer and copy numbers after rhinovirus infection compared with control subjects[15] and intercellular adhesion molecule-1, the rhinovirus major group receptor, is upregulated on the bronchial epithelium of patients with COPD.[16]

Seasonal Environmental Variations and Viral Infection

In the Northern hemisphere, COPD exacerbations are more common in the winter months and may also be more severe, because small but significant falls in lung function in patients with COPD occur with a reduction in outdoor temperature.[17] The increase in exacerbations may be caused by the increasing prevalence of respiratory viruses in low temperature winter months or increased susceptibility to upper respiratory tract virus infections in cold weather. In children, respiratory syncytial virus (RSV) outbreaks cause a significant increase in hospital admissions during the winter season[18] and increased RSV activity has been observed when temperatures decrease.[19]

RSV

Seemungal and colleagues[10] detected RSV in nasal aspirates at exacerbation, although more patients had RSV detected in the stable state than at exacerbation (23.5% vs 14.2%). Stable patients in whom RSV has been detected have elevated inflammatory markers, more severely impaired gas exchange (higher $Paco_2$) and accelerated lung function decline.[10,20] Thus, RSV may also be a cause of chronic airway infection in COPD.

Influenza Virus

Influenza has been detected relatively infrequently at COPD exacerbation,[10] though this may relate to widespread use of influenza immunization for patients with chronic lung disease. In studies of older patients with chronic lung disease, those not vaccinated with influenza had twice the hospitalization rate in the influenza season compared with the noninfluenza season.[21] This highlights the importance of influenza vaccination in patients with COPD and suggests that influenza may still be an important etiologic factor during influenza epidemics.

BACTERIAL INFECTIONS
Species

Bacteria are isolated from sputum using standard culture techniques in 40% to 60% of exacerbations.[22] The three most common species isolated in COPD exacerbations are *Haemophilus influenzae*, *Moraxella catarrhalis*, and *Streptococcus pneumoniae*. Less frequently, exacerbations may be caused by *Pseudomonas aeruginosa*, gram-negative Enterobacteriacea, *Staphylococcus aureus*, *Haemophilus parainfluenzae*, and *Haemophilus hemolyticus*.[23–25]

Sputum Characteristics

Some of the earliest evidence supporting a causative role for bacteria in COPD exacerbations came from antibiotic studies, including the seminal paper by Anthonisen and colleagues,[26] which identified exacerbation features predictive of benefit from antibiotics. Patients with increased dyspnea, sputum volume, and sputum purulence showed a significant benefit with antibiotic therapy, whereas those with only one of these three features showed none. After this paper, studies related sputum characteristics to the presence of bacteria and bacterial load. Theoretically, airway bacterial infection should be accompanied by an influx of neutrophils, resulting in a change in secretions from mucoid to purulent, because neutrophil-derived myeloperoxidase is green. Antibiotic therapy, by reducing bacterial load, should reverse this process.[27]

In studies during exacerbations of COPD, positive bacterial cultures were obtained from 84% of patients if sputum was purulent at presentation but only 38% if the sputum was mucoid (*P*<.0001). Moreover, the median bacterial load for positive purulent culture samples was significantly higher than for mucoid samples. When the same patients were reexamined in the stable state after antibiotics, sputum color improved significantly in the group who presented with purulent sputum. In purulent exacerbations a clear relationship was demonstrated between semiquantitative neutrophil count and sputum color. The presence of green (purulent) sputum was 94.4% sensitive and 77% specific for a high bacterial load ($>10^7$ colony forming units per milliliter).[27]

Colonization

Darker sputum color in stable COPD may reflect bronchial bacterial colonization,[28] which has traditionally been characterized as the isolation by culture of significant numbers of bacteria in samples obtained from the lower airways of patients with COPD when clinically stable.[29] Bacteria in the lower airways have been hypothesized to disrupt host defense mechanisms leading to a vicious cycle of epithelial cell injury, defective mucociliary clearance, chronic mucous hypersecretion, and inflammatory cell infiltration, further damaging host defenses and leading to bacterial adherence and growth.[23] This mechanism may explain why colonization in the stable state has been associated with increased exacerbation frequency (**Fig. 3**).[30] However, recent technologic advances in bacterial detection have challenged conventional thinking and definitions in the field of bacterial colonization.

Molecular Analysis Techniques

Classically, it was thought the lower airways were sterile in healthy patients; however, the development of culture-independent molecular techniques using 16S-rRNA techniques has challenged this assumption. The 16S-rRNA gene is a section of prokaryotic DNA found in all bacteria. 16S-rRNA gene sequences contain hypervariable regions that can provide species-specific signature sequences useful for bacterial identification. Consequently, 16S rRNA gene sequencing provides a potentially more accurate alternative to traditional methods of bacterial identification. Hilty and colleagues[31]

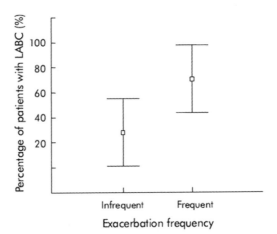

Fig. 3. Relationship between lower airway bacterial colonization (LABC) by a possible pathogen in induced sputum and frequent (>2.58 exacerbations per year; n = 14) and infrequent exacerbations (<2.58 exacerbations per year; n = 14) with 95% confidence intervals. (*From* Patel IS, Seemungal TA, Wilks M, et al. Relationship between bacterial colonisation and the frequency, character, and severity of COPD exacerbations. Thorax 2002;57(9):759–64; with permission.)

used molecular analysis of the polymorphic bacterial 16S-rRNA gene to characterize the composition of bacterial communities from the airways of patients with asthma, patients with COPD, and healthy control subjects. Over 5000 16S rRNA bacterial sequences were identified from 43 subjects and the bronchial tree of all patient groups was nonsterile. However, proteobacteria, especially *Haemophilus* sp, were much more frequently identified in the bronchi of patients with asthma and patients with COPD compared with control subjects, suggesting that the bronchial tree contains a characteristic microbial flora that differs between health and disease. Further studies using these techniques have also revealed that there are significant microanatomic differences in bacterial communities within the same lung of subjects with advanced COPD.[32] These techniques are exciting developments in the study of bacteria in patients with COPD, but should be interpreted with caution because studies using these methods have been conducted on small numbers of patients[31,32] and the clinical applicability of the results remains uncertain.

Bacterial Load

The prevalence of potentially pathogenic microorganisms and airway bacterial load in sputum have been shown to increase from stable state to exacerbation. The most frequently isolated organism is *H influenzae*, followed by *M catarrhalis* and *S pneumoniae*.[33] Studies using protected brush specimens collected in the stable state and at exacerbation have also demonstrated an increased prevalence of positive bacterial cultures at exacerbation. In the stable state, patients colonized by potentially pathogenic microorganisms on culture had greater disease severity (reduced mean forced expiratory volume in 1 second [FEV_1]% predicted) and multivariate analyses demonstrated that a high potentially pathogenic microorganism load in lower airway secretions was a major determinant of exacerbation risk and lung function impairment.[34]

Strain Changes

Strain changes may play an important role in the cause of COPD exacerbations. In a prospective study, Sethi and colleagues[25] hypothesized that acquisition of a new bacterial strain would be associated with an exacerbation of COPD and so collected sputum samples from 81 outpatients with moderate to severe COPD on a monthly basis and at exacerbation. Molecular typing of sputum showed that isolation of a new strain of a pathogen (*H influenzae*, *M catarrhalis*, and *S pneumoniae*) was associated with a significant increase in the risk of exacerbation. These findings were proposed as a mechanism to explain recurrent bacterial exacerbations of COPD, the authors speculating that after a first exacerbation, patients develop a protective immune response that is strain specific. Therefore, acquisition of a different strain from the same bacterial species may still lead to a second exacerbation. However, not all exacerbations were associated with strain change, and not all strain changes were associated with exacerbation.

Controversy exists regarding the relative contributions made by exacerbation load and strain change to the cause of COPD exacerbations. Sethi and colleagues[35] further explored this issue by examining sputum from 104 patients when stable and at exacerbation over a period of 81 months. Among preexisting strains, no differences were found between exacerbation and stable bacterial load for *H influenzae*. *M catarrhalis* was present at significantly lower concentrations during exacerbation with a similar trend observed for *S pneumoniae*. However, for *H influenzae* and *M catarrhalis* (but not *S pneumoniae*) increased load of new strains was seen during exacerbation compared with during stable visits. In the case of *H influenzae*, bacterial load increased significantly from $10^{7.28}$ to $10^{7.76}$ colony forming units per milliliter. When the same strain was isolated during stable and exacerbation visits paired analysis also showed a significant increase in load for *H influenzae*. The observed increases of around 0.5 log in magnitude, although representing a small relative change,[35] equate to a 202% or threefold increase in absolute bacterial numbers,[36] suggesting that changes in bacterial load remain an important mechanism for some exacerbations.

Interaction of Bacteria and Viruses

Frequent exacerbators have a higher incidence of lower airway bacterial colonization[30] and bacteria may also play a role in susceptibility to viral infection in COPD. *H influenzae* increases expression of intercellular adhesion molecule-1 and Toll-like receptor-3, and augments binding of rhinovirus to cultured human airway epithelial cells.[37] Therefore, patients colonized with bacteria may be more susceptible to the development of virally triggered exacerbations.

Wilkinson and colleagues[33] demonstrated a synergistic effect of viral and bacterial infections at exacerbation in patients with COPD. Exacerbation symptoms and FEV_1 decline were more severe in the presence of bacteria and colds (as a surrogate of viral infection) than with a cold or bacterial pathogen alone, and exacerbations associated with human rhinovirus and *H influenzae* exhibited a greater bacterial load and inflammation than those without both pathogens. Patients hospitalized because of COPD exacerbations also have more marked lung function impairment and increased length of stay in the context of bacterial and viral coinfection.[38]

ENVIRONMENTAL FACTORS
Air Pollution

Epidemiologic data supports a role for air pollution in the cause of some COPD exacerbations with studies showing an increased risk of hospitalization for COPD with increased levels of pollutants.[39–41] Air pollution likely causes COPD exacerbations through modulation of airway inflammation and immunity. Diesel exhaust induces airway inflammation in healthy volunteers as characterized by an increased percentage of sputum neutrophils, IL-6, and methylhistamine.[42] Furthermore, diesel exhaust reduces T-cell activation and induces migration of alveolar macrophages into the airspaces.[43]

EXACERBATION PREVENTION

There are now a wide range of pharmacologic and nonpharmacologic interventions documented to reduce exacerbation frequency or hospitalization in COPD (**Table 1**). However, there remains a real need for further novel interventions because

Table 1
Interventions to reduce exacerbation frequency or hospitalization in patients with COPD

Pharmacologic	Nonpharmacologic
Inhaled corticosteroids	Lung volume reduction surgery
Long-acting bronchodilators	Home oxygen
Phosphodiesterase inhibitors	Ventilatory support
Theophyllines	Pulmonary rehabilitation
Long-term antibiotics	
Mucolytics	
Vaccination	

current approaches are not completely effective, even when targeted and used optimally.

PHARMACOLOGIC THERAPIES

Conceptually, some pharmacotherapy (eg, a vaccine) may be delivered once with lasting effect on reducing exacerbations, whereas other interventions need to be administered continually for that effect to be maintained.

Vaccination

The largest study of the efficacy of influenza vaccination was conducted retrospectively using data pooled from 18 cohort studies of community-dwelling elderly patients over 10 influenza seasons. In this data set composed of 713,872 person-seasons of observation, influenza vaccination was associated with a 27% reduction in the risk of hospitalization for pneumonia or influenza and a 48% reduction in the risk of death.[44] The same authors also conducted a 2-year retrospective cohort study of elderly patients with diagnosis of chronic lung disease to assess the health-economic benefits of pneumococcal vaccination.[45] Pneumococcal vaccination was associated with significantly lower risks of hospitalization for pneumonia and death. However, a randomized controlled trial of pneumococcal polysaccharide vaccine in patients with COPD demonstrated no significant reduction in rates of community-acquired pneumonia when the entire study population was analyzed.[46] Subanalyses of the data showed a reduction in the incidence of community-acquired pneumonia in those patients younger than age 65 years and those with severe airflow obstruction, although no mortality benefit was demonstrated.[46] Data also suggest an additive benefit of combined influenza and pneumococcal vaccination[45] and hence both vaccines are recommended to all patients with COPD.[47] It is important to note that these studies have not specifically addressed exacerbations of COPD.

Bacterial immunostimulation has also been advocated as a method to prevent exacerbations of COPD and reduce the severity and duration of acute episodes. OM-85 BV (Bronchovaxom) is a detoxified immunoactive bacterial extract that has been examined in multiple trials; however, assessment of its efficacy is hampered by heterogeneity of study design and conflicting results.[48–51] Furthermore, it is not known if any protective effects seen are additive to other conventional treatments and thus larger and longer trials are required before this vaccine can be recommended as part of the routine clinical management of COPD.[52]

Inhaled Corticosteroids and Long-Acting Bronchodilators

The Inhaled Steroid in Obstructive Lung Disease in Europe study was performed primarily to assess the effect of inhaled corticosteroids (ICS) on the rate of FEV_1 decline in patients with moderate-to-severe COPD. Although this primary outcome was negative, a 25% reduction in exacerbation frequency was noted in the group who received fluticasone.[53] Long-acting β-agonists (LABA) also reduce exacerbation frequency and in the Toward A Revolution in COPD Health (TORCH) study, in which 6112 patients were followed over 3 years, inhaled fluticasone and salmeterol reduced exacerbation frequency when administered separately compared with placebo.[54] In the same study, the combination of fluticasone and salmeterol (SFC) reduced exacerbation frequency further still, in addition to improving health status and lung function compared with placebo. The annual rate of moderate and severe exacerbations in the placebo group was 1.13 per year, compared with 0.97 for salmeterol, 0.93 for fluticasone, and 0.85 in patients receiving SFC. The combination of ICS and LABA also resulted in fewer hospital admissions over the study period and trended toward a mortality benefit. Reduction in exacerbation frequency has been found for other ICS, and other LABA, singly and in combination. New drugs in development include once-daily ICS and LABA.

Long-acting antimuscarinics (LAMA) also reduce exacerbation frequency. In the Understanding Potential Long-Term Impacts on Function with Tiotropium trial 5993 patients were randomized to tiotropium or placebo over 4 years, with concomitant therapy allowed. Although the primary end point of the trial (a reduction in rate of decline in FEV_1) was negative, the group of patients randomized to tiotropium in addition to usual care had a significant reduction in exacerbation frequency, related hospitalizations, and respiratory failure.[55] Because this trial involved the addition of tiotropium to existing therapy, which could include combination preparations of ICS and LABA, many patients were in effect on triple combination of therapy.

Triple combination therapy is commonly prescribed in advanced COPD. This approach was examined in the OPTIMAL study, which examined whether combining tiotropium with salmeterol or SFC improved outcomes compared with tiotropium alone in patients with moderate to severe COPD.[56] The primary outcome was negative, because the addition of SFC to tiotropium therapy did not statistically influence rates of COPD exacerbation. However, triple combination therapy did improve lung function, quality of life, and hospitalization rates compared with tiotropium plus placebo. In keeping with the TORCH study, drop-outs in the placebo arm may have affected the study: more than 40% of patients who received tiotropium plus placebo and tiotropium plus salmeterol discontinued therapy prematurely, and many crossed over to treatment with open-label inhaled steroids or LABA.

An important clinical question is which combination of therapies is most effective for different patients. Network analysis techniques have assessed the relative effectiveness of competing inhaled drug regimens for the prevention of COPD exacerbations.[57] Based on 35 trials, all inhaled drug regimens (LABA, LAMA, and ICS, alone and in combination) significantly reduced exacerbations but there were no significant differences between them. In subanalyses, in patients with FEV_1 less than or equal to 40% predicted, LAMA, ICS, and combination treatment reduced exacerbations significantly compared with LABA alone, but not if FEV_1 was greater than 40% predicted. This effect modification was significant for ICS and combination treatment but not for LAMA suggesting that combination treatment may be more effective than LABA alone in patients with a low FEV_1.

Phosphodiesterase Inhibitors

There is some evidence that theophyllines reduce exacerbation frequency.[58,59] However, they are nonselective phosphodiesterase inhibitors, potentially toxic with the need to monitor plasma levels, and with potential for interaction with other medication, restricting therapeutic use. This is a particularly important consideration in elderly patients because of differences in pharmacokinetics, increased prevalence of comorbidities, and concomitant medications. Therefore, theophyllines should only be used after a trial of other more effective therapies (LABA, LAMA, or ICS), or in patients unable to use inhaled therapy. If prescribed, the theophylline dose must be monitored or reduced at exacerbation when macrolide or fluoroquinolones antibiotics are used.[47]

Selective phosphodiesterase-4 inhibitors inhibit the airway inflammatory processes associated with COPD and have a considerably better side effect profile than theophylline. Evidence from a pooled analysis of two large placebo-controlled, double-blind multicentre trials revealed a significant reduction of 17% in the frequency of moderate (glucocorticoid treated) or severe (hospitalization or death) exacerbations.[60] However, the study design of these trials limits the generalizability: patients had to have an FEV_1 less than 50% (Global Initiative for Chronic Obstructive Lung Disease stages 3 and 4); bronchitic symptoms; and a history of exacerbations. Furthermore, only LABA were allowed as maintenance therapy during the study and there are currently no comparator studies of roflumilast with ICS. Discontinuations because of adverse events were more common in the roflumilast group than in the placebo group, the most frequent adverse events leading to discontinuation (with the exception of COPD) being diarrhea, nausea, and headache. Weight loss was also noted in the roflumilast group, with a mean reduction of 2.1 kg after 1 year, which was greatest in obese patients. Concerns regarding tolerability and side effects of roflumilast therapy may have limited its clinical use.

Long-Term Antibiotics

At present there is insufficient evidence to recommend routine prophylactic antibiotic therapy in the management of stable COPD. However, recent studies have shown promise, particularly those involving macrolides, which have anti-inflammatory and antimicrobial properties. Erythromycin reduced the frequency of moderate or severe exacerbations (treated with systemic steroids or antibiotics, or hospitalized) and shortened exacerbation length when taken twice daily over 12 months by patients with moderate-to-severe COPD.[61] The macrolide azithromycin has been used as prophylaxis in patients with cystic fibrosis and is also suitable for use in patients with COPD for exacerbation prevention. A large United States trial of more than 1500 patients with COPD at high risk of exacerbations recently reported that when added to usual treatment, azithromycin taken daily for 1 year decreased the frequency of exacerbations and improved quality of life. However, patients in the azithromycin intervention group were more likely to become colonized with macrolide-resistant organisms and suffer hearing decrements.[62] Ongoing concerns regarding the development of antibiotic resistance have led to trials of alternative, pulsed antibiotic regimens. Intermittent pulsed moxifloxacin when given to stable patients significantly reduced exacerbation frequency in a per-protocol population, and in a post hoc subgroup of patients with bronchitis at baseline. However, this reduction did not meet statistical significance in the intention-to-treat analysis and further work is required in this area.[63]

Mucolytics

The routine use of these agents is not currently recommended. Some evidence exists that mucolytics, such as carbocysteine, may reduce exacerbation frequency in selected patients with viscous sputum.[64] However, it is not certain if these treatments provide additional benefit to patients already being treated with LABA or ICS.

Novel Anti-Inflammatory Drugs

COPD is an inflammatory condition associated with relative steroid resistance and approaches to restore steroid sensitivity may lead to novel future therapies.[65] Histone deacetylase-2 is reduced in airway tissue from patients with COPD compared with healthy nonsmokers and has been implicated in impaired sensitivity to corticosteroids.[66] Increasing histone deacetylase-2 expression or activation may be a potential avenue to reversing corticosteroid subsensitivity in COPD. Low doses of oral theophylline have been shown to increase histone deacetylase-2 expression in alveolar macrophages from patients with COPD[67,68] and so potentially may restore corticosteroid responsiveness in vivo.

There is evidence of significantly increased phosphoinositide-3-kinase activity in peripheral blood monocytes from patients with COPD compared with smokers and normal control subjects, a pathway that is also associated with reduced corticosteroid sensitivity.[69] The addition of a phosphoinositide-3-kinase inhibitor has been shown to restore steroid sensitivity toward normal[70] and a number of phosphoinositide-3-kinase–delta inhibitors are currently under development.

Alveolar macrophages from patients with COPD demonstrate increased p38 mitogen-activated protein kinase activity.[71] In patients with COPD, selective p38 (p38 mitogen-activated protein kinase) inhibitors reduce lipopolysaccharide-induced cytokine production in alveolar macrophages and synergistically increase the cytokine suppressive effects of dexamethasone.[72]

NONPHARMACOLOGIC THERAPIES
Lung Volume Reduction Surgery

The National Emphysema Treatment Trial reported that lung volume reduction surgery can improve morbidity and mortality in a subset of patients with COPD who have predominantly upper-lobe emphysema and low baseline exercise capacity.[73] A retrospective investigation of data from the same study also showed that lung volume reduction surgery reduces the frequency of COPD exacerbations, possibly through postoperative improvement in lung function[74] and reduction in dynamic hyperinflation. Therefore, this therapeutic option should be explored in selected eligible patients.

Home Oxygen and Ventilatory Support

Although a specific effect of oxygen on reducing exacerbations has not been demonstrated, long-term oxygen therapy has a proved mortality benefit in COPD.[75,76] Furthermore, under-prescription of long-term oxygen therapy where indicated was associated with increased hospital admissions.[77] Domiciliary noninvasive ventilation (NIV) may also improve survival for patients with COPD with hypercapneic respiratory failure[78]; however, controlled trials in this area with regard to exacerbations are also lacking.

Pulmonary Rehabilitation

There is evidence that multiprofessional exercise and education pulmonary rehabilitation programs reduce hospitalization rates in COPD, while improving health status and functional capacity.[79] Maintenance programs may be necessary to maintain these benefits.

Exacerbation therapy is administered in a step-wise model as previously mentioned (**Fig. 4**).[80] The mainstay of exacerbation therapy is an increase in the dose and frequency of short-acting bronchodilators and systemic corticosteroids. Antibiotics are reserved for exacerbations associated with increasing sputum volume or purulence.

Self Management

Patient education is vital to improved management of COPD exacerbations. Rapid recognition of exacerbation symptoms and earlier treatment improves recovery and reduces the risk of hospitalization.[81] These findings have been incorporated into many patient self-management plans and programs that are designed to enable patients to respond appropriately to the first signs of an exacerbation without leading to overtreatment of minor symptom variations. Patients at high risk of exacerbations can be provided with a course of "rescue" antibiotics and corticosteroids to keep at home for use as part of a self-management strategy and instructed to commence

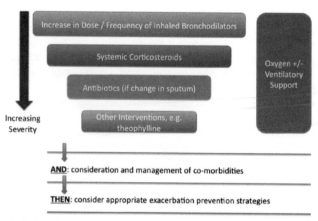

Fig. 4. General scheme for management of a chronic obstructive pulmonary disease (COPD) exacerbation. (*From* Hurst JR, Wedzicha JA. Management and prevention of chronic obstructive pulmonary disease exacerbations: a state of the art review. BMC Med 2009;7:40.)

oral corticosteroid therapy if their increased dyspnea interferes with activities of daily living, either independently or after seeking advice from a healthcare professional. Antibiotics should be started in response to increased sputum volume or purulence and bronchodilator therapy increased to control symptoms.[47] Such interventions have been shown to reduce admission rates[82,83]; however, not all patients are suitable for these strategies. Patients with COPD are frequently elderly and may have cognitive difficulties limiting their ability to self manage, particularly when acutely unwell. Further research is required in this area, with a focus on identification and management of patients at high risk of hospital admission.[84]

Inhaled or Nebulized Bronchodilators

Bronchodilators relieve dyspnea and airflow obstruction during exacerbations[85] and short-acting inhaled β_2 agonists are usually the preferred bronchodilators for the initial treatment of COPD exacerbations.[86] The addition of anticholinergics has the potential for increased therapeutic benefit; however, empiric evidence to support this combination is lacking[85] and the drugs are generally reserved for exacerbations that exhibit a suboptimal response to inhaled β_2 agonists alone.[86] Nebulizers and hand-held inhalers can be used to administer inhaled bronchodilators during exacerbations of COPD and the choice of delivery method should consider the ability of the patient to use the device and the dose of drug required.[47]

Antibiotics

There is considerable evidence to support the role of bacteria in COPD exacerbation etiology and most guidelines highlight that antibiotics are beneficial in selected patients.[86] Purulent sputum is a reasonable surrogate of bacterial infection[27] and routine antibiotic use is normally advised only in the context of exacerbations associated with an increase in sputum purulence.[86] Much of the evidence for these recommendations stems from the seminal study by Anthonisen and colleagues[26] that provided strong evidence that antibiotics had a significant effect on peak expiratory flow rate (PEFR) and led to earlier resolution of symptoms. Type 1 exacerbations (those associated with increased sputum volume, sputum purulence, and dyspnea) benefited the most with resolution of symptoms in 63% of the antibiotic-treated exacerbations and 43% of the placebo group. However, patients with type 3 exacerbations (who met just one of the three cardinal symptoms) did not show significant benefit.

Studies have also assessed the benefits of stratifying antibiotic use according to exacerbation severity. However, the concept of exacerbation severity is difficult, reflecting the severity of the initiating insult, and that of the underlying COPD. In COPD exacerbations requiring mechanical ventilation, oral ofloxacin reduced in-hospital mortality, duration of hospital stay, length of mechanical ventilation, and the need for additional courses of antibiotics.[87] Therefore, in addition to exacerbations associated with increased sputum purulence, antibiotics are recommended in severe exacerbations requiring mechanical ventilation.[86]

The choice of antibiotics remains uncertain, predominantly because of methodologic limitations hampering comparison of studies examining different antibiotics. At present, most guidelines suggest initial empiric treatment should be in the form of an aminopenicillin, a macrolide, or a tetracycline, taking into account guidance from local microbiologists and in the light of local resistance patterns.[47] In hospitalized patients, sputum should be sent for culture at exacerbation if purulent, and the appropriateness of therapy checked against sensitivities when available. In those patients at high risk of P aeruginosa, fluoroquinolones should be considered.

Antiviral Agents

Viral infections (in particular rhinovirus) play a key role in exacerbation etiology and a variety of potential therapeutic agents have been trialed for the treatment of rhinoviral infections. Compounds have attempted to target cell susceptibility, viral attachment and receptor blockade, viral uncoating, viral RNA replication, and viral protein synthesis. Unfortunately, although the neuraminidase inhibitors amantadine and zanamivir are effective against influenza, antirhinoviral compounds have failed to demonstrate a clinically significant benefit in trials and are often complicated by adverse events and lack of tolerability.[88,89]

Systemic Corticosteroids

Multiple studies have found significant short-term benefits of corticosteroids in the treatment of COPD exacerbations. Corticosteroids lead to improvements in FEV_1 in the first 3 to 5 days of treatment[90–92] and Pao_2 in the first 72 hours compared with placebo.[92,93] Corticosteroids have also been shown to reduce hospitalization length[90,91] and the likelihood of treatment failure.[94] However, treatment of exacerbations with corticosteroids has not been shown to improve mortality.[94]

Considerable debate exists regarding the optimal dose and duration of treatment for acute exacerbations, often because of the heterogeneity of treatment regimens in different clinical trials.[95] There is no clear benefit of intravenous therapy over oral preparations and most guidelines recommend a dose of 30 to 40 mg oral prednisone per day for duration of 7 to 14 days.[47,86] There is no advantage in prolonged courses of therapy[91] and shorter courses of therapy reduce the risk of adverse effects. Tapering of this regimen is not required for most patients.[96] The most common reported adverse effect of corticosteroid therapy is hyperglycemia, particularly in patients with preexisting diabetes mellitus,[91] although osteoporosis prophylaxis should also be considered in patients requiring frequent courses of treatment.

The addition of antibiotics to oral steroids as part of exacerbation treatment may have further benefits to regimens composed of oral corticosteroids alone. Epidemiologic research using data from historical cohorts found that adding antibiotics to oral corticosteroids as part of index exacerbation treatment was associated with an increased time to the next exacerbation,[97] a reduced risk of future exacerbations, and reduced risk of all-cause mortality.[98]

Methylxanthines (Theophylline)

Intravenous theophyllines seem to increase respiratory drive, act as bronchodilators, and produce small improvements in acid–base balance during COPD exacerbations.[99] However, they do not improve lung function, dyspnea, or length of hospital stay when given in addition to nebulized bronchodilators and corticosteroids.[99] Given the toxicity associated with these medications, intravenous theophyllines are reserved for patients inadequately responding to standard therapy consisting of nebulized bronchodilators, oral corticosteroids, and antibiotics where indicated.

Oxygen

Oxygen is a treatment for hypoxemia, not breathlessness. However, when patients are hospitalized for exacerbations oxygen is not uncommonly administered during ambulance transportation, at assessment, and on admission. Oxygen must be prescribed with caution in this context because the respiratory drive of some patients with COPD may depend on their degree of hypoxia rather than the usual dependence on hypercapnia. Although rarely seen, overzealous and unmonitored oxygen therapy may result in suppression of a patient's respiratory drive, CO_2 narcosis, and respiratory arrest. Therefore, on arrival at the emergency room, arterial blood gases should be measured and the inspired oxygen concentration adjusted accordingly. Patients who have had a prior episode of hypercapnic respiratory failure should be issued with an oxygen alert card and a 24% or 28% Venturi mask for use during transportation.[47] For most patients with known COPD a target saturation range of 88% to 92% is recommended pending the availability of blood gas results.[100]

NIV

NIV, usually administered as pressure-cycled bi-level positive airway pressure is the treatment of choice for hypercapnic respiratory failure at acute exacerbation of COPD that persists despite optimal medical therapy including controlled oxygen therapy. NIV has been shown to improve gas exchange and acid–base disturbances. Consequently, NIV can reduce the length of hospital stay, mortality, and the need for intubation compared with usual medical care.[101] NIV should be delivered in a dedicated setting by trained, experienced staff. Before patients commence treatment, a clear management plan must be established to determine a course of action in the event of deterioration and to define the ceiling of care.[47]

Invasive Ventilation

If patients do not respond adequately or tolerate NIV (eg, because of multiorgan failure or reduced levels of consciousness), they may require endotracheal intubation and invasive ventilation. Historically, there has been a reluctance to intubate patients with COPD because of concerns about weaning and long-term outcomes. However, patients receiving mechanical ventilation because of acute decompensation of COPD have a significantly lower mortality (estimated 22%) than patients receiving mechanical ventilation for acute respiratory failure from other etiologies.[102] Thus, patients with exacerbations of COPD should be considered eligible to receive treatment on intensive care units, including invasive ventilation when necessary. Factors to be considered before admission include premorbid functional status, body mass index, the prevalence and severity of comorbidities, stable-state oxygen requirements, and prior intensive care unit admissions, in addition to age and degree of airflow obstruction or lung function impairment.[47]

Palliative Care

Palliative care involves the active care of patients and their families by a multidisciplinary team when a patient's disease is no longer responsive to curative treatment. Palliative care focuses on symptom control and optimizing quality of life. Anxiety and depression is common in COPD and may become particularly problematic in patients with end-stage disease, and those hospitalized with exacerbations. These symptoms should be treated with conventional pharmacotherapy. Intractable dyspnea that is unresponsive to other medical therapies may be treated with opiates, benzodiazepines, and tricyclic antidepressants[47]; however, there is little evidence to support the use of oxygen to relieve dyspnea in nonhypoxemic patients.[103] Palliative care should also include consideration of admission to hospices.

SUMMARY

The mechanisms of COPD exacerbation are complex. Respiratory viruses (in particular rhinovirus) and bacteria play a major role in the causative etiology of COPD exacerbations. In some patients, noninfective environmental factors may also be important. Data recently published from a large observational study identified a phenotype of patients more susceptible to frequent exacerbations. Many current therapeutic strategies can reduce exacerbation frequency. Future studies may target the frequent exacerbator phenotype, or those patients colonized with potential bacterial pathogens, for such therapies as long-term antibiotics, thus preventing exacerbations by decreasing bacterial load or preventing new strain acquisition in the stable state. Respiratory viral infections are also an important therapeutic target for COPD. Further work is required to develop new anti-inflammatory agents for exacerbation prevention, and novel acute treatments to improve outcomes at exacerbation.

REFERENCES

1. Burden of lung disease report. 2nd edition. British Thoracic Society (BTS); 2006. Available at: http://www.brit-thoracic.org.uk/Portals/0/Library/BTSPublications/burdeon_of_lung_disease2007.pdf. Accessed September 14, 2011.
2. Hurst JR, Vestbo J, Anzueto A, et al. Susceptibility to exacerbation in chronic obstructive pulmonary disease. N Engl J Med 2010;363(12):1128–38.
3. Donaldson GC, Seemungal TA, Bhowmik A, et al. Relationship between exacerbation frequency and lung function decline in chronic obstructive pulmonary disease. Thorax 2002;57(10):847–52.
4. Kanner RE, Anthonisen NR, Connett JE. Lower respiratory illnesses promote FEV(1) decline in current smokers but not ex-smokers with mild chronic obstructive pulmonary disease: results from the Lung Health Study. Am J Respir Crit Care Med 2001;164(3):358–64.
5. Donaldson GC, Hurst JR, Smith CJ, et al. Increased risk of myocardial infarction and stroke following exacerbation of COPD. Chest 2010;137(5):1091–7.
6. Seemungal TA, Donaldson GC, Paul EA, et al. Effect of exacerbation on quality of life in patients with chronic obstructive pulmonary disease. Am J Respir Crit Care Med 1998;157(5 Pt 1):1418–22.
7. Soler-Cataluna JJ, Martinez-Garcia MA, Roman Sanchez P, et al. Severe acute exacerbations and mortality in patients with chronic obstructive pulmonary disease. Thorax 2005;60(11):925–31.

8. Garcia-Aymerich J, Farrero E, Felez MA, et al. Risk factors of readmission to hospital for a COPD exacerbation: a prospective study. Thorax 2003;58(2): 100–5.

9. Burge S, Wedzicha JA. COPD exacerbations: definitions and classifications. Eur Respir J Suppl 2003;41:46s–53s.

10. Seemungal T, Harper-Owen R, Bhowmik A, et al. Respiratory viruses, symptoms, and inflammatory markers in acute exacerbations and stable chronic obstructive pulmonary disease. Am J Respir Crit Care Med 2001;164(9): 1618–23.

11. Bhowmik A, Seemungal TA, Sapsford RJ, et al. Relation of sputum inflammatory markers to symptoms and lung function changes in COPD exacerbations. Thorax 2000;55(2):114–20.

12. Seemungal TA, Donaldson GC, Bhowmik A, et al. Time course and recovery of exacerbations in patients with chronic obstructive pulmonary disease. Am J Respir Crit Care Med 2000;161(5):1608–13.

13. Rohde G, Wiethege A, Borg I, et al. Respiratory viruses in exacerbations of chronic obstructive pulmonary disease requiring hospitalisation: a case-control study. Thorax 2003;58(1):37–42.

14. Mallia P, Message SD, Gielen V, et al. Experimental rhinovirus infection as a human model of chronic obstructive pulmonary disease exacerbation. Am J Respir Crit Care Med 2011;183(6):734–42.

15. Schneider D, Ganesan S, Comstock AT, et al. Increased cytokine response of rhinovirus-infected airway epithelial cells in chronic obstructive pulmonary disease. Am J Respir Crit Care Med 2010;182(3):332–40.

16. Di Stefano A, Maestrelli P, Roggeri A, et al. Upregulation of adhesion molecules in the bronchial mucosa of subjects with chronic obstructive bronchitis. Am J Respir Crit Care Med 1994;149(3 Pt 1):803–10.

17. Donaldson GC, Seemungal T, Jeffries DJ, et al. Effect of temperature on lung function and symptoms in chronic obstructive pulmonary disease. Eur Respir J 1999;13(4):844–9.

18. Lyon JL, Stoddard G, Ferguson D, et al. An every other year cyclic epidemic of infants hospitalized with respiratory syncytial virus. Pediatrics 1996;97(1): 152–3.

19. Meerhoff TJ, Paget JW, Kimpen JL, et al. Variation of respiratory syncytial virus and the relation with meteorological factors in different winter seasons. Pediatr Infect Dis J 2009;28(10):860–6.

20. Wilkinson TM, Donaldson GC, Johnston SL, et al. Respiratory syncytial virus, airway inflammation, and FEV1 decline in patients with chronic obstructive pulmonary disease. Am J Respir Crit Care Med 2006;173(8):871–6.

21. Nichol KL, Baken L, Nelson A. Relation between influenza vaccination and outpatient visits, hospitalization, and mortality in elderly persons with chronic lung disease. Ann Intern Med 1999;130(5):397–403.

22. Sethi S. Infectious etiology of acute exacerbations of chronic bronchitis. Chest 2000;117(5 Suppl 2):380S–5S.

23. Sethi S, Murphy TF. Bacterial infection in chronic obstructive pulmonary disease in 2000: a state-of-the-art review. Clin Microbiol Rev 2001;14(2):336–63.

24. Murphy TF, Brauer AL, Sethi S, et al. Haemophilus haemolyticus: a human respiratory tract commensal to be distinguished from Haemophilus influenzae. J Infect Dis 2007;195(1):81–9.

25. Sethi S, Evans N, Grant BJ, et al. New strains of bacteria and exacerbations of chronic obstructive pulmonary disease. N Engl J Med 2002;347(7):465–71.

26. Anthonisen NR, Manfreda J, Warren CP, et al. Antibiotic therapy in exacerbations of chronic obstructive pulmonary disease. Ann Intern Med 1987;106(2): 196–204.
27. Stockley RA, O'Brien C, Pye A, et al. Relationship of sputum color to nature and outpatient management of acute exacerbations of COPD. Chest 2000; 117(6):1638–45.
28. Miravitlles M, Marin A, Monso E, et al. Colour of sputum is a marker for bacterial colonisation in chronic obstructive pulmonary disease. Respir Res 2010; 11:58.
29. Monso E, Ruiz J, Rosell A, et al. Bacterial infection in chronic obstructive pulmonary disease. A study of stable and exacerbated outpatients using the protected specimen brush. Am J Respir Crit Care Med 1995;152(4 Pt 1):1316–20.
30. Patel IS, Seemungal TA, Wilks M, et al. Relationship between bacterial colonisation and the frequency, character, and severity of COPD exacerbations. Thorax 2002;57(9):759–64.
31. Hilty M, Burke C, Pedro H, et al. Disordered microbial communities in asthmatic airways. PLoS One 2010;5(1):e8578.
32. Erb-Downward JR, Thompson DL, Han MK, et al. Analysis of the lung microbiome in the "healthy" smoker and in COPD. PLoS One 2011;6(2):e16384.
33. Wilkinson TM, Hurst JR, Perera WR, et al. Effect of interactions between lower airway bacterial and rhinoviral infection in exacerbations of COPD. Chest 2006;129(2):317–24.
34. Rosell A, Monso E, Soler N, et al. Microbiologic determinants of exacerbation in chronic obstructive pulmonary disease. Arch Intern Med 2005;165(8):891–7.
35. Sethi S, Sethi R, Eschberger K, et al. Airway bacterial concentrations and exacerbations of chronic obstructive pulmonary disease. Am J Respir Crit Care Med 2007;176(4):356–61.
36. Abusriwil H, Stockley RA. Bacterial load and exacerbations of COPD. Am J Respir Crit Care Med 2008;177(9):1048–9 [author reply: 1049].
37. Sajjan US, Jia Y, Newcomb DC, et al. H. influenzae potentiates airway epithelial cell responses to rhinovirus by increasing ICAM-1 and TLR3 expression. FASEB J 2006;20(12):2121–3.
38. Papi A, Bellettato CM, Braccioni F, et al. Infections and airway inflammation in chronic obstructive pulmonary disease severe exacerbations. Am J Respir Crit Care Med 2006;173(10):1114–21.
39. Anderson HR, Spix C, Medina S, et al. Air pollution and daily admissions for chronic obstructive pulmonary disease in 6 European cities: results from the APHEA project. Eur Respir J 1997;10(5):1064–71.
40. Wordley J, Walters S, Ayres JG. Short term variations in hospital admissions and mortality and particulate air pollution. Occup Environ Med 1997;54(2):108–16.
41. Dominici F, Peng RD, Bell ML, et al. Fine particulate air pollution and hospital admission for cardiovascular and respiratory diseases. JAMA 2006;295(10): 1127–34.
42. Nordenhall C, Pourazar J, Blomberg A, et al. Airway inflammation following exposure to diesel exhaust: a study of time kinetics using induced sputum. Eur Respir J 2000;15(6):1046–51.
43. Rudell B, Blomberg A, Helleday R, et al. Bronchoalveolar inflammation after exposure to diesel exhaust: comparison between unfiltered and particle trap filtered exhaust. Occup Environ Med 1999;56(8):527–34.
44. Nichol KL, Nordin JD, Nelson DB, et al. Effectiveness of influenza vaccine in the community-dwelling elderly. N Engl J Med 2007;357(14):1373–81.

45. Nichol KL, Baken L, Wuorenma J, et al. The health and economic benefits associated with pneumococcal vaccination of elderly persons with chronic lung disease. Arch Intern Med 1999;159(20):2437–42.

46. Alfageme I, Vazquez R, Reyes N, et al. Clinical efficacy of anti-pneumococcal vaccination in patients with COPD. Thorax 2006;61(3):189–95.

47. National Clinical Guideline Centre. Chronic obstructive pulmonary disease: management of chronic obstructive pulmonary disease in adults in primary and secondary care. London: National Clinical Guideline Centre; 2010. Available at: http://guidance.nice.org.uk/CG101/Guidance/pdf/English. Accessed September 14, 2011.

48. Sprenkle MD, Niewoehner DE, MacDonald R, et al. Clinical efficacy of OM-85 BV in COPD and chronic bronchitis: a systematic review. COPD 2005;2(1):167–75.

49. Orcel B, Delclaux B, Baud M, et al. Oral immunization with bacterial extracts for protection against acute bronchitis in elderly institutionalized patients with chronic bronchitis. Eur Respir J 1994;7(3):446–52.

50. Collet JP, Shapiro P, Ernst P, et al. Effects of an immunostimulating agent on acute exacerbations and hospitalizations in patients with chronic obstructive pulmonary disease. The PARI-IS Study Steering Committee and Research Group. Prevention of Acute Respiratory Infection by an Immunostimulant. Am J Respir Crit Care Med 1997;156(6):1719–24.

51. Soler M, Mutterlein R, Cozma G. Double-blind study of OM-85 in patients with chronic bronchitis or mild chronic obstructive pulmonary disease. Respiration 2007;74(1):26–32.

52. Cazzola M, Rogliani P, Curradi G. Bacterial extracts for the prevention of acute exacerbations in chronic obstructive pulmonary disease: a point of view. Respir Med 2008;102(3):321–7.

53. Burge PS, Calverley PM, Jones PW, et al. Randomised, double blind, placebo controlled study of fluticasone propionate in patients with moderate to severe chronic obstructive pulmonary disease: the ISOLDE trial. BMJ 2000;320(7245):1297–303.

54. Calverley PM, Anderson JA, Celli B, et al. Salmeterol and fluticasone propionate and survival in chronic obstructive pulmonary disease. N Engl J Med 2007;356(8):775–89.

55. Tashkin DP, Celli B, Senn S, et al. A 4-year trial of tiotropium in chronic obstructive pulmonary disease. N Engl J Med 2008;359(15):1543–54.

56. Aaron SD, Vandemheen KL, Fergusson D, et al. Tiotropium in combination with placebo, salmeterol, or fluticasone-salmeterol for treatment of chronic obstructive pulmonary disease: a randomized trial. Ann Intern Med 2007;146(8):545–55.

57. Puhan MA, Bachmann LM, Kleijnen J, et al. Inhaled drugs to reduce exacerbations in patients with chronic obstructive pulmonary disease: a network meta-analysis. BMC Med 2009;7:2.

58. Rossi A, Kristufek P, Levine BE, et al. Comparison of the efficacy, tolerability, and safety of formoterol dry powder and oral, slow-release theophylline in the treatment of COPD. Chest 2002;121(4):1058–69.

59. Zhou Y, Wang X, Zeng X, et al. Positive benefits of theophylline in a randomized, double-blind, parallel-group, placebo-controlled study of low-dose, slow-release theophylline in the treatment of COPD for 1 year. Respirology 2006;11(5):603–10.

60. Calverley PM, Rabe KF, Goehring UM, et al. Roflumilast in symptomatic chronic obstructive pulmonary disease: two randomised clinical trials. Lancet 2009;374(9691):685–94.

61. Seemungal TA, Wilkinson TM, Hurst JR, et al. Long-term erythromycin therapy is associated with decreased chronic obstructive pulmonary disease exacerbations. Am J Respir Crit Care Med 2008;178(11):1139–47.
62. Albert RK, Connett J, Bailey WC, et al. Azithromycin for prevention of exacerbations of COPD. N Engl J Med 2011;365(8):689–98.
63. Sethi S, Jones PW, Theron MS, et al. Pulsed moxifloxacin for the prevention of exacerbations of chronic obstructive pulmonary disease: a randomized controlled trial. Respir Res 2010;11:10.
64. Zheng JP, Kang J, Huang SG, et al. Effect of carbocisteine on acute exacerbation of chronic obstructive pulmonary disease (PEACE Study): a randomised placebo-controlled study. Lancet 2008;371(9629):2013–8.
65. Barnes PJ. Corticosteroid resistance in airway disease. Proc Am Thorac Soc 2004;1(3):264–8.
66. Ito K, Ito M, Elliott WM, et al. Decreased histone deacetylase activity in chronic obstructive pulmonary disease. N Engl J Med 2005;352(19):1967–76.
67. Cosio BG, Tsaprouni L, Ito K, et al. Theophylline restores histone deacetylase activity and steroid responses in COPD macrophages. J Exp Med 2004; 200(5):689–95.
68. Ito K, Lim S, Caramori G, et al. A molecular mechanism of action of theophylline: induction of histone deacetylase activity to decrease inflammatory gene expression. Proc Natl Acad Sci U S A 2002;99(13):8921–6.
69. Marwick JA, Caramori G, Casolari P, et al. A role for phosphoinositol 3-kinase delta in the impairment of glucocorticoid responsiveness in patients with chronic obstructive pulmonary disease. J Allergy Clin Immunol 2010;125(5):1146–53.
70. Marwick JA, Caramori G, Stevenson CS, et al. Inhibition of PI3Kdelta restores glucocorticoid function in smoking-induced airway inflammation in mice. Am J Respir Crit Care Med 2009;179(7):542–8.
71. Renda T, Baraldo S, Pelaia G, et al. Increased activation of p38 MAPK in COPD. Eur Respir J 2008;31(1):62–9.
72. Armstrong J, Harbron C, Lea S, et al. Synergistic effects of p38 mitogen-activated protein kinase inhibition with a corticosteroid in alveolar macrophages from patients with chronic obstructive pulmonary disease. J Pharmacol Exp Ther 2011;338(3):732–40.
73. Fishman A, Martinez F, Naunheim K, et al. A randomized trial comparing lung-volume-reduction surgery with medical therapy for severe emphysema. N Engl J Med 2003;348(21):2059–73.
74. Washko GR, Fan VS, Ramsey SD, et al. The effect of lung volume reduction surgery on chronic obstructive pulmonary disease exacerbations. Am J Respir Crit Care Med 2008;177(2):164–9.
75. Continuous or nocturnal oxygen therapy in hypoxemic chronic obstructive lung disease: a clinical trial. Nocturnal Oxygen Therapy Trial Group. Ann Intern Med 1980;93(3):391–8.
76. Long term domiciliary oxygen therapy in chronic hypoxic cor pulmonale complicating chronic bronchitis and emphysema. Report of the Medical Research Council Working Party. Lancet 1981;1(8222):681–6.
77. Garcia-Aymerich J, Monso E, Marrades RM, et al. Risk factors for hospitalization for a chronic obstructive pulmonary disease exacerbation. EFRAM study. Am J Respir Crit Care Med 2001;164(6):1002–7.
78. McEvoy RD, Pierce RJ, Hillman D, et al. Nocturnal non-invasive nasal ventilation in stable hypercapnic COPD: a randomised controlled trial. Thorax 2009;64(7): 561–6.

79. Casaburi R, ZuWallack R. Pulmonary rehabilitation for management of chronic obstructive pulmonary disease. N Engl J Med 2009;360(13):1329–35.

80. Hurst JR, Wedzicha JA. Management and prevention of chronic obstructive pulmonary disease exacerbations: a state of the art review. BMC Med 2009;7:40.

81. Wilkinson TM, Donaldson GC, Hurst JR, et al. Early therapy improves outcomes of exacerbations of chronic obstructive pulmonary disease. Am J Respir Crit Care Med 2004;169(12):1298–303.

82. Bourbeau J, Julien M, Maltais F, et al. Reduction of hospital utilization in patients with chronic obstructive pulmonary disease: a disease-specific self-management intervention. Arch Intern Med 2003;163(5):585–91.

83. Casas A, Troosters T, Garcia-Aymerich J, et al. Integrated care prevents hospitalisations for exacerbations in COPD patients. Eur Respir J 2006;28(1):123–30.

84. Wedzicha JA, Seemungal TA. COPD exacerbations: defining their cause and prevention. Lancet 2007;370(9589):786–96.

85. McCrory DC, Brown CD. Anti-cholinergic bronchodilators versus beta2-sympathomimetic agents for acute exacerbations of chronic obstructive pulmonary disease. Cochrane Database Syst Rev 2002;4:CD003900.

86. Global Strategy for the Diagnosis, Management and Prevention of COPD. Global Initiative for Chronic Obstructive Lung Disease (GOLD); 2009. Available at: http://www.goldcopd.org. Accessed September 14, 2011.

87. Nouira S, Marghli S, Belghith M, et al. Once daily oral ofloxacin in chronic obstructive pulmonary disease exacerbation requiring mechanical ventilation: a randomised placebo-controlled trial. Lancet 2001;358(9298):2020–5.

88. Martinez FJ. Pathogen-directed therapy in acute exacerbations of chronic obstructive pulmonary disease. Proc Am Thorac Soc 2007;4(8):647–58.

89. Anzueto A, Niederman MS. Diagnosis and treatment of rhinovirus respiratory infections. Chest 2003;123(5):1664–72.

90. Davies L, Angus RM, Calverley PM. Oral corticosteroids in patients admitted to hospital with exacerbations of chronic obstructive pulmonary disease: a prospective randomised controlled trial. Lancet 1999;354(9177):456–60.

91. Niewoehner DE, Erbland ML, Deupree RH, et al. Effect of systemic glucocorticoids on exacerbations of chronic obstructive pulmonary disease. Department of Veterans Affairs Cooperative Study Group. N Engl J Med 1999;340(25):1941–7.

92. Thompson WH, Nielson CP, Carvalho P, et al. Controlled trial of oral prednisone in outpatients with acute COPD exacerbation. Am J Respir Crit Care Med 1996; 154(2 Pt 1):407–12.

93. Maltais F, Ostinelli J, Bourbeau J, et al. Comparison of nebulized budesonide and oral prednisolone with placebo in the treatment of acute exacerbations of chronic obstructive pulmonary disease: a randomized controlled trial. Am J Respir Crit Care Med 2002;165(5):698–703.

94. Wood-Baker RR, Gibson PG, Hannay M, et al. Systemic corticosteroids for acute exacerbations of chronic obstructive pulmonary disease. Cochrane Database Syst Rev 2005;1:CD001288.

95. McCrory DC, Brown C, Gray RN, et al. Management of acute exacerbations of chronic obstructive pulmonary disease. Evid Rep Technol Assess (Summ) 2000;(19):1–4.

96. Joint Formulary Committee. British National Formulary. 61st edition. London: British Medical Association and Royal Pharmaceutical Society; 2011.

97. Roede BM, Bresser P, Bindels PJ, et al. Antibiotic treatment is associated with reduced risk of a subsequent exacerbation in obstructive lung disease: an historical population based cohort study. Thorax 2008;63(11):968–73.

98. Roede BM, Bresser P, Prins JM, et al. Reduced risk of next exacerbation and mortality associated with antibiotic use in COPD. Eur Respir J 2009;33(2):282–8.
99. Duffy N, Walker P, Diamantea F, et al. Intravenous aminophylline in patients admitted to hospital with non-acidotic exacerbations of chronic obstructive pulmonary disease: a prospective randomised controlled trial. Thorax 2005; 60(9):713–7.
100. O'Driscoll BR, Howard LS, Davison AG. BTS guideline for emergency oxygen use in adult patients. Thorax 2008;63(Suppl 6):vi1–68.
101. Ram FS, Lightowler JV, Wedzicha JA. Non-invasive positive pressure ventilation for treatment of respiratory failure due to exacerbations of chronic obstructive pulmonary disease. Cochrane Database Syst Rev 2003;1:CD004104.
102. Esteban A, Anzueto A, Frutos F, et al. Characteristics and outcomes in adult patients receiving mechanical ventilation: a 28-day international study. JAMA 2002;287(3):345–55.
103. Clemens KE, Quednau I, Klaschik E. Use of oxygen and opioids in the palliation of dyspnoea in hypoxic and non-hypoxic palliative care patients: a prospective study. Support Care Cancer 2009;17(4):367–77.

An Integrated Approach to the Medical Treatment of Chronic Obstructive Pulmonary Disease

Sharon R. Rosenberg, MD, MS, Ravi Kalhan, MD, MS*

KEYWORDS

- Chronic obstructive pulmonary disease (COPD) • Treatment • Symptoms
- Lung function • Patient-centered outcomes

KEY POINTS

- The goals of chronic obstructive pulmonary disease (COPD) pharmacotherapy are to reduce symptoms, reduce the frequency and severity of exacerbations, improve exercise tolerance and health status, and reduce mortality.
- Recently updated guidelines recommend that the evaluation of patients with COPD includes objective symptom assessment, measurement of lung function, and determination of exacerbation history to more definitively individualize a therapeutic plan.
- Effective treatment of COPD requires that attention be paid to the therapeutic response with objective measurement of symptoms, exacerbations, and exercise capacity on an ongoing basis.
- Many treatment therapies exist that effectively treat symptoms or reduce exacerbations, including long-acting beta2 agonists (LABAs), combination LABA-inhaled corticosteroids, long-acting antimuscarinics, phosphodiesterase-4 inhibitors, and macrolides.
- Nonpharmacologic therapy, such as formal programs of rehabilitative exercise and education regarding lung disease, have substantial benefits in COPD.

INTRODUCTION

Chronic obstructive pulmonary disease (COPD) is now the third leading cause of death in the United States[1] and is the only leading cause of death that is increasing in prevalence.[2] The American Thoracic Society (ATS), the European Respiratory Society (ERS), and the Global Initiative for Obstructive Lung Disease (GOLD) define COPD as a preventable and treatable condition characterized by airflow limitation that is not completely reversible.[3,4] This definition marked an important paradigm shift

Dr Kalhan has served as a paid consultant to Boehringer-Ingelheim, Forest Laboratories, and Elevation Pharmaceuticals.
Asthma and COPD Program, Northwestern University Feinberg School of Medicine, 676 North Saint Clair Street, #1400, Chicago, IL 60611, USA
* Corresponding author.
E-mail address: r-kalhan@northwestern.edu

Med Clin N Am 96 (2012) 811–826
doi:10.1016/j.mcna.2012.05.002
medical.theclinics.com

from earlier definitions, which did not emphasize the treatable nature of COPD.[5] The treatment of patients with COPD now requires a detailed evaluation of the disease severity and the impacts beyond the measurement of lung function and then the selection of therapies in the context of individual disease severity. This review focuses on how measurements of disease severity and impacts can be integrated with therapeutic selection to improve clinical outcomes and quality of life for individuals living with COPD.

EVALUATING COPD SEVERITY IN CLINICAL PRACTICE: MORE THAN THE FORCED EXPIRATORY VOLUME IN THE FIRST SECOND OF EXPIRATION

Traditionally, COPD severity has been staged according to the degree of airflow limitation measured through forced spirometry. In fact, until the recently released 2011 update, the GOLD guidelines advocated that medical therapies be selected according to severity of airflow limitation measured by forced expiratory volume in the first second of expiration (FEV_1). Although the measurement of FEV_1 is essential to establish a diagnosis of COPD and may provide a useful starting-off point for the evaluation of disease severity and formulation of a treatment plan, it does not necessarily reflect the impact COPD has on an individual's daily experiences. In fact, FEV_1 correlates weakly with breathlessness, exercise tolerance, and overall health status.[6–8] Although no COPD pharmacotherapy has ever been shown to modify the natural history of FEV_1 decline in COPD, most COPD medications have documented benefits of not just immediately improving lung function but also improving perceived breathlessness, exercise capacity, and overall quality of life. It has also been documented that COPD exacerbations, defined as "an event in the natural course of the disease characterized by a change in the patient's baseline dyspnea, cough, and/or sputum that is beyond normal day-to-day variations that is acute in onset…" occur across the spectrum of FEV_1 impairment in COPD[9] and, therefore, must be incorporated as their own domain in the assessment of disease severity with an eye toward preventing their recurrence. In this section, the authors outline the systematic evaluation of patients with COPD in clinical practice that they think maximizes the possibility of formulating an individualized treatment plan (**Table 1**).

Table 1	
The key elements of an objective clinical assessment of COPD	
COPD Patient Assessment	
Spirometry	BODE index
mMRC dyspnea scale	
Body mass index	
6-min walk distance	
Exacerbation History	
Self-report of requiring antibiotics or steroids	
CAT	
Comorbidity Assessment	
Heart failure	
Depression	
Osteoporosis	
Individualized Pharmacotherapy Plan	
Inhaler technique and skill	
Affordability	
Exacerbation frequency and symptom burden	

COPD Symptom Assessment: Objective Approaches

The 2011 update to the GOLD COPD guidelines now recommend that COPD symptoms be assessed in an objective manner and incorporated into the selection process of a COPD treatment strategy.[4] This recommendation validates the clinical intuition that if an individual patient perceives greater breathlessness, their overall sense of well-being and functional status will be compromised more significantly than those with less shortness of breath. It is critical, therefore, for clinicians to evaluate breathlessness and related symptoms in an ongoing and objective manner. The GOLD guideline recommends use of either the 5-point modified Medical Research Council (mMRC) dyspnea scale or the more recently developed COPD Assessment Test (CAT).[4]

The mMRC dyspnea scale uses the degree of breathlessness related to the limitations associated with the completion of physical tasks, such as walking or dressing, which are self-reported by patients to place the degree of dyspnea on a 5-point scale (**Table 2**). The mMRC score is associated with 5-year mortality in COPD and, in at least one report, has greater discriminatory power than staging by FEV_1.[8,10] In the authors' clinical program, the ease of use and rapid objective assessment of impacts of breathlessness on daily activities that it provides is valuable in the initial evaluation of patients with COPD; however, it is important to recognize that the 5-point scale of the mMRC makes it difficult to detect changes in symptoms after beginning a COPD treatment or to detect a subtle worsening in symptoms.[11]

More recently, the CAT has been developed using rigorous psychometric methods and is widely available (www.catestonline.org). The CAT evaluates 8 patient-centered items and how they are impacted by COPD on a semantic 6-point differential scale (rated 0–5) for each: cough, chest congestion, chest tightness, breathlessness with ascending stairs or a hill, limitation in household activities, confidence leaving the home, quality of sleep, and energy level.[12] The test is scored from a minimum score of 0 to a maximum of 40. The CAT correlates strongly with the St George respiratory quotient (SGRQ), a detailed quality-of-life instrument that has been used in respiratory clinical trials.[12] Importantly, recent reports indicate that the CAT may be useful as a response variable following therapeutic intervention.[13–15] In addition, CAT scores worsen with the onset of a COPD exacerbation, improve over the subsequent days, and may prove useful as a marker of exacerbation severity.[15,16]

Exercise Capacity and Lung Hyperinflation in the Assessment of COPD Severity

As mentioned, FEV_1 correlates poorly with not only breathlessness but also exercise capacity. Exercise capacity in COPD is tied closely to dynamic (with exercise or other causes of tachypnea) and static (at rest) lung hyperinflation that manifests as an increase in end expiratory lung volume (EELV). At equilibrium, when an individual has

Table 2
The mMRC scale

mMRC Grade	Description
Grade 0	I only get breathless with strenuous exercise
Grade 1	I get short of breath when hurrying on the level or walking up a slight hill
Grade 2	I walk slower than people of the same age on the level because of breathlessness, or I have to stop for breath when walking at my own pace on the level
Grade 3	I stop for breath after walking about 100 m after a few minutes on the level
Grade 4	I am too breathless to leave the house or I am breathless when dressing or undressing

fully exhaled, EELV is the same as functional residual capacity (FRC); The EELV is more rigorously correct in dynamic conditions whereby equilibrium is not achieved. The difference between the total amount of air that can be contained in the lung, total lung capacity (TLC), and EELV is termed the inspiratory capacity (IC), which can viewed as the reserve a person has to breath. The IC decreases as hyperinflation worsens in COPD and the extent to which IC becomes a smaller proportion of TLC (the IC-to-TLC ratio can be thought of as the lung's version of the cardiac ejection fraction) indicates worsening hyperinflation with an IC/TLC value of less than 0.25, portending a particularly poor prognosis.[17]

Measuring the magnitude of static lung hyperinflation is feasible in the context of pulmonary function testing but not practical on a routine basis, and dynamic hyperinflation with exercise cannot be readily measured in the clinic. Hyperinflation, however, does correlate with exercise tolerance, which, through the measurement of the 6-minute walk distance (6MWD), allows for severity assessment and monitoring of disease.[18,19] The 6MWD is a straightforward simple test with standardized methods[20] that predicts survival independently in COPD.[21] Because of its ease of use, tangible results for both the provider and patients, and reflection of underlying pathophysiology (dynamic hyperinflation) the authors use the 6MWD in their clinic program as both a means to assess severity and to identify progression or improvement of COPD.

Integrative COPD Severity Indices

Several integrative measures that incorporate both traditional measures of lung function and other factors that impact an individual's health status have been developed in an effort to bring greater refinement to clinical assessments of disease severity. The most prominent of these indices is the BODE index, which is a composite of 4 parameters: body mass index, magnitude of airflow obstruction according to FEV_1, dyspnea determined by the mMRC scale, and exercise capacity via 6MWD. The BODE index is a 10-point scale in which a higher score indicates a worse prognosis (**Table 3**). In a prospective validation study, the BODE outperformed FEV_1 in predicting all-cause mortality over a 1-year period.[22] More recent studies have also pointed to the BODE index as a predictor of hospitalization (again outperforming FEV_1),[23] and data indicate that the BODE may serve as a useful parameter to assess the effect of therapeutic interventions in COPD.[24–26]

Two additional COPD integrative indices have been developed that do not require the measurement of 6MWD, which serves as a strength when that test is not practical. The ADO index includes age, dyspnea (mMRC scale), and the severity of airflow obstruction (FEV_1). The discriminatory power of ADO is similar to that of BODE,[27] but it has not been evaluated as an indicator of therapeutic response. The DOSE index incorporates dyspnea (mMRC scale), obstruction (FEV_1), smoking status (current vs

Table 3
Components and scoring of the BODE index

Variable	Points on BODE Index			
	0	1	2	3
FEV1 (% of predicted)	65	50–64	36–49	35
6 min walk distance (m)	350	250–349	150–249	149 or less
mMRC dyspnea scale	0–1	2	3	4
Body mass index	>21	21 or less		

Data from Celli BR, Cote CG, Marin JM, et al. The body-mass index, airflow obstruction, dyspnea, and exercise capacity index in chronic obstructive pulmonary disease. N Engl J Med 2004;350:1005–12.

former), and exacerbation frequency.[28] The inclusion of exacerbations and smoking status distinguishes DOSE from other integrative measures. The DOSE index predicts important future COPD outcomes, including hospital admissions, respiratory failure, and exacerbations; but, like the ADO, it has not been tested in the context of evaluating therapeutic responses. In the authors' clinical program, because of its 0-to-10 scale (something the authors have found appeals to patients who desire a rating of their COPD on a 10-point scale) and its potential responsiveness to therapeutic intervention, they have opted to measure the BODE index on a twice-yearly basis in most patients.

Evaluating for a History of COPD Exacerbations

COPD exacerbations present a great burden to both individual patients and the health care system.[29] Recent evidence indicates that exacerbations occur across a spectrum of FEV_1 impairment, although individuals with lower FEV_1 do have more frequent COPD exacerbations.[9] The most reliable predictor of COPD exacerbations in an individual is a history of prior exacerbations suggesting a stable phenotype of exacerbation susceptibility.[9,30] It is well established that COPD exacerbations lead to accelerated decline in lung function and deterioration in quality of life.[31,32] In a prospective cohort of 205 patients with COPD in the United States, individuals who experienced exacerbations of COPD had a greater decline in FEV_1, increasing (ie, worsening) mMRC scores, declining 6MWD, and worsening of the BODE index compared with individuals who did not have exacerbations.[33]

Despite their significant consequences, patients do not consistently report COPD exacerbations to health care providers. In a study conducted in the United Kingdom, patients recorded daily respiratory symptoms on diary cards. Using a precise definition of exacerbations that required worsening respiratory symptoms for 2 consecutive days, the investigators found that just less than 60% of exacerbations were actually reported to physicians.[34] The reason for underreporting of exacerbation symptoms is uncertain, but one could speculate that some patients have adapted to living with COPD such that they do not identify symptomatic variability as anything more than something they have to live with. This gap in the reporting of COPD exacerbation symptoms has been reinforced in other studies and magnifies the need to educate patients and providers alike about signs and symptoms of COPD exacerbations.[35,36] This further supports the importance of exacerbation history assessment and the prevention of future exacerbations. Because reduction of COPD exacerbations is a proven benefit of several COPD pharmacotherapies (see later discussion), the GOLD guidelines now emphasize exacerbation history as an important component in therapeutic decision making.[4] Unfortunately, the authors are not aware of any patient-completed tools that assist in the identification of prior exacerbations. In the authors' clinical program, they attempt to ascertain exacerbation history by asking patients with COPD if and, if yes, how many times they have required treatment with antibiotics or corticosteroids for a respiratory illness over the past 3 years. Although this question does not account for those who have not received treatment of exacerbations but experienced one nonetheless (ie, the unreported exacerbations described previously), this level of recall does seem reliable in predicting a frequent COPD exacerbation phenotype.[9]

Comorbidity Assessment

There has been increasing recognition of COPD as a multicomponent systemic disease associated with a variety of comorbid conditions.[37] The comprehensive approach to care in COPD mandates that comorbidities be recognized and treated. Although there is no evidence that comorbidities commonly found in COPD should be treated any differently in people with COPD that those without COPD, the recognition and treatment of comorbid conditions remains important to ensure good outcomes. Frequently occurring comorbid conditions include ischemic heart disease, heart failure with both reduced and preserved ejection fraction, atrial fibrillation, osteoporosis, anxiety and depression, lung cancer, and metabolic syndrome and diabetes.[4] In the authors' COPD program, particular attention is paid to those that frequently go undetected in routine medical care and are associated with a particularly poor prognosis in COPD if either undetected or left untreated, particularly anxiety and depression[38,39] and lung cancer.[40,41] To identify depression in their clinical practice, the authors have implemented one of the screening procedures that are recommended by the US Preventive Services Task Force. At each visit, patients are asked 2 questions (and their responses are recorded in the medical record) that assess mood and anhedonia: (1) Over the past 2 weeks, have you felt down, depressed, or hopeless? (2) Over the past 2 weeks, have you felt little interest or pleasure in doing things?[42] When patients answer affirmatively to either of these questions, they are referred for full diagnostic interviews with either their primary care doctor or a mental health provider.

COPD MEDICAL THERAPY IN CONTEXT

The goals of therapy in COPD are to reduce symptoms, reduce the frequency and severity of exacerbations, improve exercise tolerance and health status, slow disease progression, and reduce mortality. To date, no COPD pharmacologic therapy has been demonstrated to improve mortality. Supplemental oxygen improves mortality among individuals who are hypoxemic at rest; whether it should be considered pharmacotherapy is a semantic debate. Other pharmacotherapies have demonstrated trends toward improved survival. However, their rigorous assessment is difficult because a truly untreated control group is generally unacceptable and unethical because treatment has clear benefits. At present, evidence supports the use of pharmacotherapy to reduce symptoms, reduce the frequency and severity of exacerbations, and improve exercise tolerance and health status. The choice of therapeutic agents should be patient specific because the relationship between and severity among symptoms, airflow limitation, and exacerbations will differ between individual patients. Attention to inhaler technique and training is essential to effective drug delivery and should be evaluated at all subsequent clinic visits.[43] In addition to symptoms, airflow limitation and exacerbation history to guide therapeutic decision making, patient skill and ability with inhaler delivery devices, and cost may influence treatment regimens.

Selecting Pharmacotherapies Based on Disease Severity

As mentioned earlier, the most recent update of the GOLD guidelines has shifted the evaluation of COPD and the selection of therapies to include an objective evaluation of symptoms via the mMRC (see **Table 2**) or CAT, severity of airflow limitation based on postbronchodilator FEV_1 (**Table 4**), and history and frequency of exacerbations. In the current GOLD schema, patients are designated into 1 of 4 categories (A–D) and the initial treatment is designated according to this classification (**Table 5**)[4]:

GOLD group A patients
These individuals have few symptoms (defined as CAT <10 or mMRC of 0 or 1), do not have a history of more than 1 exacerbation per year (termed low risk in the GOLD guideline), and have an FEV_1 that places them in stage 1 or 2 of impairment (an FEV_1 of >50% of predicted). In these patients, an as-needed short-acting bronchodilator is recommended. Long-acting bronchodilators may be used, but it should be noted that these patients have not been typically included in trials of any long-acting (maintenance) COPD therapies.

Table 4
Classification of severity of airflow limitation based on postbronchodilator spirometry as suggested in the GOLD guidelines

GOLD Class	FEV_1 Percent Predicted
GOLD 1	Greater than 80% of predicted
GOLD 2	50%–80% of predicted
GOLD 3	30%–49% of predicted
GOLD 4	Less than 30% of predicted

Data from Global strategy for the diagnosis, management, and prevention of COPD, Global Initiative for Chronic Obstructive Lung Disease (GOLD) 2011. Available at: http://www.goldcopd.org/. Accessed April 14, 2012.

GOLD group B patients

These individuals have more COPD symptoms (CAT >10 or mMRC 2 or more), are low risk for exacerbations, and have GOLD stage 1 or 2 FEV_1 impairment. Long-acting bronchodilators, either long-acting beta$_2$-agonists (LABA) or long-acting antimuscarinics (LAMA), are the suggested therapies for these patients. A combination of long-acting bronchodilators from each of the 2 therapeutic classes may be used with a possible favorable effect on both FEV_1 and symptoms,[44,45] but there is not a robust clinical trial database to support this approach.[46]

GOLD group C patients

These patients report few COPD symptoms (CAT <10 or mMRC <2) but have history of 2 or more exacerbations per year (making them high risk for exacerbations) or GOLD stage 3 or 4 FEV_1 impairment (FEV_1 <50% of predicted). In these patients, either a fixed combination LABA and inhaled corticosteroid (LABA-ICS) or an LAMA are recommended. There is virtually no clinical evidence to support the superiority of either an LABA-ICS or LAMA in this setting, with the only direct comparator study documenting no difference in exacerbation reduction.[47]

Table 5
Categories of COPD severity and suggested therapies according to the GOLD guidelines

Patient Category	Spirometry Class	Exacerbation Frequency	Symptoms	Suggested Therapy
A	GOLD 1 or 2	0 or 1 per y	Few mMRC 0–1 CAT less than 10	As-needed, short-acting bronchodilator or long-acting bronchodilator
B	GOLD 1–2	0 or 1 per y	Significant mMRC 2 or greater CAT greater than 10	LABA or LAMA
C	GOLD 3–4	2 or more per y	Few mMRC 0–1 CAT less than 10	LAMA or LABA-ICS
D	GOLD 3–4	2 or more per y	Significant mMRC 2 or greater CAT greater than 10	LAMA or LABA-ICS or LAMA and LABA-ICS Consider Roflumilast

Data from Global strategy for the diagnosis, management and prevention of COPD, Global Initiative for Chronic Obstructive Lung Disease (GOLD) 2011. Available at: http://www.goldcopd.org/. Accessed April 14, 2012.

GOLD group D patients

These patients report a high symptom burden (CAT 10 or greater or mMRC 2 or greater) and high risk for exacerbations or GOLD stage 3 or 4 FEV_1 impairment. The first-line therapy in this group is recommended to be the same as group C: LABA-ICS or LAMA. However, it is suggested that a therapeutic approach that includes both LABA-ICS and LAMA may be of added clinical benefit.[48] When group C or D patients who are at a high risk for exacerbations report symptoms of chronic bronchitis, it is reasonable to consider a phosphodiesterase-4 (PDE4) inhibitor in addition to long-acting bronchodilators in an effort to maximize reduction in exacerbations[49,50]; although the impact of PDE4 inhibitors in addition to inhaled corticosteroids (ICS) has not been studied in a prospective study.

The effective treatment of COPD requires that attention be paid to the therapeutic response. As outlined previously, the authors find the ongoing objective measurement of symptoms and exercise capacity and monitoring for exacerbations to be essential; if uncontrolled symptoms, decreasing exercise tolerance, or recurrent exacerbations are present, escalation of therapy may be warranted. The effective treatment of COPD also depends on the addition of nonpharmacologic COPD therapy, most notably pulmonary rehabilitation, which plays an essential role in the management of COPD on top of maintenance medications.

LABAs

There are presently 3 LABAs that are approved in the United States for the treatment of COPD: salmeterol, formoterol, and indacaterol. Both salmeterol and formoterol are administered twice daily and indacaterol is administered once daily. Salmeterol has been compared directly with the short-acting anticholinergic ipratropium documenting equal efficacy in increasing FEV_1. Despite equal magnitude of FEV_1 improvement, participants receiving salmeterol reported less dyspnea and a nonstatistically significant trend toward improved health status.[51,52] Because of its twice-daily dosing, there are obvious benefits to patients from salmeterol compared with short-acting bronchodilators (including ipratropium), which are given every 6 hours. Salmeterol reduces both static and dynamic lung hyperinflation while also increasing exercise time during constant-load exercise.[53] Formoterol has a more rapid onset of action than salmeterol and has been shown to be superior to ipratropium in increasing FEV_1 and improving health status.[54] Indacaterol is a novel once-daily LABA with 24-hour duration of action. In a 12-week, randomized, double-blind study, indacaterol provided sustained bronchodilation and reduced rescue medication use compared with placebo in patients with moderate-severe COPD.[55] Comparative studies show that indacaterol is at least as effective, if not more effective, as salmeterol[56] and formoterol as a bronchodilator.[57] Indacaterol is at least as effective as tiotropium in improving both lung function and health status.[58]

LABAs are superior to short-acting bronchodilators in the treatment of COPD. We lack information regarding their comparative effectiveness with LAMA agents and the comparative effectiveness of drugs within the LABA class. For patients who do not experience exacerbations but have respiratory symptoms, LABAs are appropriate maintenance medications.

Combination LABAs and ICS

Several studies have demonstrated that inhaled LABAs in combination with ICS are more effective than either medication alone in improving IC and FEV_1.[59–62] Therapy with salmeterol and fluticasone combination (SFC) in patients with COPD can also improve exercise tolerance and is directly correlated to the improvement in inspiratory capacity.[61] SFC is more effective in relieving dyspnea, lessening the requirement for rescue inhalers, improving health status, and reducing exacerbations than monotherapy with salmeterol or fluticasone.[59] The largest placebo-controlled trial to date comparing twice-daily SFC with salmeterol and fluticasone is the Toward a Revolution in COPD Health (TORCH) trial, which evaluated SFC compared with salmeterol, fluticasone, and placebo in 6184 participants with moderate to severe COPD.[63] Data from TORCH demonstrated that the use of SFC reduced exacerbations and modestly improved health status over all other treatments and placebo.[63] A nonstatistically significant trend ($P = .052$) toward improved mortality was present for participants receiving SFC compared with placebo. However, the use of SFC or fluticasone was associated with an increased rate of pneumonia.[63] The increased risk for pneumonia with SFC, despite reducing the risk for exacerbations, was reproduced in a subsequent study.[64] The clinical significance of the risk of pneumonia when treating COPD with fluticasone-containing regimens is currently unknown but does inform the recommendation to reserve ICS therapy for individuals who are at a high risk for exacerbations.

The other LABA-ICS combination therapy approved for the treatment of COPD in the United States is formoterol/budesonide combination (FBC). A large, randomized, placebo-controlled trial of participants with severe COPD found that patients who received FBC had less dyspnea, cough, chest tightness, and severe exacerbations compared with both formoterol alone and placebo.[65] The improvement in symptoms with FBC was sustained throughout the 12-month study. Two additional studies compared FBC with formoterol or placebo and documented that FBC-treated participants had greater improvements in FEV_1 compared with other treatment regimens throughout the trials.[66,67] In these studies, IC was increased significantly with FBC, but, unlike SFC, it is not known what effect FBC has on exercise capacity in COPD. It does not seem that budesonide-containing regimens have an increased risk of pneumonia.[68] Although the formoterol/mometasone combination is available in the United States, it has not been systematically evaluated or approved for use in COPD.

Combination therapy using inhaled LABA-ICS is effective at reducing symptoms, improving exercise tolerance, and decreasing risk for exacerbations in patients with COPD. The risk for pneumonia with SFC therapy is currently of uncertain clinical significance and should be studied further. However, the available evidence on the benefits of LABA-ICS therapy is strong and as such it should be considered part of the standard of care in patients with moderate to severe COPD, particularly those with a history of exacerbations.

LAMAs

Tiotropium is currently the only LAMA approved for the treatment of COPD. Tiotropium improves both FEV_1 and health status to a greater extent than ipratropium in COPD and has the advantage of being a once-daily medication.[69] The Understanding Potential Long-Term Impacts on Function with Tiotropium trial (UPLIFT) investigated the use of tiotropium on top of existing COPD therapies (including LABA and LABA-ICS) compared with placebo in approximately 6000 patients over a 4-year period.[70] Participants receiving tiotropium had higher FEV_1 throughout the study (although the primary endpoint of slowing rate of decline in FEV_1 over the 4-year period in the tiotropium group was not met), improved health status, and fewer exacerbations.[70] Tiotropium is also associated with increased exercise endurance compared with placebo.[71,72] Tiotropium plays a role in COPD therapy as a maintenance therapy to relieve symptoms and reduce exacerbations. The comparative effectiveness of tiotropium alone relative to LABA-ICS or LABA-ICS-LAMA has not been well studied; although in those with severe disease and recurrent exacerbations, it is intuitive that triple therapy with LABA-ICS and tiotropium is warranted, but there is only limited evidence to support this practice.[48]

Methylxanthines

Controversy exists regarding the exact effects of theophylline, the most commonly prescribed methylxanthine in COPD. It may act as a nonselective phosphodiesterase inhibitor with a variety of nonbronchodilator actions.[73] There is evidence that theophylline is a modest bronchodilator compared with placebo in stable COPD, is associated with improvement in respiratory symptoms, and reduces exacerbations even at low doses.[74] There has been experimental data that low-dose theophylline enhances the antiinflammatory effects of ICS in COPD airways,[75,76] but large-scale clinical trials investigating exacerbation reduction through this mechanism have not been conducted. Because theophylline is less effective and less well tolerated than inhaled long-acting bronchodilators, it is not recommended if those drugs are available to patients. Because toxicity is dose related, only low-dose theophylline use is recommended and with caution given its many toxic effects, including the development of atrial and ventricular arrhythmias and seizures.

PDE4 Inhibitors

Roflumilast is a once-daily oral medication and the first selective PDE4 inhibitor available to patients with COPD in the United States. It reduces inflammation by inhibiting the breakdown of intracellular cyclic AMP through the inhibition of PDE4, which is expressed predominantly in the respiratory and gastrointestinal epithelium.[77] Roflumilast is recommended as an add-on to bronchodilator treatment for the maintenance of severe COPD associated with chronic bronchitis and a history of frequent exacerbations. Compared with placebo, roflumilast resulted in a 17% reduction in exacerbations[49] and improved lung function when added to either salmeterol or tiotroprium.[50] Adverse effects, such as nausea, diarrhea, reduced appetite, and abdominal pain, seem to be reversible, occur early in the treatment course and diminish over time with continued treatment. The impact of roflumilast in individuals treated with ICS containing regimens has not been systematically investigated, although benefits were observed in patients concurrently taking ICS.[78] That said, the authors typically prescribe roflumilast to individuals with recurrent severe exacerbations and chronic bronchitis symptoms in addition to the inhaled triple therapy of LABA-ICS and LAMA in an effort to maximize an exacerbation reduction strategy.

Antibiotics

Azithromycin is a macrolide antibiotic, a class of antibiotics with immunomodulatory, antiinflammatory, and antibacterial effects.[79] Macrolides have been shown to affect outcomes in 2 diseases that involve chronic airway obstruction: diffuse panbronchiolitis and cystic fibrosis. The antiinflammatory activity of macrolide antibiotics is thought to be unrelated to their antibacterial actions.[80] Human rhinovirus infections may account for the more severe COPD exacerbations,[81] and macrolides may reduce airway cytokine production caused by this virus.[82] This rationale has led to several studies evaluating whether macrolides decrease the frequency of exacerbations of COPD.[83–86] These studies have had conflicting results, but most have tested erythromycin rather than the newer-generation macrolides, clarithromycin or azithromycin. The most recent trial included participants with moderately severe COPD in whom daily treatment with azithromycin 250 mg was added to usual treatment (ICS-LABA or LAMA) for 1 year compared with placebo.[86] Treatment with azithromycin was associated with fewer exacerbations and improved quality of life. The treatment did have the significant adverse event of audiogram-confirmed hearing decrement in 25% of the participants receiving azithromycin compared with 20% receiving placebo. Azithromycin treatment also changed microbial resistance pattern, but the long-term effect (beyond 1 year) of the change is not known.[86] At present, given the lack of long-term data and the potential impact on quality of life related to hearing loss, the authors reserve daily azithromycin for those with recurrent exacerbations on maximum therapy (including roflumilast) with careful screening of the QT-interval on electrocardiogram and normal hearing.

The fluoroquinolone antibiotic moxifloxacin was evaluated for use in a pulsed fashion in patients with COPD who had chronic bronchitis symptoms and experienced 2 exacerbations in the antecedent 12 months in a proof-of-concept study.[87] Participants were treated with either moxifloxacin 400 mg daily or placebo for 5 days every 8 weeks for 48 weeks. Participants treated with moxifloxacin had a trend toward reduced risk of exacerbations, although it did not reach statistical significance in the most robust intention-to-treat analysis (the per protocol analysis did show a statistically significant benefit). In addition, moxifloxacin-treated participants had fewer respiratory symptoms and adverse effects were modest, most frequently related gastrointestinal effects.[87] Although this early evidence is promising, the currently available clinical trials data do not support that pulsed moxifloxacin be implemented in clinical practice to prevent COPD exacerbations.

Pulmonary Rehabilitation

Formal programs of rehabilitative exercise and education regarding lung disease have substantial benefits in COPD. In the National Emphysema Treatment Trial (NETT), 1218 participants underwent pulmonary rehabilitation before randomization to either lung volume reduction surgery or medical therapy. Pulmonary rehabilitation in this group of patients with severe COPD resulted in improvements in breathlessness, exercise capacity, and health-related quality of life (determined by SGRQ).[88] Similar benefits have been documented in individuals with less severe COPD than those included in the NETT, including reductions in health care use following the completion of pulmonary rehabilitation.[89,90]

Because of its safety and impressive results, the authors recommend all of their patients with COPD who require maintenance treatment with long-acting bronchodilators participate in pulmonary rehabilitation. Although access to pulmonary rehabilitation programs is an ongoing challenge in the United Sates, a recent national coverage determination by the US Centers for Medicare and Medicaid Services mandates Medicare reimbursement for such programs in patients with COPD with a spirometric severity of GOLD 2 or higher.

SUMMARY

COPD is a treatable condition for which careful and objective evaluation of patients' lung function, symptoms, exercise capacity, and exacerbation history on an ongoing basis is essential so that treatments may be individualized as much as possible. Although the comparative effectiveness of drug classes has not yet been tested completely in COPD, virtually all inhaled COPD therapies improve lung function, quality of life, and reduce COPD exacerbations, which fulfills the major goals of care. Pulmonary rehabilitation is safe, effective, and a crucial component of COPD therapy. Newer therapies have been developed with the specific purpose of reducing COPD exacerbations and should be prescribed to individuals who have evidence of recurrent exacerbations despite maximal inhaled maintenance medications.

REFERENCES

1. Kochanek K, Xu J, Murphy S, et al. Deaths: preliminary data for 2009. Hyattsville (MD): National Center for Health Statistics; 2011.
2. NHLBI morbidity and mortality chart book. Available at: http://www.nhlbi.nih.gov/resources/docs/cht-book.htm. Accessed April 14, 2012.
3. Celli BR, MacNee W, Agusti A, et al. Standards for the diagnosis and treatment of patients with COPD: a summary of the ATS/ERS position paper. Eur Respir J 2004;23:932–46.
4. Global strategy for the diagnosis, management and prevention of COPD, Global Initiative for Chronic Obstructive Lung Disease (GOLD) 2011. Available at: http://www.goldcopd.org/. Accessed April 14, 2012.
5. Pauwels RA, Buist AS, Calverley PM, et al. Global strategy for the diagnosis, management, and prevention of chronic obstructive pulmonary disease. NHLBI/WHO Global Initiative for Chronic Obstructive Lung Disease (GOLD) workshop summary. Am J Respir Crit Care Med 2001;163:1256–76.
6. Mahler DA, Harver A. A factor analysis of dyspnea ratings, respiratory muscle strength, and lung function in patients with chronic obstructive pulmonary disease. Am Rev Respir Dis 1992;145:467–70.
7. Cooper CB. The connection between chronic obstructive pulmonary disease symptoms and hyperinflation and its impact on exercise and function. Am J Med 2006;119:21–31.
8. Jones PW. Issues concerning health-related quality of life in COPD. Chest 1995; 107:187S–93S.
9. Hurst JR, Vestbo J, Anzueto A, et al. Susceptibility to exacerbation in chronic obstructive pulmonary disease. N Engl J Med 2010;363:1128–38.
10. Nishimura K, Izumi T, Tsukino M, et al. Dyspnea is a better predictor of 5-year survival than airway obstruction in patients with COPD. Chest 2002;121:1434–40.
11. Mahler DA. Mechanisms and measurement of dyspnea in chronic obstructive pulmonary disease. Proc Am Thorac Soc 2006;3:234–8.
12. Jones PW, Harding G, Berry P, et al. Development and first validation of the COPD assessment test. Eur Respir J 2009;34:648–54.
13. Dodd JW, Hogg L, Nolan J, et al. The COPD assessment test (CAT): response to pulmonary rehabilitation. A multicentre, prospective study. Thorax 2011;66: 425–9.
14. Dodd JW, Marns PL, Clark AL, et al. The COPD assessment test (CAT): short- and medium-term response to pulmonary rehabilitation. COPD 2012. [Epub ahead of print].
15. Jones PW, Harding G, Wiklund I, et al. Tests of the responsiveness of the chronic obstructive pulmonary disease (COPD) assessment test TM (CAT) following acute exacerbation and pulmonary rehabilitation. Chest 2012. [Epub ahead of print].
16. Mackay AJ, Donaldson GC, Patel AR, et al. Utility of the COPD assessment test (CAT) to evaluate severity of COPD exacerbations. Am J Respir Crit Care Med 2012;185(11):1218–24.
17. Casanova C, Cote C, de Torres JP, et al. Inspiratory-to-total lung capacity ratio predicts mortality in patients with chronic obstructive pulmonary disease. Am J Respir Crit Care Med 2005;171:591–7.
18. Ofir D, Laveneziana P, Webb KA, et al. Mechanisms of dyspnea during cycle exercise in symptomatic patients with GOLD stage I COPD. Am J Respir Crit Care Med 2008;177:622–9.

19. Garcia-Rio F, Lores V, Mediano O, et al. Daily physical activity in patients with chronic obstructive pulmonary disease is mainly associated with dynamic hyperinflation. Am J Respir Crit Care Med 2009;180:506–12.

20. ATS Committee on Proficiency Standards for Clinical Pulmonary Function Laboratories. ATS statement: guidelines for the six-minute walk test. Am J Respir Crit Care Med 2002;166:111–7.

21. Pinto-Plata VM, Cote C, Cabral H, et al. The 6-min walk distance: change over time and value as a predictor of survival in severe COPD. Eur Respir J 2004; 23:28–33.

22. Celli BR, Cote CG, Marin JM, et al. The body-mass index, airflow obstruction, dyspnea, and exercise capacity index in chronic obstructive pulmonary disease. N Engl J Med 2004;350:1005–12.

23. Ong KC, Earnest A, Lu SJ. A multidimensional grading system (BODE Index) as predictor of hospitalization for COPD. Chest 2005;128:3810–6.

24. Imfeld S, Bloch KE, Weder W, et al. The BODE index after lung volume reduction surgery correlates with survival. Chest 2006;129:873–8.

25. Cote CG, Celli BR. Pulmonary rehabilitation and the BODE index in COPD. Eur Respir J 2005;26:630–6.

26. Pompeo E, Mineo TC. Two-year improvement in multidimensional body mass index, airflow obstruction, dyspnea, and exercise capacity index after nonresectional lung volume reduction surgery in awake patients. Ann Thorac Surg 2007; 84:1862–9 [discussion: 1862–9].

27. Puhan MA, Garcia-Aymerich J, Frey M, et al. Expansion of the prognostic assessment of patients with chronic obstructive pulmonary disease: the updated BODE index and the ADO index. Lancet 2009;374:704–11.

28. Jones RC, Donaldson GC, Chavannes NH, et al. Derivation and validation of a composite index of severity in chronic obstructive pulmonary disease: the DOSE Index. Am J Respir Crit Care Med 2009;180:1189–95.

29. Anzueto A. Impact of exacerbations on COPD. Eur Respir Rev 2010;19:113–8.

30. Donaldson GC, Wedzicha JA. COPD exacerbations.1: epidemiology. Thorax 2006;61:164–8.

31. Donaldson GC, Seemungal T, Bhowmik A, et al. Relationship between exacerbation frequency and lung function decline in chronic obstructive pulmonary disease. Thorax 2002;57:847–52.

32. Spencer S, Calverley PM, Burge PS, et al. Impact of preventing exacerbations on deterioration of health status in COPD. Eur Respir J 2004;23:698–702.

33. Cote CG, Dordelly LJ, Celli BR. Impact of COPD exacerbations on patient-centered outcomes. Chest 2007;131:696–704.

34. Wilkinson TM, Donaldson GC, Hurst JR, et al. Early therapy improves outcomes of exacerbations of chronic obstructive pulmonary disease. Am J Respir Crit Care Med 2004;169:1298–303.

35. Langsetmo L, Platt RW, Ernst P, et al. Underreporting exacerbation of chronic obstructive pulmonary disease in a longitudinal cohort. Am J Respir Crit Care Med 2008;177:396–401.

36. Vijayasaratha K, Stockley RA. Reported and unreported exacerbations of COPD: analysis by diary cards. Chest 2008;133:34–41.

37. Fabbri LM, Luppi F, Beghe B, et al. Complex chronic comorbidities of COPD. Eur Respir J 2008;31:204–12.

38. Ng TP, Niti M, Tan WC, et al. Depressive symptoms and chronic obstructive pulmonary disease: effect on mortality, hospital readmission, symptom burden, functional status, and quality of life. Arch Intern Med 2007;167:60–7.

39. Eisner MD, Blanc PD, Yelin EH, et al. Influence of anxiety on health outcomes in COPD. Thorax 2010;65:229–34.
40. Schroedl C, Kalhan R. Incidence, treatment options, and outcomes of lung cancer in patients with chronic obstructive pulmonary disease. Curr Opin Pulm Med 2012;18:131–7.
41. Raviv S, Hawkins KA, DeCamp MM Jr, et al. Lung cancer in chronic obstructive pulmonary disease: enhancing surgical options and outcomes. Am J Respir Crit Care Med 2011;183:1138–46.
42. U.S. Preventive Services Task Force. Screening for depression in adults: U.S. preventive services task force recommendation statement. Ann Intern Med 2009;151:784–92.
43. Al-Showair RA, Tarsin WY, Assi KH, et al. Can all patients with COPD use the correct inhalation flow with all inhalers and does training help? Respir Med 2007;101:2395–401.
44. Tashkin DP, Pearle J, Iezzoni D, et al. Formoterol and tiotropium compared with tiotropium alone for treatment of COPD. COPD 2009;6:17–25.
45. van Noord JA, Aumann JL, Janssens E, et al. Comparison of tiotropium once daily, formoterol twice daily and both combined once daily in patients with COPD. Eur Respir J 2005;26:214–22.
46. Karner C, Cates CJ. Long-acting beta(2)-agonist in addition to tiotropium versus either tiotropium or long-acting beta(2)-agonist alone for chronic obstructive pulmonary disease. Cochrane Database Syst Rev 2012;4:CD008989.
47. Wedzicha JA, Calverley PM, Seemungal TA, et al. The prevention of chronic obstructive pulmonary disease exacerbations by salmeterol/fluticasone propionate or tiotropium bromide. Am J Respir Crit Care Med 2008;177:19–26.
48. Aaron SD, Vandemheen KL, Fergusson D, et al. Tiotropium in combination with placebo, salmeterol, or fluticasone-salmeterol for treatment of chronic obstructive pulmonary disease: a randomized trial. Ann Intern Med 2007;146:545–55.
49. Calverley PM, Rabe KF, Goehring UM, et al. Roflumilast in symptomatic chronic obstructive pulmonary disease: two randomised clinical trials. Lancet 2009; 374:685–94.
50. Fabbri LM, Calverley PM, Izquierdo-Alonso JL, et al. Roflumilast in moderate-to-severe chronic obstructive pulmonary disease treated with long acting bronchodilators: two randomised clinical trials. Lancet 2009;374:695–703.
51. Rennard SI, Anderson W, ZuWallack R, et al. Use of a long-acting inhaled beta2-adrenergic agonist, salmeterol xinafoate, in patients with chronic obstructive pulmonary disease. Am J Respir Crit Care Med 2001;163:1087–92.
52. Mahler DA, Donohue JF, Barbee RA, et al. Efficacy of salmeterol xinafoate in the treatment of COPD. Chest 1999;115:957–65.
53. O'Donnell DE, Voduc N, Fitzpatrick M, et al. Effect of salmeterol on the ventilatory response to exercise in chronic obstructive pulmonary disease. Eur Respir J 2004;24:86–94.
54. Dahl R, Greefhorst LA, Nowak D, et al. Inhaled formoterol dry powder versus ipratropium bromide in chronic obstructive pulmonary disease. Am J Respir Crit Care Med 2001;164:778–84.
55. Feldman G, Siler T, Prasad N, et al. Efficacy and safety of indacaterol 150 microg once-daily in COPD: a double-blind, randomised, 12-week study. BMC Pulm Med 2010;10:11.
56. Kornmann O, Dahl R, Centanni S, et al. Once-daily indacaterol versus twice-daily salmeterol for COPD: a placebo-controlled comparison. Eur Respir J 2011;37: 273–9.

57. Dahl R, Chung KF, Buhl R, et al. Efficacy of a new once-daily long-acting inhaled beta2-agonist indacaterol versus twice-daily formoterol in COPD. Thorax 2010; 65:473–9.

58. Donohue JF, Fogarty C, Lotvall J, et al. Once-daily bronchodilators for chronic obstructive pulmonary disease: indacaterol versus tiotropium. Am J Respir Crit Care Med 2010;182:155–62.

59. Calverley P, Pauwels R, Vestbo J, et al. Combined salmeterol and fluticasone in the treatment of chronic obstructive pulmonary disease: a randomised controlled trial. Lancet 2003;361:449–56.

60. Hanania NA, Darken P, Horstman D, et al. The efficacy and safety of fluticasone propionate (250 microg)/salmeterol (50 microg) combined in the Diskus inhaler for the treatment of COPD. Chest 2003;124:834–43.

61. O'Donnell DE, Sciurba F, Celli B, et al. Effect of fluticasone propionate/salmeterol on lung hyperinflation and exercise endurance in COPD. Chest 2006;130: 647–56.

62. Szafranski W, Cukier A, Ramirez A, et al. Efficacy and safety of budesonide/formoterol in the management of chronic obstructive pulmonary disease. Eur Respir J 2003;21:74–81.

63. Calverley PM, Anderson JA, Celli B, et al. Salmeterol and fluticasone propionate and survival in chronic obstructive pulmonary disease. N Engl J Med 2007;356: 775–89.

64. Ferguson GT, Anzueto A, Fei R, et al. Effect of fluticasone propionate/salmeterol (250/50 microg) or salmeterol (50 microg) on COPD exacerbations. Respir Med 2008;102:1099–108.

65. Calverley PM, Boonsawat W, Cseke Z, et al. Maintenance therapy with budesonide and formoterol in chronic obstructive pulmonary disease. Eur Respir J 2003;22:912–9.

66. Tashkin DP, Rennard SI, Martin P, et al. Efficacy and safety of budesonide and formoterol in one pressurized metered-dose inhaler in patients with moderate to very severe chronic obstructive pulmonary disease: results of a 6-month randomized clinical trial. Drugs 2008;68:1975–2000.

67. Rennard SI, Tashkin DP, McElhattan J, et al. Efficacy and tolerability of budesonide/formoterol in one hydrofluoroalkane pressurized metered-dose inhaler in patients with chronic obstructive pulmonary disease: results from a 1-year randomized controlled clinical trial. Drugs 2009;69:549–65.

68. Sin DD, Tashkin D, Zhang X, et al. Budesonide and the risk of pneumonia: a meta-analysis of individual patient data. Lancet 2009;374:712–9.

69. Vincken W, van Noord JA, Greefhorst AP, et al. Improved health outcomes in patients with COPD during 1 yr's treatment with tiotropium. Eur Respir J 2002; 19:209–16.

70. Tashkin DP, Celli B, Senn S, et al. A 4-year trial of tiotropium in chronic obstructive pulmonary disease. N Engl J Med 2008;359:1543–54.

71. Maltais F, Hamilton A, Marciniuk D, et al. Improvements in symptom-limited exercise performance over 8 h with once-daily tiotropium in patients with COPD. Chest 2005;128:1168–78.

72. Kesten S, Casaburi R, Kukafka D, et al. Improvement in self-reported exercise participation with the combination of tiotropium and rehabilitative exercise training in COPD patients. Int J Chron Obstruct Pulmon Dis 2008;3:127–36.

73. Murciano D, Auclair MH, Pariente R, et al. A randomized, controlled trial of theophylline in patients with severe chronic obstructive pulmonary disease. N Engl J Med 1989;320:1521–5.

74. Zhou Y, Wang X, Zeng X, et al. Positive benefits of theophylline in a randomized, double-blind, parallel-group, placebo-controlled study of low-dose, slow-release theophylline in the treatment of COPD for 1 year. Respirology 2006;11:603–10.
75. Barnes PJ. Emerging pharmacotherapies for COPD. Chest 2008;134:1278–86.
76. Ford PA, Durham AL, Russell RE, et al. Treatment effects of low-dose theophylline combined with an inhaled corticosteroid in COPD. Chest 2010;137:1338–44.
77. Rabe KF. Update on roflumilast, a phosphodiesterase 4 inhibitor for the treatment of chronic obstructive pulmonary disease. Br J Pharmacol 2011;163:53–67.
78. Rennard SI, Calverley PM, Goehring UM, et al. Reduction of exacerbations by the PDE4 inhibitor roflumilast–the importance of defining different subsets of patients with COPD. Respir Res 2011;12:18.
79. Martinez FJ, Curtis JL, Albert R. Role of macrolide therapy in chronic obstructive pulmonary disease. Int J Chron Obstruct Pulmon Dis 2008;3:331–50.
80. Peckham DG. Macrolide antibiotics and cystic fibrosis. Thorax 2002;57:189–90.
81. Seemungal T, Harper-Owen R, Bhowmik A, et al. Respiratory viruses, symptoms, and inflammatory markers in acute exacerbations and stable chronic obstructive pulmonary disease. Am J Respir Crit Care Med 2001;164:1618–23.
82. Suzuki T, Yamaya M, Sekizawa K, et al. Erythromycin inhibits rhinovirus infection in cultured human tracheal epithelial cells. Am J Respir Crit Care Med 2002;165:1113–8.
83. Banerjee D, Khair OA, Honeybourne D. The effect of oral clarithromycin on health status and sputum bacteriology in stable COPD. Respir Med 2005;99:208–15.
84. Suzuki T, Yanai M, Yamaya M, et al. Erythromycin and common cold in COPD. Chest 2001;120:730–3.
85. Seemungal TA, Wilkinson TM, Hurst JR, et al. Long-term erythromycin therapy is associated with decreased chronic obstructive pulmonary disease exacerbations. Am J Respir Crit Care Med 2008;178:1139–47.
86. Albert RK, Connett J, Bailey WC, et al. Azithromycin for prevention of exacerbations of COPD. N Engl J Med 2011;365:689–98.
87. Sethi S, Jones PW, Theron MS, et al. Pulsed moxifloxacin for the prevention of exacerbations of chronic obstructive pulmonary disease: a randomized controlled trial. Respir Res 2010;11:10.
88. Ries AL, Make BJ, Lee SM, et al. The effects of pulmonary rehabilitation in the national emphysema treatment trial. Chest 2005;128:3799–809.
89. Ries AL, Kaplan RM, Limberg TM, et al. Effects of pulmonary rehabilitation on physiologic and psychosocial outcomes in patients with chronic obstructive pulmonary disease. Ann Intern Med 1995;122:823–32.
90. Hui KP, Hewitt AB. A simple pulmonary rehabilitation program improves health outcomes and reduces hospital utilization in patients with COPD. Chest 2003;124:94–7.

Medical Pneumoplasty, Surgical Resection, or Lung Transplant

Francis C. Cordova, MD

KEYWORDS

- Bronchoscopic lung volume reduction • BioLVR • Endobronchial valves
- Airway bypass stent • Bullectomy • Giant bullous emphysema
- Lung volume reduction surgery • Lung transplant

KEY POINTS

- In patients with chronic obstructive pulmonary disease, lung hyperinflation is associated with worse health-related quality of life and confers poor prognosis for survival.
- Surgical and nonsurgical options that result in decreased hyperinflation improve outcome and may improve survival in selected patients with emphysema.
- In patients with severely compromised lung physiology and very poor functional capacity, lung transplantation remains a possible option.

INTRODUCTION

Chronic obstructive pulmonary disease (COPD) is progressive despite optimal medical management. In patients with very severe COPD who remain incapacitated by dyspnea and continue to have poor exercise tolerance and quality of life, surgical treatment such as lung volume reduction surgery (LVRS), bullectomy, and lung transplantation have been shown to improve symptoms, quality of life, and exercise capacity in carefully selected patients. More recently, medical pneumoplasty using bronchoscopic techniques for deployment of unidirectional endobronchial valves, instillation of biodegradable gel, and creation of airway bypass tracts have been developed in an attempt to decrease lung volume, attenuate the effect of dynamic hyperinflation during exercise, and attempt to replicate the clinical benefit of LVRS without the associated morbidity and mortality of surgery. In this review the rationale of lung volume reduction (LVR), the indications and outcome of different surgical treatments of COPD, and emerging techniques of medical pneumoplasty are discussed.

PATHOPHYSIOLOGIC BASIS FOR LUNG VOLUME REDUCTION

Progressive irreversible air-flow limitation caused by air-flow obstruction (due to mucus hypersecretion, airway remodeling, and bronchoconstriction) and loss of lung elastic

Lung and Heart/Lung Transplant Program, Temple University School of Medicine, 3401 North Broad Street, Philadelphia, PA 19140, USA
E-mail address: francis.cordova@temple.edu

Med Clin N Am 96 (2012) 827–847
doi:10.1016/j.mcna.2012.05.006
0025-7125/12/$ – see front matter © 2012 Elsevier Inc. All rights reserved.

recoil (due to increase in lung compliance) are the pathologic hallmark of COPD. In patients with moderate and severe COPD, the air-flow limitation is associated with hyperinflation and gas trapping because of insufficient time for adequate lung emptying. This hyperinflation is compounded during exercise as the increase in ventilatory demand leads to a progressive increase in end-expiratory lung volume and a reciprocal decrease in inspiratory capacity, resulting in an acute increase in the degree of hyperinflation, commonly referred to as dynamic hyperinflation. Breathing at elevated lung volume places the inspiratory muscles at a mechanical disadvantage, and the resulting higher elastic load in the lung and chest wall leads to increased work for breathing. Moreover, hyperinflation also leads to a decrease venous return and impairs functioning of the right ventricle, resulting in a decrease in cardiac output. Indeed dynamic hyperinflation is the primary mechanism for dyspnea on exertion, reduced exercise capacity, and poor quality of life in patients with COPD.

Lung volume reduction, by medical pneumoplasty, bullectomy, or surgical LVRS, is purported to reverse the pathophysiologic consequences of lung hyperinflation by improvement in expiratory air flow, and restoration of respiratory muscle and cardiac function. Several studies, both conceptually and with actual measurements of static lung mechanics, diaphragmatic muscle strength, and pulmonary hemodynamics, have shown that LVR leads to improvement in lung elastic recoil, diaphragm muscle strength, and right ventricular function.

MEDICAL PNEUMOPLASTY

Several bronchoscopic techniques have been developed to reduce lung volume and improve clinical outcomes without the attendant morbidity and mortality associated with LVRS. Bronchoscopic techniques that have shown promising results include: (1) the deployment of unidirectional endobronchial valves (Zephyr valve [Pulmonx, Redwood City, CA, USA]; Spiration valve [Spiration Inc, Redmond, WA, USA]) to collapse the targeted lobe and decrease its lung volume; (2) instillation of biodegradable gel into subsegmental bronchi, to initiate local inflammatory response to the targeted lung parenchyma thus inducing scar formation and reduction of lung volume (BioLVR); and (3) creation of extra-anatomic fenestrations between the emphysematous lung and bronchial tree to allow deflation of the hyperinflated lung (airway bypass tract). Other techniques in development include bronchoscopic thermal vapor ablation (Update Inc, Seattle, WA, USA), the use of thermal vapor to achieve ablation of the emphysematous lung, and the deployment of the nitinol endobronchial coil system (PneumRx Inc, Mountain View, CA, USA) in the distal airway to limit hyperinflation of the emphysematous lung segment.[1,2] At present, none of the endobronchial devices are approved by the Food and Drug Administration for use in the treatment of emphysema in the United States. One of the endobronchial valves (Spiration Inc, Redmond, WA, USA) received a Humanitarian Device Exemption for the treatment of persistent air leaks following lobectomy, segmentectomy, and LVRS. The Zephyr valve is approved in Europe for the treatment of emphysema.

Endobronchial Valves

The endobronchial valve is the first device developed to attempt bronchoscopic lung reduction. There are 2 endobronchial valve systems available, the Zephyr valve (Pulmonx) and the Spiration valve (Spiration). The endobronchial valves are designed to facilitate distal airway collapse by limiting air flow to the emphysematous lung segments, leading to a decrease in segmental and lobar hyperinflation. The resulting segmental and lobar atelectasis leads to compensatory lobar enlargement of the adjacent, more functional lung, improving expiratory air flow and alveolar ventilation.

The Zephyr valve consists of a one-way duck-billed valve inside a stainless-steel cage attached to a nickel-titanium (nitinol) self-expanding retainer. The framework of the valve is covered with silicone to create a seal between the valve and the bronchial wall. The valve is designed to allow outflow of air and prevent inflow of air during respiration (**Fig. 1**), and is available in different sizes to fit different bronchial-lumen sizes. The valve is delivered via a catheter and deployed into the targeted segment or subsegment of the lung using the bronchoscope. The Spiration valve consists of an umbrella-shaped valve made of a nitinol frame with 5 outer and 1 inner struts. The outer struts are flexible and are covered with a thin membrane, which abuts the airway wall. Once the valve is properly deployed in the distal airway, it prevents inflow of air but allows outflow of air, fluid, and mucus during exhalation or coughing (**Fig. 2**). Delivery of the Spiration device is similar to that of the Zephyr valve, but it is recommended that the valves be deployed under general anesthesia with endotracheal intubation.

Several initial case series reported the feasibility, safety, and clinical utility of the Zephyr valve in patients with emphysema. In general, selection criteria for bronchoscopic LVR are similar to those for surgical LVR, limiting the procedure to patients with upper lobe–predominant emphysema. In a pilot study of 10 patients with upper lobe–predominant emphysema, Snell and colleagues[3] showed that placement of multiple endobronchial valves (Nitinol bronchial stent; Emphasys Medical, Redwood, CA) was feasible and safe. Postprocedure complications included COPD exacerbation in 3 patients, pneumothorax (n = 1), and lower lobe pneumonia (n = 1). Four patients (40%) reported improvement in symptoms. However, there were no improvements in air flow, lung volume, and 6-minute walk distance. Using the same endobronchial valve in 8 patients with severe emphysema, Toma and colleagues[4] reported a 34% improvement in forced expiratory volume in 1 second (FEV_1) (0.79 vs 1.06 L, $P = .028$) and 29% improvement in diffusion capacity. Follow-up computed tomography (CT) scan of the chest showed significant atelectasis in the treated upper lobe region in 50% of the patients. The procedure was complicated by ipsilateral pneumothorax in 2 patients and COPD exacerbations in 3 patients. Other investigators reported not only improvement in air-flow obstruction but also significant improvement in exercise capacity and quality of life up to 24 months of follow-up.

A   B

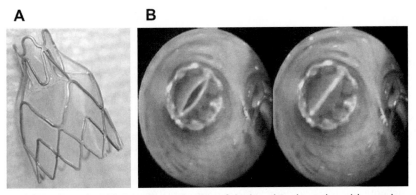

Fig. 1. (A) Zephyr valve. (B) Bronchoscopic view of deployed Zephyr valve with opening and closing of the inner valve during expiration and inspiration, respectively. (*From* Strange C, Herth FJ, Kovitz KL, et al. Design of the Endobronchial Valve for Emphysema Palliation Trial (VENT): a non-surgical method of lung volume reduction. BMC Pulm Med 2007,7:10.)

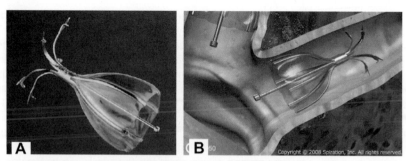

Fig. 2. (A) Spiration valve. (B) Schematic picture of Spiration valve seated in the airway. (*Courtesy of* Spiration Inc, Olympus Respiratory America, Redmond, WA; with permission.)

In a combined analysis of the first 98 patients with severe emphysema who were treated with endobronchial valve, there were significant increases in forced vital capacity (FVC) (9% $\pm$ 23.9%, P = .024), FEV_1 (10.7% $\pm$ 26.2%, $P<.007$), and 6-minute walk distance (23% $\pm$ 55.3%, P = .001). In addition, diffusion capacity also improved (17.2% $\pm$ 52%, P = .063).[5] Patients who received unilateral treatment of the entire lobe were more likely to have greater improvement in lung function than patients who received bilateral treatment or were treated with only 1 or 2 bronchopulmonary segments. Indeed the greatest improvement in static lung function, exercise capacity, was seen in patients with unilateral and lobar endobronchial valve placement. In this subgroup of patients, the FEV_1 increased by 16% and the exercise capacity improved by 40%. Other predictors of good response to endobronchial valve treatment include FEV_1 less than 30% and residual volume (RV) greater than 225% of predicted. Serious complications reported within 90 days included 1 (1%) death, 3 (3.1%) pneumothoraces requiring surgical intervention, and 4 (4.1%) patients with prolonged air leak. The most common complications were COPD exacerbations (17%) and pneumonia in nontreated lobes (5%). These early efficacy trials on endobronchial valve were limited by its open-label design, evolving endobronchial valve design and development, small number of patients, and short-term follow-up.

The Valve for Emphysema Palliation Trial (VENT)[6] is a randomized, prospective, multicenter study designed to evaluate the safety and efficacy of unilateral (Zephyr) endobronchial valve treatment (n = 220) in patients with severe emphysema in comparison with standard medical therapy (n = 101). The coprimary end points were percent change in FEV_1 and distance on the 6-minute walk test (6MWT) at 6 months between the 2 treatment arms. The primary safety end point was a composite of 6 major complications at 6 months after the procedure. These composite major complications included death, empyema, massive hemoptysis, pneumonia distal to valves, pneumothorax or air leak of more than 7 days' duration, and ventilator-dependent respiratory failure of more than 24 hours' duration. Secondary end points in the analysis include exercise capacity, dyspnea, and quality-of-life measures. Patients with very severe emphysema with profound hypoxemia (Pao_2 <45 mm Hg), hypercapnia ($Paco_2$ >50 mm Hg), and poor functional status (6MWT <140 m) were excluded. In addition, patients with severe impairment of diffusion capacity (<20%), presence of giant bullae, α1-antitrypsin deficiency, previous thoracotomy, excessive sputum production, and severe pulmonary hypertension were also excluded. At baseline, patients who were randomized to endobronchial valve therapy had severe air-flow obstruction (FEV_1 −30% $\pm$ 8%), hyperinflation (total lung capacity [TLC] −124% $\pm$ 15%), and air trapping (RV −216% $\pm$ 44%). The mean number of valves deployed was 3.8 per patient (range, 1–9). The right upper lobe was targeted in the majority of patients (52.3%), followed by left upper lobe (24.3%), left lower lobe (14%), and right lower lobe (9.3%). At 6 months, there was a modest improvement in lung function (FEV_1 +4.3%) in the endobronchial valve group (EBV group) compared with a 2.5% decrease in FEV_1 in the control group, a difference in mean FEV_1 of 6.8% between the 2 groups. Similarly, there was a small improvement in exercise capacity. The 6MWT in the EBV group increased by 2.5% compared with a 3.2% decrease in the control group, representing an increase of 9.3 m in 6-minute walk distance in the EBV group compared with a 10.7-m decline in the control group. Two factors, the degree of heterogeneity of emphysema between lobes and fissure integrity, were important in predicting which patients would likely have clinically significant improvement in lung function and exercise capacity following treatment with the endobronchial valve. Patients in the EBV group who had 15% or higher heterogeneity score on high resolution of the chest had greater improvements in both FEV_1 (10.7%, $P = .004$) and 6MWT (12.4%, $P = .002$). Similarly, patients who were treated with the endobronchial valve who had complete fissures had incremental improvements in FEV_1 of 16.2% at 6 months and 17.9% at 12 months. By contrast, patients with incomplete fissure had no significant improvement in air flow at the same follow-up times. There were small improvements in health-quality measures, and no difference in the rate of composite major complications. However, there were 6 deaths in the EBV group compared with no deaths in the control group ($P = .19$).

Overall, the endobronchial valve has been shown to improve lung function, exercise capacity, and quality of life, and to ameliorate dyspnea in carefully selected patients with severe heterogeneous emphysema. Most of the patients experienced improvement in dyspnea and quality of life despite minimal improvement in expiratory air flow and lung volume. Incomplete fissure between the treated lobes can decrease the effectiveness of the endobronchial valve in inducing segmental and lobar collapse, as well as its clinical efficacy.[7] It appeared to be safer than LVRS, with a lower 6-month mortality rate (VENT −2.8% vs National Emphysema Treatment Trial [NETT] non–high-risk group −5.2%). Future studies need to further define which subgroup of patients with emphysema will have the best response to endobronchial valve treatment, the optimal valve design, the number of valves needed, and the durability of the clinical improvement.

Biological Lung Volume Reduction

BioLVR is a novel endoscopic therapy that reduces lung volume by instillation of a biodegradable gel to induce localized inflammation, scarring, and reduction of emphysematous lung volume.[8] The gel is also thought to fill the alveoli and blocks collateral ventilation. The biodegradable gel is a mixture of chondroitin sulfate and poly-L-lysine in a fibrin-based solution that is delivered in conjunction with thrombin solution via a dual-lumen catheter. In a phase 2, open-label, dose-ranging study involving 50 patients with predominantly upper lobe emphysema, patients received either high-dose (20 mL/subsegment) or low-dose (10 mL/subsegment) biogel on 4 subsegments on each upper lobe.[9] The high-dose biogel regimen was found to be more efficacious, resulting in greater improvement in spirometry (ΔFEV_1, +15%; ΔFVC, +9.1%) compared with patients who received low-dose biogel at 6 months' follow-up (ΔFEV_1, +6.7%; ΔFVC, +5.1%). Both treatment groups achieved a significant reduction in gas trapping, and improved symptom scores and health-related quality-of-life measures. Follow-up CT scan of the chest showed localized scarring of the treated sites that was sustained at 6 months in patients in the high-dose group (**Fig. 3**). The efficacy of the high-dose BioLVR regimen was confirmed in a separate study involving patients with homogeneous emphysema.

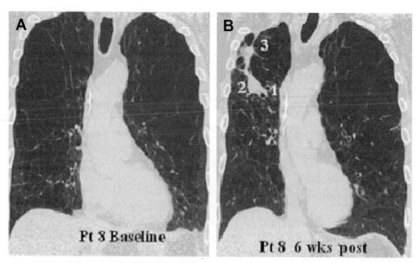

Fig. 3. CT scan of the chest before (*A*) and 6 weeks after (*B*) BioLVR on the right upper lobe. There is focal atelectasis, volume loss, and apical pleural thickening on the treated right upper lobe of the lung. (Reprinted with permission of the American Thoracic Society. Copyright © 2012 American Thoracic Society. *From* Criner GJ, Pinto-Plata V, Strange C, et al. Biologic lung volume reduction in advanced upper lobe emphysema: phase 2 results. Am J Respir Crit Care Med 2009;179(9):791–8. Official journal of the American Thoracic Society. This reproduction is a portion of the original image.)

Common reactions within 24 hours of the BioLVR procedure include pleuritic chest pain, nausea, headache, malaise, and leukocytosis. The reactions resolved with 24 to 48 hours. There were no reported deaths or procedure-related complications. Thus, it appears that BioLVR, if confirmed in larger randomized controlled trials, is a safer alternative to surgical LVR in improving lung function and quality of life.

Airway Bypass Tracts

The creation of airway bypass via transbronchial fenestration is based on the role of collateral ventilation in emphysema. Collateral ventilation occurs through interalveolar pores, accessory bronchoalveolar connections, accessory respiratory bronchioles, and interlobar pathways across fissures. The importance of collateral ventilation is minimal in normal lungs because the resistance to air flow is higher in collateral channels than in the airways. Because of increased airway resistance in emphysematous lung, collateral ventilation provides an important channel for alveolar gas distribution. In creating an endoscopic airway bypass between the emphysematous lung and bronchial airways, gas emptying is enhanced by bypassing obstructed airways and through collateral ventilation.[10] Interlobar collateral ventilation occurred more commonly in homogeneous than in heterogeneous emphysema patterns, lending support to the concept that this procedure, unlike other LVR procedures, should work better in patients with homogeneous emphysema.[11] Indeed, the degree of collateral ventilation is correlated with the degree of homogeneity of emphysema. In a proof-of-concept study using 12 human lungs explanted during lung transplant, the placement of multiple airway bypass tracts significantly increased FEV_1 from 245 ± 107 mL to 666 ± 284 mL.[12] A follow-up in vivo animal study showed the benefit of using paclitaxel-eluting stents in maintaining bypass tract patency in a comparison with bare-metal stents.[13]

The bronchoscopic procedure entailed identification of a suitable area of segmental bronchi free of blood vessels using a Doppler probe, followed by fenestration of the airways using a transbronchial needle with balloon dilatation, and placement of a paclitaxel-eluting stent (**Fig. 4**). In an open-label study of 35 patients with homogeneous emphysema, creation of airway bypass tracts in both lungs (median of 8 stents, range 2–12) showed initial improvement in spirometry (FVC +17.2%, $P<.001$; FEV_1 7.3%, $P = .038$), lung volume (RV −0.75 L, $P<.001$), dyspnea score (modified Medical Research Council dyspnea [mMRC] score −0.6, $P = .003$), functional capacity (6MWT +37.2 m, $P<.001$), and quality of life (St. George Respiratory Questionnaire [SGRQ] score −4.7, $P = .008$) at 1-month follow-up.[14] However, at 6-month follow-up only reduction in RV and improvement in dyspnea score remained statistically significant. There were no changes in spirometry, 6MWT, and quality-of=life measures. On post hoc analysis, patients with RV/TLC greater than 0.67, signifying severe hyperinflation and gas trapping, appeared to benefit the most from the procedure. The most common adverse events were COPD exacerbations and infections. Three patients (7.9%) had experienced intraoperative serious adverse events (1 death, 2 pneumomediastinum).

In a randomized, sham-controlled, multicenter trial of bronchoscopic LVR with exhale airway stents for emphysema (EASE trial), 315 patients who had severe homogeneous emphysema and severe hyperinflation (RV/TLC $\geq$0.65) were enrolled to either airway bypass (n = 208) or sham (n = 107).[15] The coprimary end points were a 12% improvement in FVC and 1-point or greater decrease in the mMRC dyspnea score from baseline at 6 months' follow-up. The patients who received airway bypass had transient improvement in FVC, FEV_1, and reduction in RV on day 1 postprocedure, which were attenuated at 1 month. More importantly, there were no differences in the coprimary end points between the treated and the sham group. There was no significant difference in composite primary safety end point (pulmonary hemorrhage that required blood transfusion or embolization or transfusion, acute respiratory failure requiring mechanical ventilation, COPD exacerbation requiring hospitalization >7 days, pneumothorax >7 days or needing drainage, or death with 30 days) between the 2 groups (14.4% vs 11.2%). The transient improvement in static lung function was attributed to loss of stent function over time because of stent expectoration, loss of stent patency because of mucus plug, growth of granulation tissue, or insufficient collateral ventilation to maintain flow through the stents. Future studies need to address these problems to improve the durability of reduction in RV after an airway bypass procedure.[16]

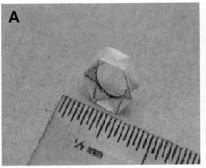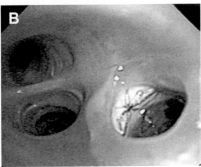

Fig. 4. (*A*) Airway bypass tract valve. (*B*) Bronchoscopic view of seated airway bypass valve. (*From* Cardoso PF, Snell GI, Hopkins P, et al. Clinical application of airway bypass with paclitaxel-eluting stents: early results. J Thorac Cardiovasc Surg 2007;134(4):974–81; with permission.)

SURGICAL RESECTION
Bullectomy

Before the concept of lung reduction surgery was introduced, surgical resection of giant bullae was used to ameliorate symptoms and improve lung function in patients with giant bullous emphysema. Bullae are defined as air spaces in the lung greater than 1 cm in diameter. The bullae may enlarge progressively over time, trapping more air and consequently occupying a larger proportion of the thorax. Giant bullae commonly refer to bullae occupying more than 30% of a hemithorax. Bullae are usually the consequence of paraseptal, centrilobular, or panacinar emphysema. Bullae have been classified into 3 morphologic subtypes based on the degree of destruction of the lung parenchyma. Type I bullae are located along the subpleural surface of the lung. Pathologically they have a narrow neck and the sacs are devoid of parenchymal remnants. Type I bullae are associated with paraseptal emphysema and can become severely overinflated. This type of bulla is associated with vanishing lung syndrome or idiopathic giant bullous emphysema. Type II bullae are also located on the subpleural surface but have a broader neck and usually contain destroyed emphysematous lung. Type II bullae have been associated with a higher risk for spontaneous pneumothorax. Type III bullae are located deep in the lung parenchyma toward the hilum and are associated with the least degree of hyperinflation. This type of bulla has no well-defined neck, and contains emphysematous lung throughout the sac. Both Type II and III bullae are caused by centrilobular or panacinar emphysema, and are more difficult to resect surgically than type I bullae.

Radiographically, bullae are recognized as regions of hyperlucency with absent vascular markings often subtended by a thin linear shadow, and depending on their size may compress the surrounding lung tissue. Bullae are often seen in the upper lung zones with 2:1 preponderance in the right lung. Giant bullae are often seen associated with diffuse emphysema. Bullous emphysema without concomitant diffuse emphysema may represent the extreme end of the heterogeneous emphysema phenotype. The presence of giant bullae often manifests as air-flow obstruction, and the severity of air-flow obstruction depends on the presence or absence of concomitant generalized emphysema. CT of the chest is the best method to characterize the bullae and to evaluate the viability of the surrounding lung tissue (**Fig. 5**).

Rationale for bullectomy

Giant bullae, depending on their size, can occupy a large volume of the chest cavity and compress adjacent normal lung tissue. The compression of the surrounding lung tissue leads to decreased alveolar ventilation and reduced elastic recoil of the lung. Similar to diffuse emphysema, the giant bullae can lead lung hyperinflation, loss of normal diaphragm curvature, and apposition with the chest wall, resulting in reduced mechanical contractile efficiency of the diaphragm. During exercise, dynamic hyperinflation can lead to further enlargement of the bullae because of its high compliance, and impaired emptying of the bullae because of a floppy airway (ball-valve effect), which further impairs lung function.

Surgical resection of the bullae results in reexpansion of the compressed normal lung tissue, and reduces the size mismatch between the lung and chest cavity (**Fig. 6**). In turn this leads to an increase in elastic recoil of lung, improvement in expiratory air flow, and reduction of air trapping.[17] The resultant decrease in hyperinflation and air trapping and the concomitant expansion of the compressed normal lung tissue improve diaphragm function and gas exchange. The surgical technique for bullectomy depends on the surgeon's preference and experience,[18] the patient's condition, and whether bilateral or unilateral bullectomy are considered. Thoracotomy or video-assisted thoracoscopy

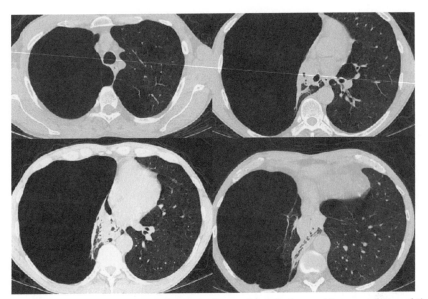

Fig. 5. CT scan of the chest showing giant bulla on the right lung with compression of the surrounding lung parenchyma medially. Note the presence of paraseptal emphysema on the left lung.

(VATS) are the usual surgical approaches for unilateral bullectomy, and median sternotomy is used for bilateral bullectomy. VATS is generally used in patients with limited pulmonary function who are otherwise considered at high risk for thoracotomy. Simple resection of the bullae with sparing of the surrounding compressed but functional tissue is the goal of bullectomy. However, segmentectomy or lobectomy may be needed some patients with diffuse involvement of a segment or lobe, to decrease the likelihood of prolonged and severe air leak.

Patient selection for bullectomy

The most common indications for bullectomy are persistent dyspnea in patients who have moderate to severe air-flow obstruction and have giant bullae on chest radiography, or secondary spontaneous pneumothorax. Patients who are likely to

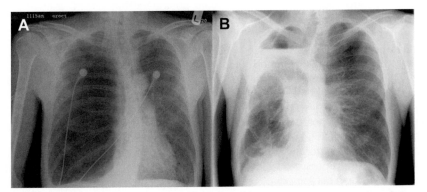

Fig. 6. Chest radiograph before (A) and after (B) bullectomy. Before surgery, there is hyperlucency of the right lung, hyperinflation, and shifting of the mediastinum to the contralateral side. After bullectomy, there is expansion of the compressed lung level of and apical air fluid.

benefit from a bullectomy typically have a pulmonary function test that shows evidence of moderate to severe air-flow obstruction (FEV$_1$ $\geq$40%), hyperinflation (TLC >100%), and air trapping (RV >150% of predicted).[19–21] Because most bullae communicate poorly with the airways, the volume of the nonventilated lung can be estimated by the difference in the measured TLC obtained from the body plethysmography and helium-dilution techniques. The larger the volume of the sequestered gas (>500 mL), the more likely the patient will have good clinical response after surgery. An important predictor of good surgical outcome is giant bullae occupying more than 30% to 50% of a hemithorax with radiographic evidence of normal compressed lung tissue adjacent to the bullae. Patients with concomitant diffuse emphysema can also benefit from bullectomy, with a similar degree of short-term improvement in lung function and functional capacity. However, the effect on lung function is not as durable as that in patients without diffuse emphysema. In addition, the presence of diffuse emphysema portends a poorer long-term outcome. In a study of 41 patients who underwent elective bullectomy, patients who had concomitant emphysema were sicker and had accelerated decline in lung function after the second postoperative year, and a higher 5-year mortality compared with patients without concomitant emphysema.[19] Other predictors of poor outcome include very low FEV$_1$ (<30% of predicted), and the presence of chronic hypercapnia or cor pulmonale.

Effects of bullectomy on lung function and exercise

The extent of improvement in lung function after bullectomy depends on the size of the bullae and the health of the surrounding compressed lung. In patients with giant bullous emphysema occupying less than 30% of a hemithorax who underwent bullectomy for spontaneous pneumothorax, there was no significant improvement in lung function, and may be associated with a transient decline in spirometry in the immediate postoperative period. In carefully selected patients with giant bullae occupying more than 30% to 50% of the hemithorax, the FEV$_1$ has been shown to increase between 20% and 58% with an associated significant decrease in TLC and RV.[19,21,22] The patients also reported significant decrease in dyspnea, and improvement in exercise capacity and quality of life. In addition, bullectomy may decrease the need for supplemental oxygen at rest and during exercise in the majority of patients. Long-term study of up to 5 years of follow-up showed that there is a gradual decline in lung function at 3 years after surgery, albeit remaining significantly higher than baseline. In patients with concomitant diffuse emphysema the decline in lung function occurred earlier, starting at 2 years postoperatively and at a more rapid rate in comparison with patients with diffuse emphysema.[19]

Complications

Similar to LVRS, the most common complication following bullectomy is prolonged air leak, which occurs in more than half of the patients. The presence of very severe air-flow obstruction preoperatively increases the risk of prolonged air leak postoperatively. Surgical techniques, such as using a bovine pericardial strip along the staple line of lung resection and the creation of a pleural tent, are designed to minimize postoperative leak. Other postoperative complications include atrial fibrillation (12%), postoperative respiratory failure (9%), and pneumonia (5%). The postoperative mortality rate from published reports ranges from 0% to 22.5% with a weighted mean of 8.0%. In a contemporary report on long-term outcome following bullectomy, the 1-, 3-, and 5-year survival was 97.7%, 92.1%, and 88.5%, respectively.[18,19,21–23] Postoperative imaging showed no evidence of recurrence of the giant bullae or progressive enlargement of surrounding small bullae after surgery.

Lung Volume Reduction Surgery

The concept of LVRS through standard thoracotomy was first introduced by Brantigan and colleagues[24] in 1957. In this study, partial pulmonary resection led to subjective and functional improvement in 75% of the patients. However, no objective physiologic data were reported and because of the high mortality rate (16%), the procedure was not widely accepted. With advances in thoracic surgery, Cooper and colleagues[25] revived the concept of LVRS in patients with COPD. In this pivotal study, bilateral LVRS was performed in 20 carefully selected patients via median sternotomy whereby 20% to 30% of each lung was resected. After surgery a significant increase in lung function, gas exchange, relief of dyspnea, and quality of life were reported. Since the initial report, several studies from different centers have reported similar but varying degrees of improvement in lung function, exercise performance, and quality of life. A follow-up report from the same surgical group showed that the physiologic and functional improvements following LVRS are sustained for up to 5 years in some patients.[26] However, most of the studies were limited by variability in patient selection, surgical techniques, complications, and outcomes. The NETT was a multicenter, randomized controlled trial that was designed to answer the question regarding the effects of LVRS in comparison with optimal medical therapy on lung function, exercise performance, quality of life, and survival.[27] The results of the NETT provided the current guidance on the proper selection of patients with COPD who are likely to benefit from LVRS. Moreover, the NETT provided not only important data on perioperative morbidity and mortality but also on long-term follow-up on the durability of the physiologic and functional improvement following LVRS.

Patient selection for LVRS

Before NETT, the selection of patients with severe COPD who would likely benefit from LVRS with acceptable perioperative morbidity and mortality was not clearly defined. The current selection guidelines for LVRS are largely based on NETT inclusion criteria and outcome data. At the minimum, patients who are referred for LVRS evaluation should have severe COPD (FEV_1 $\leq$45%), with significant hyperinflation (TLC $\geq$100%) and air trapping (RV $\geq$150% predicted), with only mild to moderate hypercapnia ($Paco_2$ <60 mm Hg) and without severe hypoxemia (Pao_2 >45 mm Hg). The patient should have bilateral, heterogeneous, upper lobe–predominant emphysema on high-resolution CT of the chest.[28–30] In addition, the patient should stop smoking for at least 6 months prior, have no significant cardiac comorbidity, and be able to participate in outpatient pulmonary rehabilitation.

In the original report by Cooper and colleagues,[25] patients who had heterogeneous, predominantly upper lobe emphysema were thought to be ideal candidates for LVRS because resection of functional lung tissue is avoided or minimized. In a report of 250 consecutive patients who underwent bilateral LVRS, patients were carefully selected to have heterogeneously distributed, predominantly upper lobe emphysema to provide a target zone for surgical resection (n = 229), with only 21 patients having predominantly lower lobe emphysema, 12 of whom had α1-antityrpsin deficiency.[26] At 6 months following surgery, there were no significant differences in the degree of improvement in spirometry and functional capacity between the upper lobe–predominant and lower lobe–predominant emphysema. However, beyond 6 months the patients with lower lobe emphysema had accelerated decline in lung function compared with those with upper lobe emphysema. The mean FEV_1 at 5 years in patients with lower lobe emphysema was below baseline whereas the mean FEV_1 in the patients with upper lobe emphysema was 9% above baseline. Moreover, there was a similar rapid decline in the 6MWT in the group with lower lobe emphysema compared with patients with upper lobe emphysema. In NETT, 16 (1.3%) patients had emphysema that was due to severe α1-antitrypsin deficiency, and 10 patients underwent LVRS. The patients with α1-antitrypsin deficiency had lower and shorter duration of increases in FEV$_1$ and exercise capacity, and compared with LVRS had higher mortality than patients without α1-antitrypsin deficiency at 2-year follow-up.

In the NETT trial, 16 prognostic factors were preidentified as possibly important in affecting clinical outcome. Only 2 baseline factors, the distribution of emphysema on CT scan of the chest (upper lobe versus non–upper lobe predominant emphysema) and the exercise performance after rehabilitation were associated with differences in clinical outcome including mortality. Based on the combination of these parameters the patients were divided into 4 subgroups, namely, upper lobe emphysema with either low or high exercise, and non–upper lobe emphysema with either low or high exercise capacity.

Patients with upper lobe–predominant emphysema and low exercise capacity had a lower risk of death (relative risk [RR], 0.47; $P = .005$), and were likely to have more than 10-W improvement in exercise capacity (30% vs 0%, $P<.001$) and a more than 8-point improvement in the SGRQ score (48% vs 10%, $P<.001$) in 24 months. In patients with upper lobe emphysema but with high exercise capacity, LVRS conferred no survival advantage (RR, 0.98; $P = .7$). However, the LVRS group was more likely to have improvement in exercise capacity (15% vs 3%, $P = .001$) and significant improvement in SGRQ at 24 months (41% vs 11%, $P<.001$).

In patients with non–upper lobe disease and low exercise capacity, LVRS conferred significant improvement only in quality of life (37% vs 7%, $P = .001$), with no significant improvement in survival (RR, 0.81; $P = .49$) or exercise capacity (12 vs 7%, $P = .5$). In the last group of patients with non–upper lobe emphysema and high exercise capacity, the LVRS-treated group had a greater risk of death than the medically treated group (RR, 2.06, $P = .02$), with no improvement in exercise capacity (3% vs 3%, $P = 1.0$) and SGRQ score (15% vs 12%, $P = .61$).

Another group of patients were identified early during NETT enrollment as at high risk for perioperative death, and were subsequently excluded from the study.[31] These patients had very severe emphysema characterized by FEV$_1$ 20% or less predicted, and with a diffusion capacity of 20% or less or a homogeneous pattern of emphysema on chest CT. The postoperative mortality after LVRS was not only high, there were also no clinically meaningful improvements in lung function, exercise capacity, and quality of life. A total of 140 patients were identified as high risk. In 70 patients who had LVRS, the 30-day mortality was 16% compared with no deaths in the medical group. In patients with all 3 high-risk physiologic and radiographic characteristics, the 30-day mortality rate was 25%. The most common cause of death was respiratory failure, with 60% of the patients on mechanical ventilatory support at the time of death.

Based on these data, 3 COPD phenotypes should not be considered for LVRS: patients with severe emphysema with FEV$_1$ less than 20% and with either homogeneous emphysema on chest CT or very low diffusion capacity (<20%), patients with non–upper lobe emphysema and high exercise capacity, and patients with α1-antitrypsin deficiency. These patients not only do not benefit from LVRS but have a high mortality rate after surgery, and are best referred to a lung transplant center.

Long-term effects of LVRS
The short-term effects of LVRS on lung function, exercise capacity, and quality of life have been well described. Because COPD is a progressive disease, there has been some concern about the long-term effects of LVRS and whether LVRS contributes to a rapid decline in lung function. Overall, the yearly decline in FEV$_1$ was

approximately 60 mL per year. At 5 years of follow-up, the mean change in FEV_1 compared with baseline was 7%, and 53% of the patients had FEV_1 values higher than baseline.[32] For RV, 79% of the patients still showed lower RV compared with baseline, with the mean RV still 14% lower than baseline. A significant increase in diffusion capacity was only maintained for the first year after LVRS. A significant number of patients continue to be off oxygen at rest and during exercise. Close to 80% of the patients continued to show improvement in quality-of-life measures up to 5 years. In an updated long-term follow-up from NETT with up to 5 years of follow-up, the patients in the upper lobe–predominant emphysema group with either low exercise or high exercise capacity were likely to have sustained improvements in exercise capacity and quality of life.[32] More importantly, the survival advantage in the patients with upper lobe–predominant emphysema initially reported was confirmed on long-term follow-up. The improvement in quality of life in the patients with non–upper lobe predominant emphysema wanes after 3 years of follow-up.

Postoperative morbidity and mortality

In a single study of 250 LVRS patients, the postoperative mortality was 4.8% with a median follow-up of 4.4 years (range 1.8–9.1 years).[26] The most common complications was prolonged air leak (>7 days) occurring in 45% of the patients. Postoperative respiratory failure requiring reintubation and mechanical ventilatory support occurred in 7% of the patients. In NETT, where 17 Academic Medical Centers participated in the study, the mortality in the immediate postoperative period was higher in the LVRS group (7.9%) than in the medically treated group (1.3%).[27] However, at mean follow-up of 29.2 months after randomization, there was no difference in mortality between the 2 treatment groups. In the subsequent long-term follow-up report with a median follow-up of 4.3 years, the total mortality rate was 0.11 deaths per person-year in the LVRS group compared with 0.13 person-years in the medical group (RR, 0.85; P = .02), favoring the LVRS group. This improvement in survival in the LVRS group in comparison with the medically treated group occurred despite the expected higher immediate postoperative mortality, and was mainly driven by the patients with upper lobe–predominant emphysema with low exercise capacity. Air leaks are a common postoperative complication, and can be prolonged in some patients. Of 552 patients in whom detailed data on air leaks were recorded, 496 (90%) had air leaks within the first 30 days after surgery.[33] The median duration of air leaks was 7 days, and 66 (12%) patients had prolonged air leaks of more than 30 days' duration. The type of surgery (median sternotomy versus VATS), the use of buttressing materials, and the type of stapler have no impact on the frequency and duration of air leaks. Preoperative factors that were associated with prolonged air leaks include white race, lower FEV_1, low diffusion capacity, inhaled corticosteroids, upper lobe–predominant emphysema, and moderate to severe pleural adhesions. The most common cause of death for both the LVRS and medically treated groups was respiratory failure, with 69% and 43% of the patients on mechanical ventilatory support at the time of death. Nosocomial pneumonia was common in the high-risk LVRS patients (30%) within the first 30 postoperative days.

The predictors of postoperative pulmonary and cardiac morbidity were analyzed in 511 non–high-risk patients who had LVRS.[34] Major pulmonary morbidity was defined as tracheostomy, failure to wean from mechanical ventilation, pneumonia, reintubation, and mechanical ventilation for longer than 3 days within 30 days of surgery. Major cardiovascular morbidity was defined as myocardial infarction, pulmonary embolus, and cardiac arrhythmias requiring treatment. Major pulmonary and cardiovascular morbidity occurred in 29.8% and 20% of the patients, respectively. The incidence of postoperative 90-day mortality was 5.5%. Cardiac arrhythmia was the most common cardiac complication, occurring in 23.5% of the patients, of whom 18.6% required treatment. The major pulmonary complications included reintubation (21.8%), pneumonia (18.2%), and need for mechanical ventilation for longer than 2 days (13.6%). The sole predictor of operative mortality was the presence of non–upper lobe emphysema (relative odds, 2.99; P = .009). Predictors of pulmonary morbidity include older age, lower FEV_1, and lower diffusion capacity. Cardiovascular morbidity was higher in older patients, those who used of oral steroids, and those with non–upper lobe predominant emphysema.

Lung Transplantation

Lung transplantation is an accepted surgical treatment option for patients with end-stage lung disease who are not candidates for LVR or bullectomy procedure, because of either a homogeneous emphysema pattern or absence of giant bullae suitable for surgical resection. As previously discussed, patients with very severe COPD with FEV_1 20% or less of predicted and with diffusion capacity of 20% or less of predicted have a high postoperative mortality following LVRS, and lung transplantation is the optimal surgical procedure for these patients. COPD is the most common indication for lung transplantation worldwide, accounting for approximately one-third of lung transplants performed each year. With the implementation in May 2005 of the lung allocation system based on severity of illness, idiopathic pulmonary fibrosis has over-taken COPD as the leading indication for lung transplantation in the United States.

Candidate selection

Generally recommended absolute and relative contraindications to lung transplanta-tion are outlined in **Box 1**.[35] Transplant for patients older than 65 years with no signif-icant comorbidities has been shown to have a comparable outcome with that in younger patients. Early referral to lung transplant centers has been advocated to allow time for diagnosis and treatment of comorbidities. It is not uncommon to diagnose unsuspected coronary artery disease or valvular heart disease, or uncover new pulmo-nary nodules at the time of transplant evaluation. Successful coronary artery bypass surgery at the time of lung transplantation has been reported. However, patients who have concomitant coronary artery disease and who are treated with percuta-neous angioplasty and placement of coronary stents are often put on hold for trans-plant while they receive intensive antiplatelet therapy (aspirin and plavix) for a few months. Similarly, workup of the pulmonary nodule may entail time-consuming serial CT scan of the chest. In addition, some patients require time for outpatient pulmonary rehabilitation for reconditioning, whereas others require time to lose weight to achieve a body mass index of less than 30 kg/m^2 before transplant. The capacity to abstain from continued cigarette smoking for a minimum of 6 months is required in most trans-plant programs. In addition, ability and willingness to participate in an outpatient pulmonary rehabilitation program is also required. Exercise capacity as measured by 6-minute walk has been shown to be a reliable predictor of both waiting-list and posttransplant mortality. Patients with advanced COPD who are referred late to a transplant program have a narrow transplant window, and may decompensate rapidly, which may preclude adequate optimal reconditioning and optimal treatment of comorbidities.

The guidelines published by the International Society of Heart and Lung Transplan-tation (ISHLT) for lung transplantation in COPD[35] are shown in **Box 2**. The guidelines incorporate different factors that have been shown to be good indicators of poor prog-nosis: an FEV_1 20% or less of predicted, the presence of severe hypoxemia at rest and

Box 1
Absolute and relative contraindications to lung transplantation

Absolute Contraindications

Malignancy in the last 2 years, except squamous and basal cell carcinoma

Advanced extrapulmonary organ dysfunction

Noncurable chronic extrapulmonary infections including hepatitis B, hepatitis C, and human immunodeficiency virus infection

Significant chest wall/spinal deformity

Medical noncompliance

Untreatable psychiatric or psychological conditions

Poor social support

Substance addiction within the last 6 months

Relative Contraindications

Age 65 years or older

Critical or unstable clinical condition (mechanical ventilation, extracorporeal membrane oxygenation)

Colonization with highly resistant organism

Severe obesity with body mass index greater than 30 kg/m^2

Severe or symptomatic osteoporosis

Mechanical ventilation

Suboptimal treatment of chronic medical illness such as diabetes mellitus, gastroesophageal reflux

Adapted from Orens JB, Estenne M, Arcasoy S, et al. International guidelines for the selection of lung transplant candidates: 2006 update—a consensus report from the Pulmonary Scientific Council of the International Society for Heart and Lung Transplantation. J Heart Lung Transplant 2006;25(7):745–55; with permission.

Box 2
Guidelines for lung transplantation in patients with severe COPD

It is recommended to refer the patient early to a transplant center to give time for proper evaluation and treatment of comorbidities before transplantation

Guideline for Referral

BODE index greater than 5

Guideline for Transplantation

Bode index 7 to 10

History of hospitalization because of acute hypercapnia

Presence of pulmonary hypertension despite oxygen therapy

FEV$_1$ less than 20% with either diffusion capacity less than 20% or homogeneous emphysema pattern

Adapted from Orens JB, Estenne M, Arcasoy S, et al. International guidelines for the selection of lung transplant candidates: 2006 update—a consensus report from the Pulmonary Scientific Council of the International Society for Heart and Lung Transplantation. J Heart Lung Transplant 2006;25(7):745–55; with permission.

during ambulation, a history of multiple hospitalizations due to acute or chronic hypercapnic respiratory failure, the presence of moderate to severe secondary pulmonary hypertension, or a high BODE score. The BODE index (Body mass index/air-flow Obstruction/Dyspnea/Exercise) is a simple multidimensional, validated index that has been shown to be more accurate than FEV_1 in predicting all-cause and respiratory-related mortality in patients with COPD.[36] The 4 domains that are included in the calculation of the BODE index include the severity of air-flow obstruction (FEV_1), the patient's perception of dyspnea (the mMRC dyspnea scale), assessment of functional capacity (6MWT), and the patient's body mass index. The BODE index score ranges from 0 to 10, with each quartile increase in score associated with higher mortality. Patients with a high BODE score (7–10) have a mortality rate of 80% at 4 years with a median survival of only 3 years.

In general, transplantation should be performed when the predicted posttransplant survival exceeds the predicted disease-related survival of 50% or less in 2 to 3 years. In comparison, in the recent ISHLT registry data in 2011 encompassing the period between 1990 and 2009, the overall median survival for posttransplant recipients with a diagnosis of COPD was 5.3 years, with the median survival approaching 7 years in patients who received a double lung transplant.

Lung allocation

Previously, allocation of donor lungs was based on the candidate's accrued time on the waiting list without consideration for the severity of illness. This allocation scheme resulted in increased waiting time to transplantation and increased mortality while on the waiting list, and was deemed inequitable. The new lung allocation scheme, implemented in May 2005, is based on the lung allocation score (LAS), which is a measure that accounts for medical urgency (predicted survival during the following year on the waiting list) and transplant benefit (predicted survival 1 year posttransplant). Thus, the aim of the LAS is to improve waiting-list survival by performing transplantation in patients who are at high risk of death before transplant and to avoid lung transplantation in marginal patients who are unlikely to survive after transplant. The prediction model of the lung allocation scheme was derived from retrospective analysis of the United Network for Organ Sharing (UNOS) national database using Cox proportional hazards models to predict 1-year survival without and with transplantation. Several parameters that represent the patient's pathophysiologic and functional states are used in the model, but is heavily weighted toward the patient's underlying diagnosis. Accordingly, patients with idiopathic pulmonary fibrosis have higher LAS score than those with COPD because of higher waiting-list mortality, reflecting higher medical urgency.

Since the implementation of the LAS system, the median waiting time has decreased from 2 to 3 years to less than 200 days, about 25% of the patients being transplanted within 35 days. Because the sickest patients received the highest priority within the geographic area of the Organ Procurement Organization, there has been a significant reduction in the death rate of patients on the waiting list. As a consequence of the LAS system, the number of patients with idiopathic pulmonary fibrosis transplanted has increased, and idiopathic pulmonary fibrosis has surpassed COPD as the most common indication for lung transplantation.

Over the last several years, bilateral lung transplantation has become favored over single lung transplant as a procedure of choice, and the number of lung transplants performed in carefully selected patients older than 65 years continues to increase, with several programs reporting outcomes comparable with those of younger transplant recipients.

Posttransplant outcomes

Lung transplantation in patients with end-stage COPD improves lung function, health-related quality of life, and survival. Unlike patients with suppurative lung diseases such as cystic fibrosis or bronchiectasis, patients with COPD can receive either single or bilateral lung transplantation. There is continued controversy as to the optimal procedure for patients with COPD. Pochettino and colleagues[37] compared the outcome of single (n = 84) versus bilateral lung transplant (n = 46) in patients with COPD. Patients who received a single lung were older than those who received a bilateral lung transplant (56.2 ± 0.7 vs 51.1 ± 1.2 years, P<.0001). The improvements in lung function and exercise capacity as measured by 6MWT were significantly better following bilateral lung transplant compared with single lung transplant. With a mean follow-up of 32.4 months, the incidence of chronic allograft rejection manifesting as bronchiolitis obliterans syndrome was similar in both groups (22.2% vs 22.4%). There was no difference in 90-day mortality; however, the actuarial survival rates at 1 (82.6% vs 72.2%), 3 (74.6% vs 63.4%), and 5 (61.9% vs 57.4%) years were higher in bilateral lung transplant recipients, although it did not reach statistical significance. Based on this study, it is unclear whether the improved survival was due to age difference between the 2 groups or was attributable to higher pulmonary reserve in recipients of bilateral lung transplant. In a retrospective review of the UNOS database of 9883 patients with COPD who had either single (n = 3523) or bilateral (n = 6358) lung transplant, the median survival time (6.41 vs 4.59 years, P<.0001) was significantly longer after bilateral lung transplant than with single lung transplant even after adjustment of pretransplant confounding variables.[38] In patients who were 60 years or older, bilateral lung transplant conferred no additional benefits.

The question of whether lung transplantation confers survival benefit in patients with COPD remains controversial. Previous studies comparing observed survival of COPD patients on the waiting list with posttransplant survival showed conflicting results, with European studies showing survival advantage with transplantation in contrast to studies in the United States. These conflicting results have been attributed to differences in listing practices between the United States and European countries. At the time the studies were published, the lung allocation scheme in the United States was based on waiting-list time, and it was common practice to list patients early in anticipation of 2 to 3 years of waiting time before actual transplantation. By contrast, the European allocation scheme was based on medical urgency, suggesting that patients were sicker at the time of transplant than were transplant recipients in the United States. In a recent analysis of the UNOS database of 8182 COPD patients who were transplanted between 1986 and 2004, patients who received a bilateral lung transplant were more likely to derive survival benefit of at least 1 year in comparison with recipients of a single lung transplant.[39] In addition, survival benefit was also influenced by the severity of air-flow obstruction. Approximately 80% of COPD patients with FEV_1 of 16% or less were predicted to gain at least 1 year of life after bilateral lung transplant, compared with only 11% of patients with an FEV_1 25% or more of predicted. Thus, survival advantage can be expected following bilateral lung transplant in carefully selected patients with COPD.

Complications

Common complications include primary graft dysfunction (PGD), airway complications, infections, and acute and chronic rejection. PGD is primarily caused by ischemia/reperfusion injury manifesting as noncardiogenic pulmonary edema within 72 hours of transplantation. Both donor-related (female sex, African-American race, older age, low Pao_2/Fio_2 ratio, ischemia time >6 hours) and recipient-related factors (pulmonary hypertension) have been associated with increased risk of PGD. Treatment of severe PGD is supportive and includes the use of protective lung-ventilator strategy to minimize volutrauma, the use of inhaled nitric oxide to minimize Fio_2 requirement, and early use of an extracorporeal membrane oxygenator. Severe PGD is the leading cause of death during the perioperative period, and is associated with excess short-term and long-term mortality.

Airway complications after transplant include airway ischemia, bronchial anastomotic dehiscence, and bronchial stenosis. Bronchial artery circulation is not reestablished after lung transplantation. Blood flow to the lung allograft is largely dependent on retrograde blood flow through low-pressure pulmonary veins to vascular collaterals. Because of this less than optimal blood supply, the airway is at risk of ischemic injury. Ischemic airway injury commonly appears as patchy areas of bronchial mucosal necrosis with pseudomembrane formation on bronchoscopic examination during the immediate postoperative period. Bronchial stenosis at the anastomosis site is the most common airway complication, with a reported prevalence of 4% to 24%. It is thought to be a delayed manifestation of the initial ischemic injury often occurring several weeks after transplant. Bronchial stenosis can be due to fibrotic stricture, bronchomalacia, or excessive growth of granulation tissue. Bronchial stenosis is commonly treated with bronchial balloon dilatation, with or without placement of an endobronchial airway stent. Bronchial dehiscence is uncommon but is associated with poor outcome, even after surgical repair. An uncovered endobronchial stent has been used successfully in severe airway dehiscence to promote growth of granulation tissue.

Infection is a common cause of death after lung transplantation. Bacterial infection caused by hospital-acquired pathogens such as *Pseudomonas aeruginosa* and *Staphylococcus aureus* are common in the first months after transplant. Cytomegalovirus (CMV) infection is the most common pathogen occurring after lung transplantation, occurring in up to 30% of lung transplant recipients even with widespread use of universal CMV prophylaxis. *Aspergillus* is the most common opportunistic fungal pathogen during the first month to 6 months after lung transplantation. Most transplant programs incorporate antifungal prophylaxis with either voriconazole or inhaled amphotericin in the first 3 to 6 months after transplant.

Acute allograft rejection is common, especially after the first 6 months after lung transplantation. Routine surveillance transbronchial biopsy is used to detect early histologic signs of acute cellular rejection, which can be asymptomatic in 40% of cases. Common manifestations of acute rejection include dyspnea, cough, low-grade fever, and malaise. Decline in spirometry and oxygenation with or without radiographic changes are a common finding during acute rejection. Acute cellular rejection is commonly treated with a 3-day pulse of high-dose methylprednisolone followed by a tapering course of prednisone. Recently, acute humoral rejection attributable to the production of donor-specific anti-HLA alloantibodies has emerged as an important form of acute rejection, especially in patients who are sensitized and have high levels of panel-reactive antibodies before lung transplant. Treatment of acute humoral rejection includes intravenous immunoglobulin, plasmapheresis, and anti-CD20 monoclonal antibodies.

Chronic allograft rejection remains a major impediment to long-term survival following lung transplantation. To date, despite advances in immunosuppression regimens and increasing use of induction immunosuppression therapy at the time of transplant, the incidence of bronchiolitis obliterans syndrome or chronic rejection is approximately 50%. Unfortunately, effective therapy for chronic rejection remains elusive.

SUMMARY

Over the last decade, advances in bronchoscopic and surgical techniques have expanded our treatment armamentarium for patients with severe emphysema who previously would have received a pessimistic outlook from their physician. Advances in our understanding of the different COPD phenotypes and its natural history has refined our selection process as to which group of emphysema patients will derive maximum benefit from LVR, bullectomy, or lung transplantation. Because emphysema is a progressive disease, initial treatment with bronchoscopic or surgical LVR or bullectomy does not preclude lung transplantation in the future.

REFERENCES

1. Herth FJ, Eberhard R, Gompelmann D, et al. Bronchoscopic lung volume reduction with a dedicated coil: a clinical pilot study. Ther Adv Respir Dis 2010;4(4): 225–31.
2. Herth FJ, Gompelmann D, Ernst A, et al. Endoscopic lung volume reduction. Respiration 2010;79(1):5–13.
3. Snell GI, Holsworth L, Borrill ZL, et al. The potential for bronchoscopic lung volume reduction using bronchial prostheses: a pilot study. Chest 2003;124(3): 1073–80.
4. Toma TP, Hopkinson NS, Hillier J, et al. Bronchoscopic volume reduction with valve implants in patients with severe emphysema. Lancet 2003;361(9361):931–3.
5. Wan IY, Toma TP, Geddes DM, et al. Bronchoscopic lung volume reduction for end-stage emphysema: report on the first 98 patients. Chest 2006;129(3): 518–26.
6. Sciurba FC, Ernst A, Herth FJ, et al. A randomized study of endobronchial valves for advanced emphysema. N Engl J Med 2010;363(13):1233–44.
7. Herth FJ, Noppen M, Valipour A, et al. Efficacy predictors of lung volume reduction with Zephyr valves in a European cohort. Eur Respir J 2012;39(6):1334–42.
8. Reilly J, Washko G, Pinto-Plata V, et al. Biological lung volume reduction: a new bronchoscopic therapy for advanced emphysema. Chest 2007;131(4):1108–13.
9. Criner GJ, Pinto-Plata V, Strange C, et al. Biologic lung volume reduction in advanced upper lobe emphysema: phase 2 results. Am J Respir Crit Care Med 2009;179(9):791–8.
10. Choong CK, Cardoso PF, Sybrecht GW, et al. Airway bypass treatment of severe homogeneous emphysema: taking advantage of collateral ventilation. Thorac Surg Clin 2009;19(2):239–45.
11. Higuchi T, Reed A, Oto T, et al. Relation of interlobar collaterals to radiological heterogeneity in severe emphysema. Thorax 2006;61(5):409–13.
12. Lausberg HF, Chino K, Patterson GA, et al. Bronchial fenestration improves expiratory flow in emphysematous human lungs. Ann Thorac Surg 2003;75(2):393–7 [discussion: 398].
13. Choong CK, Phan L, Massetti P, et al. Prolongation of patency of airway bypass stents with use of drug-eluting stents. J Thorac Cardiovasc Surg 2006;131(1):60–4.
14. Cardoso PF, Snell GI, Hopkins P, et al. Clinical application of airway bypass with paclitaxel-eluting stents: early results. J Thorac Cardiovasc Surg 2007;134(4): 974–81.
15. Shah PL, Slebos DJ, Cardoso PF, et al. Bronchoscopic lung-volume reduction with Exhale airway stents for emphysema (EASE trial): randomised, sham-controlled, multicentre trial. Lancet 2011;378(9795):997–1005.

16. Ingenito EP, Wood DE, Utz JP. Bronchoscopic lung volume reduction in severe emphysema. Proc Am Thorac Soc 2008;5(4):454–60.
17. Snider GL. Reduction pneumoplasty for giant bullous emphysema. Implications for surgical treatment of nonbullous emphysema. Chest 1996;109(2):540–8.
18. Shah SS, Goldstraw P. Surgical treatment of bullous emphysema: experience with the Brompton technique. Ann Thorac Surg 1994;58(5):1452–6.
19. Palla A, Desideri M, Rossi G, et al. Elective surgery for giant bullous emphysema: a 5-year clinical and functional follow-up. Chest 2005;128(4):2043–50.
20. Meyers BF, Patterson GA. Chronic obstructive pulmonary disease. 10: Bullectomy, lung volume reduction surgery, and transplantation for patients with chronic obstructive pulmonary disease. Thorax 2003;58(7):634–8.
21. Schipper PH, Meyers BF, Battafarano RJ, et al. Outcomes after resection of giant emphysematous bullae. Ann Thorac Surg 2004;78(3):976–82 [discussion: 976–82].
22. Neviere R, Catto M, Bautin N, et al. Longitudinal changes in hyperinflation parameters and exercise capacity after giant bullous emphysema surgery. J Thorac Cardiovasc Surg 2006;132(5):1203–7.
23. Sharma N, Justaniah AM, Kanne JP, et al. Vanishing lung syndrome (giant bullous emphysema): CT findings in 7 patients and a literature review. J Thorac Imaging 2009;24(3):227–30.
24. Brantigan OC, Mueller E, Kress MB. A surgical approach to pulmonary emphysema. Am Rev Respir Dis 1959;80(1 Pt 2):194–206.
25. Cooper JD, Trulock EP, Triantafillou AN, et al. Bilateral pneumectomy (volume reduction) for chronic obstructive pulmonary disease. J Thorac Cardiovasc Surg 1995;109(1):106–16 [discussion: 116–9].
26. Ciccone AM, Meyers BF, Guthrie TJ, et al. Long-term outcome of bilateral lung volume reduction in 250 consecutive patients with emphysema. J Thorac Cardiovasc Surg 2003;125(3):513–25.
27. Fishman A, Martinez F, Naunheim K, et al. A randomized trial comparing lung-volume-reduction surgery with medical therapy for severe emphysema. N Engl J Med 2003;348(21):2059–73.
28. Criner GJ, Mamary AJ. Lung volume reduction surgery and lung volume reduction in advanced emphysema: who and why? Semin Respir Crit Care Med 2010;31(3):348–64.
29. Criner GJ, Cordova F, Sternberg AL, et al. The National Emphysema Treatment Trial (NETT): part I: lessons learned about emphysema. Am J Respir Crit Care Med 2011;184(7):763–70.
30. Criner GJ, Cordova F, Sternberg AL, et al. The National Emphysema Treatment Trial (NETT) part II: lessons learned about lung volume reduction surgery. Am J Respir Crit Care Med 2011;184(8):881–93.
31. National Emphysema Treatment Trial Research Group. Patients at high risk of death after lung-volume-reduction surgery. N Engl J Med 2001;345(15):1075–83.
32. Naunheim KS, Wood DE, Mohsenifar Z, et al. Long-term follow-up of patients receiving lung-volume-reduction surgery versus medical therapy for severe emphysema by the National Emphysema Treatment Trial Research Group. Ann Thorac Surg 2006;82(2):431–43.
33. DeCamp MM, Blackstone EH, Naunheim KS, et al. Patient and surgical factors influencing air leak after lung volume reduction surgery: lessons learned from the National Emphysema Treatment Trial. Ann Thorac Surg 2006;82(1):197–206 [discussion: 206–7].

34. Naunheim KS, Wood DE, Krasna MJ, et al. Predictors of operative mortality and cardiopulmonary morbidity in the National Emphysema Treatment Trial. J Thorac Cardiovasc Surg 2006;131(1):43–53.
35. Orens JB, Estenne M, Arcasoy S, et al. International guidelines for the selection of lung transplant candidates: 2006 update—a consensus report from the Pulmonary Scientific Council of the International Society for Heart and Lung Transplantation. J Heart Lung Transplant 2006;25(7):745–55.
36. Celli BR, Cote CG, Marin JM, et al. The body-mass index, airflow obstruction, dyspnea, and exercise capacity index in chronic obstructive pulmonary disease. N Engl J Med 2004;350(10):1005–12.
37. Pochettino A, Kotloff RM, Rosengard BR, et al. Bilateral versus single lung transplantation for chronic obstructive pulmonary disease: intermediate-term results. Ann Thorac Surg 2000;70(6):1813–8 [discussion: 1818–9].
38. Thabut G, Christie JD, Ravaud P, et al. Survival after bilateral versus single lung transplantation for patients with chronic obstructive pulmonary disease: a retrospective analysis of registry data. Lancet 2008;371(9614):744–51.
39. Thabut G, Ravaud P, Christie JD, et al. Determinants of the survival benefit of lung transplantation in patients with chronic obstructive pulmonary disease. Am J Respir Crit Care Med 2008;177(10):1156–63.

Smoking Cessation and Environmental Hygiene

Cheryl Pirozzi, MD, Mary Beth Scholand, MD*

KEYWORDS

- Smoking cessation • Air pollution • Occupational exposure • Environmental hygiene
- COPD

KEY POINTS

- Modifiable risk factors for chronic obstructive pulmonary disease (COPD) include tobacco smoking, secondhand smoke (SHS), outdoor air pollution, biomass smoke, and occupational exposures.
- Tobacco cigarette smoking is the most important risk factor for development of COPD and is the single most preventable cause of death worldwide.
- SHS contains the same respiratory irritants encountered in personal smoking and may lead to development of COPD in unaffected individuals and produce adverse health effects in persons with COPD.

Chronic obstructive pulmonary disease (COPD) represents an important public health challenge that is both preventable and treatable.[1,2] Tobacco smoking is the most important risk factor for COPD. However, a significant proportion of COPD cases cannot be fully attributed to tobacco smoke. Individual variations in the development and progression of COPD occur as a result of both host factors and environmental risks.[3]

There are several nonmodifiable risk factors that likely alter a person's susceptibility to the development of COPD. Genetic susceptibility is among the most important of these. The most well documented of these genetics factors is the hereditary deficiency of α1-antitrypsin.[4] Family aggregation studies and multiple genetic association studies have yielded several potential genes that likely contribute to the susceptibility of COPD development or progression.[5] These genetic relationships are complex and COPD susceptibility likely involves multiple genes as well as epigenetic factors.[6–8] Gender also likely affects susceptibility to COPD. Women may be more susceptible to the effects of tobacco smoke than are men.[9,10]

Despite these intrinsic susceptibilities, most known risk factors for development of COPD are modifiable. Reduction of these risk factors is critical to the prevention and management of COPD.[2] Modifiable risk factors include tobacco smoking, secondhand

Pulmonary Division, Department of Internal Medicine, University of Utah, Salt Lake City, UT, USA
* Corresponding author.
E-mail address: scholand@genetics.utah.edu

Med Clin N Am 96 (2012) 849–867
doi:10.1016/j.mcna.2012.04.014
0025-7125/12/$ – see front matter © 2012 Elsevier Inc. All rights reserved.

smoke (SHS), outdoor air pollution, biomass smoke, and occupational exposures. By identifying and understanding these factors, action can be taken to improve the environment and mitigate risks for COPD.

CIGARETTE SMOKING AND SMOKING CESSATION

Tobacco cigarette smoking is the most important risk factor for development of COPD and is the single most preventable cause of death worldwide.[11] Smoking cessation may prevent the development of COPD by reducing the accelerated rate of decline associated with smoking to the normal age-related decline rate.[12] In the setting of COPD, smoking cessation remains the only intervention proven to meaningfully reduce the rate of decline of forced expiratory volume in 1 second (FEV_1) in patients with COPD.[13] In a series of studies, smoking cessation showed improvements in respiratory symptoms,[14] FEV_1,[13] and health-related quality of life measures in smokers both with and without COPD.[15,16]

The Lung Health Study was a landmark study that defined many of the benefits of smoking cessation. This study examined the effects of smoking cessation and inhaled bronchodilators in 5887 smokers with mild-to-moderate COPD. Smoking cessation significantly reduced decline in lung function.[13] At 11-year follow-up, sustained quitters had a mean FEV_1 decline of less than 27 mL/y, compared with an FEV_1 decline of 60 mL/y in continuing smokers.[17] Sustained quitters also had less severe airway obstruction compared with continuing smokers, In sustained quitters, only 3.3% of the subjects showed an FEV_1 value less than 50% of predicted, versus 18% of the subjects who continued to smoke.[17] Further, subjects showed improvement in respiratory symptoms of chronic cough, sputum production, wheezing, and shortness of breath after 5 years of smoking cessation, with the greatest improvement seen within the first year after smoking cessation.[14] Sustained quitters also had fewer lower respiratory illnesses than continuing smokers.[18] The number of COPD exacerbations also decline after smoking cessation.[19]

Although smoking cessation mitigates the impact of COPD, sustained quitters persist with residual negative health effects. In smokers with mild-to-moderate COPD, smoking cessation improves the FEV_1 and decreases the rate of FEV_1 decline back to the age-related decline seen in nonsmokers; however, the FEV_1 does not fully recover to that predicted for nonsmokers. After smoking cessation, mortalities are less than in those who continue to smoke, but ex-smokers continue to have a higher mortality risk than never-smokers, even many years after smoking cessation.[20]

Despite clear evidence linking smoking with morbidity and mortality in COPD, a third or more of patients with moderate and severe COPD continue to smoke.[21] It is possible that patients with COPD are more resistant to smoking cessation interventions. Smokers with COPD have higher nicotine dependence scores than those without COPD.[22] Educating patients with COPD about their disease state is important. Smokers who are diagnosed with COPD and subsequently counseled regarding their lung disease have higher rates of successful smoking cessation than smokers without COPD.[23,24]

SMOKING CESSATION TECHNIQUES

Multiple pharmacologic and nonpharmacologic interventions are effective for smoking cessation. Physician advice to quit smoking during an office visit improves quit rates from 1% to 3%.[25] Telephone quitlines and mobile text messaging increase the likelihood of continuous absence.[26,27] Several studies have shown the effectiveness of group and individual counseling programs.[13,28] However, the composition of the group has a significant impact on the effectiveness of this approach.[29] Two reviews of smoking cessation strategies in patients with COPD concluded that the most effective intervention for prolonged smoking cessation is the combination of pharmacologic interventions and psychosocial interventions.[30,31]

Nicotine replacement therapy is effective for smoking cessation. Silagy and colleagues[32] reviewed 123 randomized trials and concluded that the composite odds ratio (OR) for abstinence from smoking of at least 6 months is 1.77 for nicotine replacement therapy compared with control. All forms of nicotine replacement (gum, transdermal patch, nasal spray, inhaler, and sublingual tablets/lozenges) were equally effective.[32]

Bupropion was the first non-nicotine pharmacologic agent approved for smoking cessation. It is thought to work by inhibiting uptake of dopamine and norepinephrine, which may help reduce craving and withdrawal symptoms.[33] Bupropion as much as doubles the rates of smoking cessation compared with placebo in smokers[34,35] and is particularly effective in patients with COPD.[28,36,37] Side effects include insomnia and lowering of the seizure threshold, and a black box warning was issued by the US Food and Drug Administration (FDA) in 2009 about risk of serious neuropsychiatric symptoms of depression, agitation, and suicidal thoughts and behavior (www.fda.gov). Nortriptyline, another antidepressant, has also been used effectively for smoking cessation.[37]

Varenicline is a partial agonist for the $\alpha4\beta2$ nicotinic acetylcholine receptor. Use of varenicline generates 1-year abstinence rates of 22% to 23%, compared with 8.4% to 10.3% for placebo and 14.6% to 16.1% for bupropion.[38,39] In patients with COPD, abstinence rates were higher for the varenicline group compared with placebo at 12 weeks (42.3% vs 8.8%, respectively) and at 52 weeks (18.6% vs 5.6%, respectively).[40] A black box warning for varenicline was issued by the FDA in 2009 about the risk of serious neuropsychiatric symptoms of depression, agitation, and suicidal thoughts and behavior.

Combination pharmacotherapy may be more effective than monotherapy for smoking cessation in the general smoking population. Nicotine replacement has been shown to be more effective when it is used in combination with another agent, including another form of nicotine replacement therapy or bupropion.[41] Among patients with COPD, a meta-analysis concluded that the most effective smoking cessation strategy to achieve sustained abstinence is the combination of smoking cessation counseling and nicotine replacement therapy. Less effective strategies are smoking cessation counseling combined with an antidepressant or counseling alone.[42]

An encouraging new approach to smoking cessation is with immunization against nicotine. Nicotine conjugate vaccines work by stimulating production of nicotine-specific antibodies that bind to nicotine molecules, resulting in nicotine-antibody complexes that are too large to cross the blood-brain barrier, thus preventing nicotine from entering the brain and lowering the reinforcing effects of nicotine.[21,43] Three nicotine vaccines are currently in advanced stages of clinical development and early studies are promising but not conclusive.[43,44] In one study, the higher dose created a higher antibody response to the vaccine and was associated with increased 8-week abstinence rates compared with placebo (24.6% vs 12.0%),[43] suggesting that the antinicotine antibodies are important components to smoking cessation.

Nonpharmacologic therapies are widely used as an aid for smoking cessation. Hypnotherapy is designed to weaken the desire to smoke and strengthen the will to quit. A randomized trial of 286 smokers did not show significantly higher rates of smoking cessation when hypnosis was combined with nicotine patch compared with behavioral counseling and nicotine patch.[45] A meta-analysis of randomized controlled trials failed to show effectiveness for hypnotherapy based on insufficient evidence.[46]

Acupuncture, acupressure, laser therapy, and electrostimulation have all been used to reduce nicotine withdrawal symptoms. Acupuncture was superior to sham acupuncture immediately after the intervention, but the effect was not sustained at long-term follow-up and the evidence was limited by bias.[47] Electrostimulation was not more effective than placebo, and there is insufficient evidence to support effectiveness of acupressure or laser therapy for smoking cessation.[47]

Exercise may be helpful for smoking cessation by decreasing nicotine cravings and helping manage weight gain. One randomized controlled trial comparing a cognitive-behavioral smoking cessation program with and without vigorous exercise in 281 women showed improved continuous abstinence in the exercise group persisting to 12 months after treatment (11.9% vs 5.4% $P = .05$).[48] A meta-analysis concluded that exercise is valuable in reducing tobacco withdrawal cravings, but there is insufficient evidence to recommend exercise as a specific aid to smoking cessation.[49]

NONSMOKING RISK FACTORS IN COPD

In the United States, it is estimated that as many as 30% of people with COPD were never-smokers.[50] There may be even more in developing countries, where up to 50% of the COPD population has never smoked.[51–53] Nonsmoking risk factors that contribute to the development of COPD include secondhand smoke, outdoor air pollution, biomass smoke, and occupational exposures.

SHS

SHS contains the same respiratory irritants encountered in personal smoking and may lead to development of COPD in unaffected individuals and produce adverse health effects in persons with COPD. Although the levels of tobacco smoke encountered through passive smoking are lower than those in personal smoking, exposure to tobacco smoke in the environment likely leads to respiratory disease by the same mechanisms.[3] Homes with smokers living in them have higher levels of ambient nitrogen dioxide, endotoxin, and particles less than 2.5 μm in diameter (particulate matter 2.5 μm [$PM_{2.5}$] levels).[54] Epidemiologic studies performed throughout the world support an association between exposure to environmental tobacco smoke and COPD.[55–61] Among nonsmoking housewives in Turkey, those who had lived with a smoker for greater than 30 years had an almost 5-times greater risk for developing COPD.[62] A meta-analysis of 12 studies calculated a summary OR of 1.56 for SHS exposure and risk of COPD.[3]

Among patients with COPD, exposure to SHS is associated with poorer health status, including increased respiratory symptoms and more COPD exacerbations. Persons with COPD living in smoking areas report increased respiratory symptoms.[54] Higher levels of SHS exposure levels are associated with more serious clinical effects including worse COPD severity, greater dyspnea, and reduced disease-specific quality of life.[63] Exposure to passive smoking increases the risk of emergency department visits and hospitalization for COPD exacerbations.[64] Following admission for COPD exacerbations, exposure to environmental tobacco smoke was a risk factor for readmission for COPD.[65]

Much of our knowledge of SHS risks comes from high-risk groups such as airline attendants and hospitality workers who have been exposed to high levels of environmental tobacco smoke. Airliner cabin air quality before smoking bans on planes was abysmal. Levels of respirable suspended particles on smoking flights was 3 times higher than federal air quality standards for $PM_{2.5}$ and 10 to 100 times greater than the irritation thresholds.[66] Studies of urinary cotinine concentration revealed flight attendants' exposure to SHS in aircraft cabins to be approximately 6-fold that of the average US worker and 14-fold that of the average person.[66–68] This SHS exposure was associated with diagnosis of respiratory disease, airway obstruction, and decreased diffusing capacity,[69] with 69.7% diagnosed with at least 1 respiratory disease, including 2% who developed COPD.[70] Hospitality workers in restaurants and bars are also exposed to high levels of environmental tobacco smoke. Before smoking bans, 74% of a cohort of bartenders in California reported respiratory symptoms and 77% had sensory irritation symptoms.[71] Among casino workers in London, 84% reported respiratory symptoms. Exposure to high levels of SHS at work was associated with the presence of respiratory symptoms (OR 2.24).[72]

To protect the public and employees from the harmful effects of SHS, smoking bans have been implemented in many settings. A series of regulations were imposed to make airplanes a smoke-free environment. In 1973, the US Civil Aeronautics Board established nonsmoking sections on airplanes. In 1988, the US Congress mandated a smoking ban on domestic airline flights scheduled for 2 hours or less, which was extended to 6 hours the following year. By 1999, 97% of flights to and from the United States were smoke free.[66]

In 1998, California became the first state in the United States to enact a comprehensive state-wide smoking ban prohibiting smoking in all workplaces including restaurants and bars. Since then, similar legislation has been implemented in most American states. In 2004, Ireland was the first European country to ban tobacco smoking in all workplaces and, since that time, many other countries have passed national workplace smoking bans.[73] In a systematic review of 50 studies evaluating effects of legislative smoking bans, the investigators found consistent evidence that smoking bans reduced exposure to environmental tobacco smoke in public places and improved health outcomes.[73] Following the bans, bar workers in California, New York, Scotland, and Ireland showed decreased serum cotinine levels and reported fewer respiratory symptoms. Moreover, physiologic testing revealed improvements in FEV_1 and forced expiratory vital capacity.[71,74–76] In a 2006 report, the Surgeon General reported that policies prohibiting smoking in the workplace have also reduced tobacco use by smokers and changed general public attitudes about tobacco use. Despite the significant progress that has been made, SHS exposure remains an important public health problem, and further protection of nonsmokers is needed through restriction of smoking in public places and workplaces as well as voluntary restriction of smoking at home. These restrictions are particularly necessary for vulnerable populations such as children and people with respiratory disease.

OUTDOOR AIR POLLUTION

Outdoor air pollutants originate from fuel combustion produced by motor vehicles, power stations, factories, heating, and other sources. Many pollutants contribute to outdoor air pollution, including gaseous pollutants such as nitrogen dioxide (NO_2), ozone (O_3), sulfur dioxide (SO_2), and carbon monoxide (CO), as well as particulate matter.[77] Particulate matter is categorized by aerodynamic diameter, such as less than 10 μm (PM_{10}) or less than 2.5 μm ($PM_{2.5}$). The smaller particles are particularly concerning because these can be inhaled deeply into the lungs and deposited in the alveoli.[78] The role of ultrafine particles, which are less than 0.25 μm ($PM_{.25}$) has recently attracted attention. These particles are usually not reflected in standard measures of air pollution, which reflect total mass, but may be particularly toxic.

Long-term exposure to outdoor air pollution likely contributes to the development of COPD. Increased levels of outdoor air pollution is associated with a population level reduction in pulmonary function and increased prevalence of COPD.[3] Studies in multiple countries, including Germany, Switzerland, and the United States, indicate that high levels of both gaseous and PM_{10} exposures are associated with an increased risk for COPD and a decreased FEV_1, forced vital capacity (FVC), and FEV_1/FVC.[79–81] The Swiss study showed an FVC decrease of 3.4% for every 10 $\mu g/m^3$ increase in PM_{10}.[81] Long-term exposure to traffic-related air pollution has been associated with increased incidence of COPD,[82,83] and higher traffic density was associated with decreased FEV_1 and FVC in women.[84,85] COPD is 1.6 to 1.8 times more likely in those living less than 100 m from a major road.[79,86] Outdoor air pollution has also been associated with decreased growth of pulmonary function among children and adolescents.[87,88]

Outdoor air pollution affects patients with COPD adversely. Increased levels of outdoor air pollution are associated with increased respiratory symptoms in patients with COPD.[83] Short-term increases in pollution are also associated with decreased FEV_1 and FVC in adults with COPD.[89] Among patients with COPD in the Lung Health Study, acute increases in PM_{10} of 100 $\mu g/m^3$ were associated with an approximately 2% decline in FEV_1.[90]

Many epidemiologic studies have shown an association between air pollution and COPD exacerbations. Throughout the world, increased ambient concentrations of SO_2, NO_2, O_3, PM_{10}, and $PM_{2.5}$ are consistently associated with increased emergency department visits and hospital admissions for COPD or respiratory disease.[77,91–99] Among 8 European cities, every 10 $\mu g/m^3$ increase in PM_{10} was associated with an approximately 1% increase in mean number of daily admissions for COPD.[100]

Outdoor air pollution is also associated with increased mortality, both in the general population and among people with COPD.[101] Long-term exposure to traffic-related air pollution, including black smoke, NO_2, and $PM_{2.5}$, is associated with increased natural-cause and respiratory mortality in the general population.[102–104] Long-term exposure to ozone has also been associated with increased risk of death from respiratory causes.[105] Among patients with COPD in Spain, levels of particulate pollutants, but not gaseous pollutants, were associated with increased all-cause mortality (OR 1.11) and mortality from respiratory causes.[106,107] Increased PM_{10} has been associated with increased mortality among patients with COPD following hospital discharge.[108]

The global impact of outdoor air pollution is significant. The World Health Organization (WHO) estimates that approximately 1.4% of all deaths and 0.8% of disability-adjusted life-years can be attributed to particulate air pollution. Given the large global impact of outdoor air pollution, efforts have been underway for many years to decrease levels of air pollutants, with some success. Governments worldwide have introduced air quality guidelines. The Clean Air Act of 1970 requires the US Environmental Protection Agency administrator to set National Ambient Air Quality Standards (NAAQS) for what are now known as criteria pollutants (particulate matter, ozone, carbon monoxide, nitrogen dioxide, sulfur dioxide, and lead), and regulates emissions of major polluting sectors. Worldwide, the Convention on Long-range Transboundary Air Pollution was established in 1979 and includes 51 countries in Europe, Asia, and North America (United Nations Economic Commission for Europe, www.unece.org). Aggressive air quality standards exist in Europe and other developed countries. With these efforts to reduce emissions, ambient air pollution concentrations in the United States and other developed countries have been declining in recent decades.[109]

Health outcome improvements have mirrored these changes. In an 11-year prospective study in Switzerland, improved air pollution was associated with improved lung function. For every 10 $\mu g/m^3$ reduction in PM_{10}, the rate of FEV_1 decline was decreased by 3 mL/y or approximately 9%.[110] In Germany, improvements in air quality were associated with improved lung function in children, and attenuated age-related increase in chronic respiratory diseases and symptoms in elderly women.[111–113] Decreasing fine particulate air pollution in the United States during the 1980s and 1990s correlated with improvements in life expectancy, with an estimated increase in life expectancy of 0.77 years associated with every 10-μg/m^3 decrease in PM$_{2.5}$ concentration.[114] However, cities in developing countries suffer from disproportionately high levels of outdoor air pollution because of many factors, including weak governance, geographic vulnerability, low income, and increasing populations, and have not experienced these same recent improvements.

BIOMASS SMOKE

Biomass fuels are used extensively for domestic cooking and home heating in developing countries throughout the world. Biomass fuel includes wood, animal dung, and crop residues. Biomass stoves emit high levels of many pollutants, most of which are in the inhalable size range (<10 μm, or PM$_{10}$) and similar to those present in tobacco smoke. These fuels are used by approximately half of the world's population as the main domestic energy source, and by more than 80% of households in China, India, and sub-Saharan Africa.[115,116]

In these developing countries, biomass smoke is associated with the large proportion of COPD observed in never-smokers. Studies consistently detect associations between biomass smoke exposure and decreased pulmonary function[117–119] as well as rates of COPD.[120–122] Women and children are disproportionately affected by the exposure to biomass smoke because of time spent cooking or helping in the kitchen. In a study of 841 rural Mexican women, particulate matter concentration was measured in homes using biomass stoves. PM$_{10}$ levels often exceeded 2 mg/m^3, and occasionally exceed 3 mg/m^3 (approximately 60 times the maximum levels recommended by the 2005 WHO Air Quality Guidelines).[117] The women with COPD caused by biomass smoke tend to be older, shorter, have a greater body mass index, and less severe airway obstruction than those with COPD caused by smoking; however, they have similar clinical characteristics, quality of life, and mortality.[53] There seems to be a greater risk for development of COPD and chronic bronchitis with exposure to wood smoke compared with other fuels.[121]

The burden of disease attributable to biomass smoke exposure is considerable. The WHO has ranked indoor air pollution as the 10th most important preventable risk factor causing burden of disease, and the fourth most important in developing countries. Thus, interventions to reduce biomass smoke exposure are imperative. Strategies used to this end include improving ventilation; modifying stoves to high-efficiency/low-emission models with chimneys; transition to high-efficiency/low-emission fuels such as petroleum-derived fuels or industrially processed biomass; introduction of other energy sources such as thermoelectric energy, electricity, or solar cookers; or the changing of habits, such as keeping children far away from the fire or opening doors and windows during and after cooking.[116]

Introduction of improved (high-efficiency and low-emission) cookstoves reduced levels of indoor particulate matter and carbon monoxide by up to 85% in Mexico, Guatemala, Kenya, and Pakistan.[123–126] In the Randomized Exposure Study of Pollution Indoors and Respiratory Effects (RESPIRE) trial in Guatemala, 504 rural Mayan women were randomized to either receive a chimney woodstove (plancha) or continue using the traditional indoor open fire. Use of a plancha reduced carbon monoxide exposure and respiratory symptoms but did not change lung function at 12-month to 18-month follow-up.[127] Transition to cleaner fuels, such as kerosene or liquid petroleum gas, reduces particulate indoor pollution but is costly.[124] Charcoal is inexpensive, cleaner than biomass, and reduces household PM_{10} levels by 88% compared with open wood fires.[128] Despite these efforts to improve exposures, biomass fuel persists. Almost a decade after the introduction of electricity in wood-burning regions of South Africa, the mean household consumption of fuelwood has not changed, with more than 90% of households still using fuelwood for thermal purposes like cooking.[129] Decreasing biomass smoke inhalation is a complex process and must involve education and cultural modification.[116]

OCCUPATIONAL EXPOSURES

Considerable evidence exists supporting an association between occupational exposures and development of COPD. In an official statement, The American Thoracic Society concluded that the evidence was sufficient to infer a causal relationship between occupational exposures and COPD.[3] An estimated 15% of COPD may be attributed to occupational exposures.[130]

Occupational risk for the development of COPD spans a range of occupations and is related to a large numbers of vapors, dusts, gases, and fumes.[131–133] Exposure to silica dust in multiple occupations (construction, tunneling, cement, brick manufacturing, pottery and ceramic work, silica sand, granite and diatomaceous earth industries, gold mining, and iron and steel founding) is associated with increased risk of developing COPD independently of the presence of silicosis.[134,135] Increased rates of COPD have been shown among coal miners,[136] hard-rock miners,[137] tunnel workers,[138] concrete manufacturing workers,[139] nonmining industrial workers,[140] coke oven workers,[141] and cotton textile workers.[142] Using survey data from National Health and Nutrition Examination Survey (NHANES) III, increased ORs for COPD were found to be associated with freight, stock, and material handlers; records processing and distribution clerks; sales staff; transportation-related occupations; machine operators; construction trades; and waitresses, with a fraction of COPD attributable to work estimated as 19.2% overall and 31.1% among never-smokers.[143] Increased COPD mortality has been observed among construction workers,[144] railroad workers,[145] and female cotton and silk textile workers.[146] Agricultural workers have also been found to have higher rates of COPD and obstructive lung disease.[147] Ammonia, hydrogen sulfide, and inorganic dust are strongly associated with chronic bronchitis, COPD, and reduced FEV_1, and therefore may have causal roles.[148]

In patients with COPD, exposure to occupational dusts and fumes is associated with morbidity and negative COPD-related health effects. Among smokers with COPD enrolled in the Lung Health Study, ongoing exposure to occupational fumes was associated with an increased rate of decline of FEV_1.[149] Occupational exposure to vapors, gas, dust, or fumes in patients with COPD is associated with restricted activity because of breathing (OR 3.8), emergency department visits (OR 3.9), and hospitalization (OR 7.6).[132]

Acute intense workplace exposures may also be linked to development of COPD. After the World Trade Center collapse on September 11, 2001, rescue workers and residents were exposed to high levels of airborne pollutants, including particulate matter containing pulverized building materials and combustion products. In a longitudinal study of 12,079 New York City Fire Department (FDNY) rescue workers, adjusted average FEV_1 declined significantly by 372 mL during the year after exposure. The degree of FEV_1 reduction was associated with duration of exposure and respiratory symptoms.[150] Among 1720 FDNY rescue workers exposed to the World Trade Center collapse who were referred for subspecialty pulmonary evaluation, 59% had evidence of obstructive airways disease.[151] Thirty-two percent of symptomatic workers, residents, rescue workers, and clean-up workers exposed to World Trade Center dust had reduced FVC and FEV_1.[152] Exposure to dusts in the World Trade Center collapse may be a risk factor for the development of COPD; long-term follow-up is necessary.

The large burden of occupation-related COPD has affected public policy decision making. The Occupational Safety and Health Act was passed in 1970, requiring employers to provide working conditions free of known dangers (http://www.osha. gov/). The Mine Safety and Health Administration regulates hazards and exposure standards related to mining (http://www.msha.gov). As a result of these measures, levels of respirable dust exposures in coal mines after 1980 were significantly lower than levels reported in 1970 to 1971. However, a 1991 study of US underground coal mines showed that, although 89% of the occupational exposures of underground mining personnel were less than the 2.0 mg/m^3 mandated respirable dust standard, a high percentage of occupations directly associated with the coal-getting processes continued to have exposures more than 2.0 mg/m^3.[153] Thus, continued surveillance and restrictions are necessary for the protection of workers.

AMATEUR EXPOSURES

Given the well established link between occupational exposure to dusts, vapors, gases, and fumes and COPD risk, similar exposures related to amateur activities can also increase risk for COPD. Furthermore, exposures levels associated with hobbies are not limited by the regulations. Amateur woodworking exposes artisans to wood dust, which may adversely affect workers in a similar manner to professional carpenters. Many amateur rock or mineral collectors use a mechanical rock saw to cut, trim, or abrade rocks and fossil, generating high concentrations of rock dust. Although a dust mask, respirator, or dust collection system is recommended, this is not regulated in the same way that it is for professional hard-rock miners. Other dust and fume exposures may exist for amateur cavers, boatbuilders, artists, craftspeople, or hobbyists who work with paint, sculpture, welding, soldering, glass, textiles, leather, ceramics, or jewelry. When assessing a patient for COPD risk, amateur exposures should be considered.

MARIJUANA AND OTHER INHALED ILLICIT AGENTS

Any regularly inhaled substance has the potential for negative pulmonary consequences. Worldwide, marijuana is the most commonly used illegal substance.[154] Marijuana smoke contains particulate and gas components similar to those in tobacco smoke, and is associated with a greater respiratory burden of smoke particulates than tobacco smoke.[155–157]

There has been considerable study of the relationship between marijuana smoking and COPD. Marijuana smokers suffer from chronic cough, wheezing, sputum production, and frequent respiratory tract infections.[158–160] Habitual marijuana smoking is associated with evidence of airway inflammation on bronchoscopy and bronchial lavage, and with abnormal histopathology on endobronchial biopsy.[161,162] Several small case series report upper lung zone bullous emphysema in marijuana smokers.[163,164] However, the long-term effects of marijuana smoking on lung function are less clear. In a New Zealand study, both marijuana and tobacco were associated with airflow obstruction and hyperinflation in a dose-dependant manner.[165] Conversely, over an 8-year period, heavy regular marijuana smoking was not associated with an accelerated decline in FEV_1.[166] The effect of marijuana smoking on lung function and respiratory complications was evaluated in a systematic review, which found consistent associations of long-term marijuana smoking with respiratory symptoms of cough, phlegm, and wheeze, but no consistent association with airflow obstruction.[167]

Crack cocaine is the third most commonly smoked substance and can cause many acute pulmonary complications. However, studies have not shown any consistent adverse long-term effects on pulmonary function.[168–170] Similarly, there is no clear evidence to suggest that long-term inhalational use of heroin, methamphetamine, or other inhaled recreational drugs lead to development or progression of COPD.[168]

SUMMARY

Although there are nonmodifiable genetic risk factors for COPD, most known risk factors for development and progression of COPD can be corrected. Continued efforts to encourage smoking cessation and measures to reduce exposure to SHS, outdoor air pollution, biomass smoke, and occupational and related amateur exposures will have a significant impact on worldwide health.

REFERENCES

1. Celli BR, MacNee W. Standards for the diagnosis and treatment of patients with COPD: a summary of the ATS/ERS position paper. Eur Respir J 2004;23:932–46.
2. Rabe KF, Hurd S, Anzueto A, et al. Global strategy for the diagnosis, management, and prevention of chronic obstructive pulmonary disease: GOLD executive summary. Am J Respir Crit Care Med 2007;176:532–55.
3. Eisner MD, Anthonisen N, Coultas D, et al. An official American Thoracic Society public policy statement: novel risk factors and the global burden of chronic obstructive pulmonary disease. Am J Respir Crit Care Med 2010;182:693–718.
4. Stoller JK, Aboussouan LS. Alpha1-antitrypsin deficiency. Lancet 2005;365: 2225–36.
5. Castaldi PJ, Cho MH, Cohn M, et al. The COPD genetic association compendium: a comprehensive online database of COPD genetic associations. Hum Mol Genet 2010;19:526–34.
6. Soler Artigas M, Wain LV, Repapi E, et al. Effect of 5 genetic variants associated with lung function on the risk of COPD, and their joint effects on lung function. Am J Respir Crit Care Med 2011;184(7):786–95.
7. Yang IV, Schwartz DA. Epigenetic control of gene expression in the lung. Am J Respir Crit Care Med 2011;183:1295–301.
8. Sakao S, Tatsumi K. The importance of epigenetics in the development of chronic obstructive pulmonary disease. Respirology 2011;16(7):1056–63.
9. Dransfield MT, Davis JJ, Gerald LB, et al. Racial and gender differences in susceptibility to tobacco smoke among patients with chronic obstructive pulmonary disease. Respir Med 2006;100:1110–6.
10. Sorheim IC, Johannessen A, Gulsvik A, et al. Gender differences in COPD: are women more susceptible to smoking effects than men? Thorax 2010;65:480–5.
11. Deaths from chronic obstructive pulmonary disease–United States, 2000-2005. MMWR Morb Mortal Wkly Rep 2008;57:1229–32.
12. Lokke A, Lange P, Scharling H, et al. Developing COPD: a 25 year follow up study of the general population. Thorax 2006;61:935–9.
13. Anthonisen NR, Connett JE, Kiley JP, et al. Effects of smoking intervention and the use of an inhaled anticholinergic bronchodilator on the rate of decline of FEV1. The Lung Health Study. JAMA 1994;272:1497–505.
14. Kanner RE, Connett JE, Williams DE, et al. Effects of randomized assignment to a smoking cessation intervention and changes in smoking habits on respiratory

symptoms in smokers with early chronic obstructive pulmonary disease: the Lung Health Study. Am J Med 1999;106:410–6.

15. Tashkin DP, Rennard S, Taylor Hays J, et al. Lung function and respiratory symptoms in a 1-year randomized smoking cessation trial of varenicline in COPD patients. Respir Med 2011;105(11):1682–90.

16. Willemse BW, Postma DS, Timens W, et al. The impact of smoking cessation on respiratory symptoms, lung function, airway hyperresponsiveness and inflammation. Eur Respir J 2004;23:464–76.

17. Anthonisen NR, Connett JE, Murray RP. Smoking and lung function of Lung Health Study participants after 11 years. Am J Respir Crit Care Med 2002;166:675–9.

18. Kanner RE, Anthonisen NR, Connett JE. Lower respiratory illnesses promote FEV(1) decline in current smokers but not ex-smokers with mild chronic obstructive pulmonary disease: results from the Lung Health Study. Am J Respir Crit Care Med 2001;164:358–64.

19. Au DH, Bryson CL, Chien JW, et al. The effects of smoking cessation on the risk of chronic obstructive pulmonary disease exacerbations. J Gen Intern Med 2009;24:457–63.

20. Godtfredsen NS, Lam TH, Hansel TT, et al. COPD-related morbidity and mortality after smoking cessation: status of the evidence. Eur Respir J 2008; 32:844–53.

21. Tashkin DP, Murray RP. Smoking cessation in chronic obstructive pulmonary disease. Respir Med 2009;103:963–74.

22. Jimenez-Ruiz CA, Masa F, Miravitlles M, et al. Smoking characteristics: differences in attitudes and dependence between healthy smokers and smokers with COPD. Chest 2001;119:1365–70.

23. Stratelis G, Molstad S, Jakobsson P, et al. The impact of repeated spirometry and smoking cessation advice on smokers with mild COPD. Scand J Prim Health Care 2006;24:133–9.

24. Bednarek M, Gorecka D, Wielgomas J, et al. Smokers with airway obstruction are more likely to quit smoking. Thorax 2006;61:869–73.

25. Morgan MD, Britton JR. Chronic obstructive pulmonary disease 8: nonpharmacological management of COPD. Thorax 2003;58:453–7.

26. Stead LF, Perera R, Lancaster T. A systematic review of interventions for smokers who contact quitlines. Tob Control 2007;16(Suppl 1):i3–8.

27. Free C, Knight R, Robertson S, et al. Smoking cessation support delivered via mobile phone text messaging (txt2stop): a single-blind, randomised trial. Lancet 2011;378:49–55.

28. Christenhusz L, Pieterse M, Seydel E, et al. Prospective determinants of smoking cessation in COPD patients within a high intensity or a brief counseling intervention. Patient Educ Couns 2007;66:162–6.

29. Crowley TJ, Macdonald MJ, Walter MI. Behavioral anti-smoking trial in chronic obstructive pulmonary disease patients. Psychopharmacology (Berl) 1995; 119:193–204.

30. van der Meer RM, Wagena EJ, Ostelo RW, et al. Smoking cessation for chronic obstructive pulmonary disease. Cochrane Database Syst Rev 2003;2: CD002999.

31. Wagena EJ, van der Meer RM, Ostelo RJ, et al. The efficacy of smoking cessation strategies in people with chronic obstructive pulmonary disease: results from a systematic review. Respir Med 2004;98:805–15.

32. Silagy C, Lancaster T, Stead L, et al. Nicotine replacement therapy for smoking cessation. Cochrane Database Syst Rev 2004;3:CD000146.

33. Lerman C, Shields PG, Wileyto EP, et al. Effects of dopamine transporter and receptor polymorphisms on smoking cessation in a bupropion clinical trial. Health Psychol 2003;22:541–8.

34. Jorenby DE, Leischow SJ, Nides MA, et al. A controlled trial of sustained-release bupropion, a nicotine patch, or both for smoking cessation. N Engl J Med 1999; 340:685–91.

35. Schapira RM, Reinke LF. The outpatient diagnosis and management of chronic obstructive pulmonary disease: pharmacotherapy, administration of supplemental oxygen, and smoking cessation techniques. J Gen Intern Med 1995; 10:40–55.

36. Tashkin D, Kanner R, Bailey W, et al. Smoking cessation in patients with chronic obstructive pulmonary disease: a double-blind, placebo-controlled, randomised trial. Lancet 2001;357:1571–5.

37. Wagena EJ, Knipschild PG, Huibers MJ, et al. Efficacy of bupropion and nortriptyline for smoking cessation among people at risk for or with chronic obstructive pulmonary disease. Arch Intern Med 2005;165:2286–92.

38. Gonzales D, Rennard SI, Nides M, et al. Varenicline, an alpha4beta2 nicotinic acetylcholine receptor partial agonist, vs sustained-release bupropion and placebo for smoking cessation: a randomized controlled trial. JAMA 2006; 296:47–55.

39. Jorenby DE, Hays JT, Rigotti NA, et al. Efficacy of varenicline, an alpha4beta2 nicotinic acetylcholine receptor partial agonist, vs placebo or sustained-release bupropion for smoking cessation: a randomized controlled trial. JAMA 2006;296:56–63.

40. Tashkin DP, Rennard S, Hays JT, et al. Effects of varenicline on smoking cessation in patients with mild to moderate COPD: a randomized controlled trial. Chest 2011;139:591–9.

41. Shah SD, Wilken LA, Winkler SR, et al. Systematic review and meta-analysis of combination therapy for smoking cessation. J Am Pharm Assoc (2003) 2008;48: 659–65.

42. Strassmann R, Bausch B, Spaar A, et al. Smoking cessation interventions in COPD: a network meta-analysis of randomised trials. Eur Respir J 2009;34:634–40.

43. Hatsukami DK, Jorenby DE, Gonzales D, et al. Immunogenicity and smoking-cessation outcomes for a novel nicotine immunotherapeutic. Clin Pharmacol Ther 2011;89:392–9.

44. Cornuz J, Zwahlen S, Jungi WF, et al. A vaccine against nicotine for smoking cessation: a randomized controlled trial. PLoS One 2008;3:e2547.

45. Carmody TP, Duncan C, Simon JA, et al. Hypnosis for smoking cessation: a randomized trial. Nicotine Tob Res 2008;10:811–8.

46. Barnes J, Dong CY, McRobbie H, et al. Hypnotherapy for smoking cessation. Cochrane Database Syst Rev 2010;10:CD001008.

47. White AR, Rampes H, Liu JP, et al. Acupuncture and related interventions for smoking cessation. Cochrane Database Syst Rev 2011;1:CD000009.

48. Marcus BH, Albrecht AE, King TK, et al. The efficacy of exercise as an aid for smoking cessation in women: a randomized controlled trial. Arch Intern Med 1999;159:1229–34.

49. Ussher MH, Taylor A, Faulkner G. Exercise interventions for smoking cessation. Cochrane Database Syst Rev 2008;4:CD002295.

50. Mannino DM, Gagnon RC, Petty TL, et al. Obstructive lung disease and low lung function in adults in the United States: data from the National Health and Nutrition Examination Survey, 1988-1994. Arch Intern Med 2000;160:1683–9.

51. Caballero A, Torres-Duque CA, Jaramillo C, et al. Prevalence of COPD in five Colombian cities situated at low, medium, and high altitude (PREPOCOL study). Chest 2008;133:343–9.
52. Menezes AM, Perez-Padilla R, Jardim JR, et al. Chronic obstructive pulmonary disease in five Latin American cities (the PLATINO study): a prevalence study. Lancet 2005;366:1875–81.
53. Ramirez-Venegas A, Sansores RH, Perez-Padilla R, et al. Survival of patients with chronic obstructive pulmonary disease due to biomass smoke and tobacco. Am J Respir Crit Care Med 2006;173:393–7.
54. Osman LM, Douglas JG, Garden C, et al. Indoor air quality in homes of patients with chronic obstructive pulmonary disease. Am J Respir Crit Care Med 2007; 176:465–72.
55. Eisner MD, Balmes J, Katz PP, et al. Lifetime environmental tobacco smoke exposure and the risk of chronic obstructive pulmonary disease. Environ Health 2005;4:7.
56. Robbins AS, Abbey DE, Lebowitz MD. Passive smoking and chronic respiratory disease symptoms in non-smoking adults. Int J Epidemiol 1993;22:809–17.
57. Leuenberger P, Schwartz J, Ackermann-Liebrich U, et al. Passive smoking exposure in adults and chronic respiratory symptoms (SAPALDIA Study). Swiss Study on Air Pollution and Lung Diseases in Adults, SAPALDIA Team. Am J Respir Crit Care Med 1994;150:1222–8.
58. Iribarren C, Friedman GD, Klatsky AL, et al. Exposure to environmental tobacco smoke: association with personal characteristics and self reported health conditions. J Epidemiol Community Health 2001;55:721–8.
59. Maziak W, Ward KD, Rastam S, et al. Extent of exposure to environmental tobacco smoke (ETS) and its dose-response relation to respiratory health among adults. Respir Res 2005;6:13.
60. Simoni M, Baldacci S, Puntoni R, et al. Respiratory symptoms/diseases and environmental tobacco smoke (ETS) in never smoker Italian women. Respir Med 2007;101:531–8.
61. Yin P, Jiang CQ, Cheng KK, et al. Passive smoking exposure and risk of COPD among adults in China: the Guangzhou Biobank Cohort Study. Lancet 2007;370: 751–7.
62. Sezer H, Akkurt I, Guler N, et al. A case-control study on the effect of exposure to different substances on the development of COPD. Ann Epidemiol 2006;16:59–62.
63. Eisner MD, Balmes J, Yelin EH, et al. Directly measured secondhand smoke exposure and COPD health outcomes. BMC Pulm Med 2006;6:12.
64. Eisner MD, Iribarren C, Yelin EH, et al. The impact of SHS exposure on health status and exacerbations among patients with COPD. Int J Chron Obstruct Pulmon Dis 2009;4:169–76.
65. Garcia-Aymerich J, Farrero E, Felez MA, et al. Risk factors of readmission to hospital for a COPD exacerbation: a prospective study. Thorax 2003;58:100–5.
66. Repace J. Flying the smoky skies: secondhand smoke exposure of flight attendants. Tob Control 2004;13(Suppl 1):i8–19.
67. Mattson ME, Boyd G, Byar D, et al. Passive smoking on commercial airline flights. JAMA 1989;261:867–72.
68. Lindgren T, Willers S, Skarping G, et al. Urinary cotinine concentration in flight attendants, in relation to exposure to environmental tobacco smoke during intercontinental flights. Int Arch Occup Environ Health 1999;72:475–9.
69. Arjomandi M, Haight T, Redberg R, et al. Pulmonary function abnormalities in never-smoking flight attendants exposed to secondhand tobacco smoke in the aircraft cabin. J Occup Environ Med 2009;51:639–46.

70. Ebbert JO, Croghan IT, Schroeder DR, et al. Association between respiratory tract diseases and secondhand smoke exposure among never smoking flight attendants: a cross-sectional survey. Environ Health 2007;6:28.
71. Eisner MD, Smith AK, Blanc PD. Bartenders' respiratory health after establishment of smoke-free bars and taverns. JAMA 1998;280:1909–14.
72. Pilkington PA, Gray S, Gilmore AB. Health impacts of exposure to second hand smoke (SHS) amongst a highly exposed workforce: survey of London casino workers. BMC Public Health 2007;7:257.
73. Callinan JE, Clarke A, Doherty K, et al. Legislative smoking bans for reducing secondhand smoke exposure, smoking prevalence and tobacco consumption. Cochrane Database Syst Rev 2010;4:CD005992.
74. Allwright S, Paul G, Greiner B, et al. Legislation for smoke-free workplaces and health of bar workers in Ireland: before and after study. BMJ 2005;331:1117.
75. Farrelly MC, Nonnemaker JM, Chou R, et al. Changes in hospitality workers' exposure to secondhand smoke following the implementation of New York's smoke-free law. Tob Control 2005;14:236–41.
76. Menzies D, Nair A, Williamson PA, et al. Respiratory symptoms, pulmonary function, and markers of inflammation among bar workers before and after a legislative ban on smoking in public places. JAMA 2006;296:1742–8.
77. Ko FW, Hui DS. Outdoor air pollution: impact on chronic obstructive pulmonary disease patients. Curr Opin Pulm Med 2009;15:150–7.
78. Ling SH, van Eeden SF. Particulate matter air pollution exposure: role in the development and exacerbation of chronic obstructive pulmonary disease. Int J Chron Obstruct Pulmon Dis 2009;4:233–43.
79. Schikowski T, Sugiri D, Ranft U, et al. Long-term air pollution exposure and living close to busy roads are associated with COPD in women. Respir Res 2005;6: 152.
80. Detels R, Tashkin DP, Sayre JW, et al. The UCLA population studies of chronic obstructive respiratory disease. 9. Lung function changes associated with chronic exposure to photochemical oxidants; a cohort study among never-smokers. Chest 1987;92:594–603.
81. Ackermann-Liebrich U, Leuenberger P, Schwartz J, et al. Lung function and long term exposure to air pollutants in Switzerland. Study on Air Pollution and Lung Diseases in Adults (SAPALDIA) Team. Am J Respir Crit Care Med 1997; 155:122–9.
82. Karakatsani A, Andreadaki S, Katsouyanni K, et al. Air pollution in relation to manifestations of chronic pulmonary disease: a nested case-control study in Athens, Greece. Eur J Epidemiol 2003;18:45–53.
83. Peacock JL, Anderson HR, Bremner SA, et al. Outdoor air pollution and respiratory health in patients with COPD. Thorax 2011;66:591–6.
84. Kan H, Heiss G, Rose KM, et al. Traffic exposure and lung function in adults: the Atherosclerosis Risk in Communities study. Thorax 2007;62:873–9.
85. Sekine K, Shima M, Nitta Y, et al. Long term effects of exposure to automobile exhaust on the pulmonary function of female adults in Tokyo, Japan. Occup Environ Med 2004;61:350–7.
86. Lindgren A, Stroh E, Montnemery P, et al. Traffic-related air pollution associated with prevalence of asthma and COPD/chronic bronchitis. A cross-sectional study in southern Sweden. Int J Health Geogr 2009;8:2.
87. Gauderman WJ, Vora H, McConnell R, et al. Effect of exposure to traffic on lung development from 10 to 18 years of age: a cohort study. Lancet 2007;369: 571–7.

88. Rojas-Martinez R, Perez-Padilla R, Olaiz-Fernandez G, et al. Lung function growth in children with long-term exposure to air pollutants in Mexico City. Am J Respir Crit Care Med 2007;176:377–84.

89. Trenga CA, Sullivan JH, Schildcrout JS, et al. Effect of particulate air pollution on lung function in adult and pediatric subjects in a Seattle panel study. Chest 2006;129:1614–22.

90. Pope CA 3rd, Kanner RE. Acute effects of PM10 pollution on pulmonary function of smokers with mild to moderate chronic obstructive pulmonary disease. Am Rev Respir Dis 1993;147:1336–40.

91. Pope CA 3rd. Respiratory hospital admissions associated with PM10 pollution in Utah, Salt Lake, and Cache Valleys. Arch Environ Health 1991;46:90–7.

92. Sunyer J, Saez M, Murillo C, et al. Air pollution and emergency room admissions for chronic obstructive pulmonary disease: a 5-year study. Am J Epidemiol 1993;137:701–5.

93. Morgan G, Corbett S, Wlodarczyk J. Air pollution and hospital admissions in Sydney, Australia, 1990 to 1994. Am J Public Health 1998;88:1761–6.

94. Chen L, Yang W, Jennison BL, et al. Air particulate pollution and hospital admissions for chronic obstructive pulmonary disease in Reno, Nevada. Inhal Toxicol 2000;12:281–98.

95. Dominici F, Peng RD, Bell ML, et al. Fine particulate air pollution and hospital admission for cardiovascular and respiratory diseases. JAMA 2006;295:1127–34.

96. Ko FW, Tam W, Wong TW, et al. Temporal relationship between air pollutants and hospital admissions for chronic obstructive pulmonary disease in Hong Kong. Thorax 2007;62:780–5.

97. Halonen JI, Lanki T, Yli-Tuomi T, et al. Urban air pollution, and asthma and COPD hospital emergency room visits. Thorax 2008;63:635–41.

98. Arbex MA, de Souza Conceicao GM, Cendon SP, et al. Urban air pollution and chronic obstructive pulmonary disease-related emergency department visits. J Epidemiol Community Health 2009;63:777–83.

99. Peng RD, Bell ML, Geyh AS, et al. Emergency admissions for cardiovascular and respiratory diseases and the chemical composition of fine particle air pollution. Environ Health Perspect 2009;117:957–63.

100. Atkinson RW, Anderson HR, Sunyer J, et al. Acute effects of particulate air pollution on respiratory admissions: results from APHEA 2 project. Air Pollution and Health: a European Approach. Am J Respir Crit Care Med 2001;164:1860–6.

101. Izzotti A, Parodi S, Quaglia A, et al. The relationship between urban airborne pollution and short-term mortality: quantitative and qualitative aspects. Eur J Epidemiol 2000;16:1027–34.

102. Pelucchi C, Negri E, Gallus S, et al. Long-term particulate matter exposure and mortality: a review of European epidemiological studies. BMC Public Health 2009;9:453.

103. Brunekreef B, Beelen R, Hoek G, et al. Effects of long-term exposure to traffic-related air pollution on respiratory and cardiovascular mortality in the Netherlands: the NLCS-AIR study. Res Rep Health Eff Inst 2009;(139):5–71 [discussion: 3–89].

104. Krewski D, Jerrett M, Burnett RT, et al. Extended follow-up and spatial analysis of the American Cancer Society study linking particulate air pollution and mortality. Res Rep Health Eff Inst 2009;(140):5–114 [discussion: 5–36].

105. Jerrett M, Burnett RT, Pope CA 3rd, et al. Long-term ozone exposure and mortality. N Engl J Med 2009;360:1085–95.

106. Sunyer J, Basagana X. Particles, and not gases, are associated with the risk of death in patients with chronic obstructive pulmonary disease. Int J Epidemiol 2001;30:1138–40.

107. Sunyer J, Schwartz J, Tobias A, et al. Patients with chronic obstructive pulmonary disease are at increased risk of death associated with urban particle air pollution: a case-crossover analysis. Am J Epidemiol 2000;151:50–6.

108. Zanobetti A, Bind MA, Schwartz J. Particulate air pollution and survival in a COPD cohort. Environ Health 2008;7:48.

109. Samet JM. The Clean Air Act and health–a clearer view from 2011. N Engl J Med 2011;365:198–201.

110. Downs SH, Schindler C, Liu LJ, et al. Reduced exposure to PM10 and attenuated age-related decline in lung function. N Engl J Med 2007;357:2338–47.

111. Sugiri D, Ranft U, Schikowski T, et al. The influence of large-scale airborne particle decline and traffic-related exposure on children's lung function. Environ Health Perspect 2006;114:282–8.

112. Frye C, Hoelscher B, Cyrys J, et al. Association of lung function with declining ambient air pollution. Environ Health Perspect 2003;111:383–7.

113. Schikowski T, Ranft U, Sugiri D, et al. Decline in air pollution and change in prevalence in respiratory symptoms and chronic obstructive pulmonary disease in elderly women. Respir Res 2010;11:113.

114. Pope CA 3rd, Ezzati M, Dockery DW. Fine-particulate air pollution and life expectancy in the United States. N Engl J Med 2009;360:376–86.

115. Rehfuess E, Mehta S, Pruss-Ustun A. Assessing household solid fuel use: multiple implications for the Millennium Development Goals. Environ Health Perspect 2006;114:373–8.

116. Torres-Duque C, Maldonado D, Perez-Padilla R, et al. Biomass fuels and respiratory diseases: a review of the evidence. Proc Am Thorac Soc 2008;5: 577–90.

117. Regalado J, Perez-Padilla R, Sansores R, et al. The effect of biomass burning on respiratory symptoms and lung function in rural Mexican women. Am J Respir Crit Care Med 2006;174:901–5.

118. Saha A, Rao NM, Kulkarni PK, et al. Pulmonary function and fuel use: a population survey. Respir Res 2005;6:127.

119. Rinne ST, Rodas EJ, Bender BS, et al. Relationship of pulmonary function among women and children to indoor air pollution from biomass use in rural Ecuador. Respir Med 2006;100:1208–15.

120. Hu G, Zhou Y, Tian J, et al. Risk of COPD from exposure to biomass smoke: a metaanalysis. Chest 2010;138:20–31.

121. Kurmi OP, Semple S, Simkhada P, et al. COPD and chronic bronchitis risk of indoor air pollution from solid fuel: a systematic review and meta-analysis. Thorax 2010;65:221–8.

122. Po JY, FitzGerald JM, Carlsten C. Respiratory disease associated with solid biomass fuel exposure in rural women and children: systematic review and meta-analysis. Thorax 2011;66:232–9.

123. Cynthia AA, Edwards RD, Johnson M, et al. Reduction in personal exposures to particulate matter and carbon monoxide as a result of the installation of a Patsari improved cook stove in Michoacan Mexico. Indoor Air 2008;18:93–105.

124. Albalak R, Bruce N, McCracken JP, et al. Indoor respirable particulate matter concentrations from an open fire, improved cookstove, and LPG/open fire combination in a rural Guatemalan community. Environ Sci Technol 2001;35: 2650–5.

125. Ezzati M, Saleh H, Kammen DM. The contributions of emissions and spatial microenvironments to exposure to indoor air pollution from biomass combustion in Kenya. Environ Health Perspect 2000;108:833–9.
126. Khushk WA, Fatmi Z, White F, et al. Health and social impacts of improved stoves on rural women: a pilot intervention in Sindh, Pakistan. Indoor Air 2005;15:311–6.
127. Smith-Sivertsen T, Diaz E, Pope D, et al. Effect of reducing indoor air pollution on women's respiratory symptoms and lung function: the RESPIRE Randomized Trial, Guatemala. Am J Epidemiol 2009;170:211–20.
128. Bailis R, Ezzati M, Kammen DM. Greenhouse gas implications of household energy technology in Kenya. Environ Sci Technol 2003;37:2051–9.
129. Madubansi M, Shackleton CM. Changes in fuelwood use and selection following electrification in the Bushbuckridge lowveld, South Africa. J Environ Manage 2007;83:416–26.
130. Balmes J, Becklake M, Blanc P, et al. American Thoracic Society statement: occupational contribution to the burden of airway disease. Am J Respir Crit Care Med 2003;167:787–97.
131. Govender N, Lalloo UG, Naidoo RN. Occupational exposures and chronic obstructive pulmonary disease: a hospital based case-control study. Thorax 2011;66:597–601.
132. Blanc PD, Iribarren C, Trupin L, et al. Occupational exposures and the risk of COPD: dusty trades revisited. Thorax 2009;64:6–12.
133. Dement JM, Welch L, Ringen K, et al. Airways obstruction among older construction and trade workers at Department of Energy nuclear sites. Am J Ind Med 2010;53:224–40.
134. Hnizdo E, Vallyathan V. Chronic obstructive pulmonary disease due to occupational exposure to silica dust: a review of epidemiological and pathological evidence. Occup Environ Med 2003;60:237–43.
135. Rushton L. Chronic obstructive pulmonary disease and occupational exposure to silica. Rev Environ Health 2007;22:255–72.
136. Santo Tomas LH. Emphysema and chronic obstructive pulmonary disease in coal miners. Curr Opin Pulm Med 2011;17:123–5.
137. Hnizdo E, Baskind E, Sluis-Cremer GK. Combined effect of silica dust exposure and tobacco smoking on the prevalence of respiratory impairments among gold miners. Scand J Work Environ Health 1990;16:411–22.
138. Ulvestad B, Bakke B, Melbostad E, et al. Increased risk of obstructive pulmonary disease in tunnel workers. Thorax 2000;55:277–82.
139. Mwaiselage J, Bratveit M, Moen BE, et al. Respiratory symptoms and chronic obstructive pulmonary disease among cement factory workers. Scand J Work Environ Health 2005;31:316–23.
140. Bala S, Tabaku A. Chronic obstructive pulmonary disease in iron-steel and ferrochrome industry workers. Cent Eur J Public Health 2010;18:93–8.
141. Hu Y, Chen B, Yin Z, et al. Increased risk of chronic obstructive pulmonary diseases in coke oven workers: interaction between occupational exposure and smoking. Thorax 2006;61:290–5.
142. Christiani DC, Wang XR, Pan LD, et al. Longitudinal changes in pulmonary function and respiratory symptoms in cotton textile workers. A 15-yr follow-up study. Am J Respir Crit Care Med 2001;163:847–53.
143. Hnizdo E, Sullivan PA, Bang KM, et al. Association between chronic obstructive pulmonary disease and employment by industry and occupation in the US population: a study of data from the Third National Health and Nutrition Examination Survey. Am J Epidemiol 2002;156:738–46.

144. Bergdahl IA, Toren K, Eriksson K, et al. Increased mortality in COPD among construction workers exposed to inorganic dust. Eur Respir J 2004;23:402–6.

145. Hart JE, Laden F, Eisen EA, et al. Chronic obstructive pulmonary disease mortality in railroad workers. Occup Environ Med 2009;66:221–6.

146. Cui L, Gallagher LG, Ray RM, et al. Unexpected excessive chronic obstructive pulmonary disease mortality among female silk textile workers in Shanghai, China. Occup Environ Med 2011;68(12):883–7.

147. Monso E, Riu E, Radon K, et al. Chronic obstructive pulmonary disease in never-smoking animal farmers working inside confinement buildings. Am J Ind Med 2004;46:357–62.

148. Eduard W, Pearce N, Douwes J. Chronic bronchitis, COPD, and lung function in farmers: the role of biological agents. Chest 2009;136:716–25.

149. Harber P, Tashkin DP, Simmons M, et al. Effect of occupational exposures on decline of lung function in early chronic obstructive pulmonary disease. Am J Respir Crit Care Med 2007;176:994–1000.

150. Banauch GI, Hall C, Weiden M, et al. Pulmonary function after exposure to the World Trade Center collapse in the New York City Fire Department. Am J Respir Crit Care Med 2006;174:312–9.

151. Weiden MD, Ferrier N, Nolan A, et al. Obstructive airways disease with air trapping among firefighters exposed to World Trade Center dust. Chest 2010;137: 566–74.

152. Reibman J, Liu M, Cheng Q, et al. Characteristics of a residential and working community with diverse exposure to World Trade Center dust, gas, and fumes. J Occup Environ Med 2009;51:534–41.

153. Tomb. Study to assess respirable dust exposures in underground U.S. Coal Mines. Appl Occup Environ Hyg 1998;13:62–72.

154. Leggett T. A review of the world cannabis situation. Bull Narc 2006;58:1–155.

155. Novotny M, Lee ML, Low CE, et al. High-resolution gas chromatography/mass spectrometric analysis of tobacco and marijuana sterols. Steroids 1976;27: 665–73.

156. Wu TC, Tashkin DP, Djahed B, et al. Pulmonary hazards of smoking marijuana as compared with tobacco. N Engl J Med 1988;318:347–51.

157. Moir D, Rickert WS, Levasseur G, et al. A comparison of mainstream and side-stream marijuana and tobacco cigarette smoke produced under two machine smoking conditions. Chem Res Toxicol 2008;21:494–502.

158. Tashkin DP, Coulson AH, Clark VA, et al. Respiratory symptoms and lung function in habitual heavy smokers of marijuana alone, smokers of marijuana and tobacco, smokers of tobacco alone, and nonsmokers. Am Rev Respir Dis 1987;135:209–16.

159. Taylor DR, Poulton R, Moffitt TE, et al. The respiratory effects of cannabis dependence in young adults. Addiction 2000;95:1669–77.

160. Moore BA, Augustson EM, Moser RP, et al. Respiratory effects of marijuana and tobacco use in a U.S. sample. J Gen Intern Med 2005;20:33–7.

161. Roth MD, Arora A, Barsky SH, et al. Airway inflammation in young marijuana and tobacco smokers. Am J Respir Crit Care Med 1998;157:928–37.

162. Fligiel SE, Roth MD, Kleerup EC, et al. Tracheobronchial histopathology in habitual smokers of cocaine, marijuana, and/or tobacco. Chest 1997;112:319–26.

163. Johnson MK, Smith RP, Morrison D, et al. Large lung bullae in marijuana smokers. Thorax 2000;55:340–2.

164. Hii SW, Tam JD, Thompson BR, et al. Bullous lung disease due to marijuana. Respirology 2008;13:122–7.

165. Aldington S, Williams M, Nowitz M, et al. Effects of cannabis on pulmonary structure, function and symptoms. Thorax 2007;62:1058–63.
166. Tashkin DP, Simmons MS, Sherrill DL, et al. Heavy habitual marijuana smoking does not cause an accelerated decline in FEV1 with age. Am J Respir Crit Care Med 1997;155:141–8.
167. Tashkin DP. Does cannabis use predispose to chronic airflow obstruction? Eur Respir J 2010;35:3–5.
168. Tashkin DP. Airway effects of marijuana, cocaine, and other inhaled illicit agents. Curr Opin Pulm Med 2001;7:43–61.
169. Tashkin DP, Khalsa ME, Gorelick D, et al. Pulmonary status of habitual cocaine smokers. Am Rev Respir Dis 1992;145:92–100.
170. Itkonen J, Schnoll S, Glassroth J. Pulmonary dysfunction in 'freebase' cocaine users. Arch Intern Med 1984;144:2195–7.

Index

Note: Page numbers of article titles are in **boldface** type.

Med Clin N Am 96 (2012) 869–880
doi:10.1016/S0025-7125(12)00114-9
0025-7125/12/$ – see front matter © 2012 Elsevier Inc. All rights reserved.

medical.theclinics.com

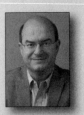
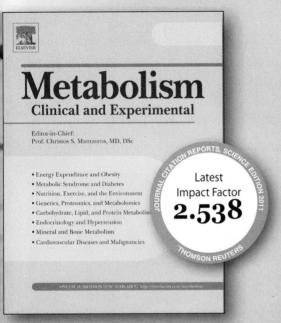
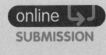

ELSEVIER
presents

...titles from our
ENDOCRINOLOGY
& METABOLISM
portfolio

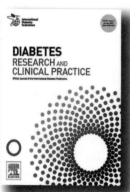

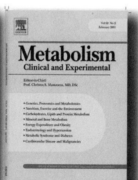

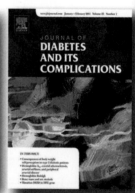

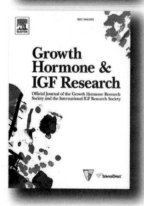

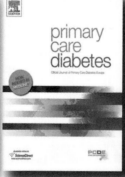

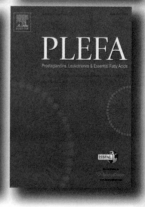

For more information please visit:
www.elsevier.com

ELSEVIER

ENDOCRINOLOGY & METABOLISM